DIVERSITY AND WOMEN'S HEALTH

A *National Women's Studies Association Journal* Reader

OTHER BOOKS IN THE SERIES

Feminist Pedagogy: Looking Back to Move Forward, edited by Robbin D. Crabtree, David Alan Sapp, and Adela C. Licona

Diversity and Women's Health

EDITED BY **Sue V. Rosser**

The Johns Hopkins University Press
Baltimore

© 2009 The Johns Hopkins University Press
All rights reserved. Published 2009
Printed in the United States of America on acid-free paper
9 8 7 6 5 4 3 2 1

The Johns Hopkins University Press
2715 North Charles Street
Baltimore, Maryland 21218-4363
www.press.jhu.edu

ISBN 10: 0-8018-9280-5
ISBN 13: 978-0-8018-9280-6

Library of Congress Control Number: 2008936106

A catalog record for this book is available from the British Library.

*Special discounts are available for bulk purchases of this book. For more informa-
tion, please contact Special Sales at 410-516-6936 or specialsales@press.jhu.edu.*

The Johns Hopkins University Press uses environmentally friendly book materials,
including recycled text paper that is composed of at least 30 percent post-consumer
waste, whenever possible. All of our book papers are acid-free, and our jackets and
covers are printed on paper with recycled content.

Contents

DIVERSITY AND WOMEN'S HEALTH

Introduction: Moving Diversity from the Margins to the Center of Women's Health

SUE V. ROSSER

The title of a book I wrote in the mid-1990s, *Women's Health: Missing from U.S. Medicine* (Rosser 1994), accurately depicted the status of women's health at the time from the point of view of most consumers of health care, as well as most formal and informal practitioners. In the book, I suggested that women had begun to critique the male-centered focus of clinical research that led to the insufficient study and funding of diseases of women, the exclusion of women from experimental drug trials, and the failure to understand the health of the majority of the population. This exclusion of women from experimental research and clinical trials translated into misdiagnoses of some conditions, such as cardiovascular disease, which manifest differently in men and women, and ultimately into less access to treatment and fewer successful interventions, with women being referred less often for procedures and with higher death rates for women after angioplasty (Kelsey et al. 1993) and coronary bypass. Not only did women suffer from male definitions of health and disease and studies that excluded them or did not extrapolate appropriately to their bodies and conditions, but the health care practitioner also was placed in a difficult position. "Because of the dearth of clinical research on those groups that now constitute the majority of the American population s/he possesses inadequate information on the etiology, symptoms, and progress of many diseases in a population which is increasingly elderly, minority, and female" (vii–viii).

As a solution to this problem, I proposed that women's studies might serve as a model for transforming health and medical research and curriculum to integrate women. Institutions successful in transforming the curriculum to include women's studies developed phase models that reflected the idea that integrating information about women into the curriculum is a process. In the first phase, women are absent from the curriculum; the final phase is the gender-balanced curriculum. McIntosh's (1984) model will be elaborated and expanded here to illustrate the process of transformation for women's health.

Phase I: Absence of Women and Women's Health Is Not Noted

This phase describes the status of most medical research and medical curricula before the late 1980s.

Research. Before a General Accounting Office audit (National News and Development 1986) drew attention to the exclusion of women as experimental subjects from research protocols in studies funded by the National Institutes of Health (NIH), the omission of women from research protocols was rarely noted. Congress, led by women such as Pat Schroeder and Barbara Mikulski, began to question the absence of substantial research devoted to women's health concerns at the time and to lead the fight for funding and focus on such research on the national level. This realization uncovered gender bias, which had distorted some medical research. Women's health had become synonymous with reproductive health and obstetrics/gynecology. This meant that many diseases that occurred in both sexes had been studied in males only or were treated with a male-as-norm approach. Cardiovascular diseases serve as a case in point. Research protocols for large-scale studies (MRFIT 1990; Steering Committee of the Physician's Health Study Group 1989; Grobbee et al. 1990) of cardiovascular diseases failed to assess gender differences. Women were excluded from clinical trials of drugs because of fear of litigation from possible teratogenic effects on fetuses.

Excessive focus on male research subjects and definition of cardiovascular diseases as "male" led to underdiagnosis and undertreatment of the disease in women. A 1991 study in Massachusetts and Maryland (Ayanian and Epstein) demonstrated that women were significantly less likely than men to undergo coronary angioplasty, angiography, or surgery when admitted to the hospital with a diagnosis of myocardial infarction, unstable or stable angina, chronic ischemic heart disease, or chest pain. This significant difference remained even when variables such as race, age, economic status, and other chronic diseases such as diabetes and heart failure were controlled. A similar study (Steingart et al. 1991) revealed that women had angina before myocardial infarction as frequently as, and with more debilitating effects than, men, yet women were referred for cardiac catheterization only half as often. These and other similar studies led Bernadine Healy, a cardiologist and first woman director of NIH, to characterize the diagnosis of coronary heart disease in women as the Yentl syndrome: "Once a woman showed that she was just like a man, by having coronary artery disease or a myocardial infarction, then she was treated as a man should be" (Healy 1991, 274). The male-as-norm approach in research and diagnosis, unsurprisingly, was translated into bias in treatments for women. Women exhibited higher death rates from angioplasty (Kelsey et al. 1993) and coronary bypass surgery (Kahn, Nessin, and Gray 1990).

Curriculum. The lecturer who used without question the 70 kilogram male as the norm and emphasized diagnosis and disease processes as they occur in the white man's body (without stating explicitly that this is the perspective from which the course is taught) exemplified this phase in the health curriculum. The specialty of obstetrics/gynecology and the illusion that it traditionally included women's health beyond the reproductive system made the absence of women and women's health from the rest of the curriculum pass without notice or seem reasonable when questioned.

Phase II: Add-and-Stir Approaches to Women and Women's Health Are Attempted

Even before the attention drawn by Congress and the NIH to the absence of women, many researchers, teachers, and practitioners became aware that their experimental designs, explanations, and diagnoses suffered from the exclusion of women. They sought to remedy the situation by adding women on to a model or explanation that assumed the male norm; the question was not raised whether the experimental design, lecture, or procedure might need to be modified because of their addition.

Research. The 18 percent of clinical trials between 1960 and 1991 for medications to prevent myocardial infarctions that included women of the same age as the men included represents this phase. By using women and men of the same age, these studies assumed the male norm for myocardial infarction. They failed to take into account its later onset in women, who constitute 24 percent of those younger than sixty-five and 64 percent of those age eighty-five or older who died of acute myocardial infarction. By choosing the male body as the norm for the experiment and simply adding women subjects, these experiments fed the myth of heart disease as a male disease rather than revealing the fact that heart disease strikes men and women with similar frequencies but at different ages.

Curriculum. Faculty often present lectures at the phase II stage. After explaining anatomy, physiology, or disease processes using the male body as the norm, the faculty member may note a slight variation that occurs in females, without explaining its possible implications or ramifications. For example, in a lecture on the use of oral antibiotics such as penicillin to fight streptococcus infections in the throat, the lecturer might note that women may experience vaginal yeast infections after using the antibiotics. If the lecturer fails to explain that the oral administration of the antibiotic kills bacteria all over the body, not just in the throat, the source of the yeast infection may not be understood. The lecturer also misses an opportunity to explain the mechanism by which bacteria and yeast normally function to limit each other's growth in the vaginal area.

Phase III: Women as a Problem, Anomaly, or Deviant from the Male Norm

At this stage, faculty recognize that simply adding women and women's health to research and lectures designed using the white male as the standard of normality often yields only inadequate, partial explanations for women.

Research. Cardiac researchers at this phase couple this recognition with the obvious statistical evidence that women live an average of 7.5 years longer than men and that heart disease is the major killer of older women. This enables these investigators to rethink experimental protocols. They begin to question including only males under the age of seventy-five as subjects for myocardial infarction experiments and begin to explore the flaws introduced into experiments when variables such as gender, age, and menstrual status are not included in experimental design.

Curriculum. Instructing students in gross anatomy to cut off the breasts of female cadavers and discard them constitutes a most dramatic example of phase III teaching in the classroom. As Dr. Fugh-Berman asked: "How many . . . students . . . take away the message that despite the epidemic of breast cancer, women's breasts had no medical significance?" (Lewin 2008). The lectures on AIDS diagnosis using the revised Centers for Disease Control (CDC) surveillance case definition predating the January 1993 revised definition also exemplify phase III classroom teaching. From their own practice, reading, and anecdotal information learned from colleagues, most faculty knew that the earlier revised CDC definition was inadequate for diagnosing AIDS in women. The most evident problem was the omission of gynecologic conditions and their numerous complications—higher rates of cervical cancer, abnormal Pap smears, increased incidence of pelvic inflammatory disease, and vaginal infections resistant to cure—thought to be manifestations of the disease in women. Since the revised definition included no gynecologic conditions, women were seen as a problem or anomaly for AIDS diagnosis.

Phase IV: Women as the Focus

Once the pervasiveness of women's exclusion from research designs and curricula and the bias that exclusion introduces into research, teaching, and practice were understood, women became a new focal point for research and curricula. By this phase, a substantial group of investigators, lecturers, and practitioners evolved who committed their efforts and careers to studying women. These individuals designed experiments that not only included women as experimental subjects but for which women's health, diseases, and issues also served as the central topic of study. The topics led to the development of experimental methods particularly appropriate for the female body and lifecycle and the experiences of women. At this phase, race and class are understood to be interlocking phenomena that must also be integrated into research design, teaching, and practice with gender in the health and disease of women.

Research. The Women's Health Initiative and other studies collect data on cardiovascular diseases using the female body as norm. The establishment of the Office of Research on Women's Health within NIH (1990) and the Women's Health Initiative (Healy 1992) demonstrate early efforts to place women's health in central focus. The collection of baseline data sought in the Women's Health Initiative on the three major causes of death and frailty in women age forty-five years and older—"cardiovascular diseases, cancers of the breast, lung, and colorectal tract, and osteoporosis" (Pinn and LaRosa 1992)—underlines the extent to which the absence of women had not been noted previously in research and curricula in specialties outside of obstetrics/gynecology. Because obstetrics/gynecology is a surgical specialty that revolves around women of reproductive age and issues of reproduction, particularly sexually transmitted diseases, contraception, infertility, pregnancy, childbirth, and menopause, this information had not been collected and explored by researchers or practitioners in the field. Women constitute the primary focus of study under the Women's Health Initiative designed to collect these data and stimulate further research on cardiovascular disease, cancers, and osteoporosis.

Curriculum. This phase leads to courses and curricula focused solely on women's health at various levels of medical and health curricula. Early courses, residencies, and continuing medical education curricula represented initial attempts to focus on women's health at all levels of the curriculum. The individuals who develop and enhance the new research and curricula must be properly trained in order to advance the field to phase V.

Phase V: Research and Curricula to Include Us All

The ultimate goal is to integrate the information on women's health into research in all medical specialties and to transform all aspects of the health curriculum to include women and their health. Patterned on women's studies and the Office of Research on Women's Health at NIH, this would aid other disciplines and specialties in understanding the importance of including women in research and teaching, while simultaneously providing trained specialists to undertake more focused research in this interdisciplinary field. Far from creating a ghetto, this phase model of the both/and approach includes women in all aspects of health.

At the time that the book was published (Rosser 1994), I identified much research and some curricula at phase III, women as a problem, anomaly, or absence, although many individuals and institutions remained at phase II and even phase I in their research and curricular designs. I noted that "phase IV is the stage at which some forward-looking national leaders thinking about women's health currently find themselves" (156).

In 2003, I co-edited a special issue of *Women's Studies Quarterly: Women, Health, and Medicine: Transforming Perspectives and Practice* (Dan and Rosser 2003). In the introductory editorial to that issue, we identified phase IV as "the phase in which the leaders of women's health and women's studies currently find themselves" (16), suggesting some advancement in research and curriculum on women's health in the nine-year interval between the two volumes.

In the editorial we also described the importance of the interaction between women's studies and women's health:

> The field of women's health serves as a model for positive interactions be-tween women's studies and disciplinary research and curriculum, changing institutions, and activism in several ways:
>
> 1) It identified major gaps in research and practice and initiated a critique of the current health care system at all levels.
>
> 2) It originated from, and remains connected with, the non-medical community.
>
> 3) It is interdisciplinary and requires interdisciplinary teams for research and clinical practice, as well as collaboration with colleagues in non-medical academic fields.
>
> 4) It developed new curriculum focused on women's health and elaborated the women's studies model for integrating gender into curriculum into all aspects and levels of health education.
>
> 5) It emphasizes race, class, sexual orientation, and other diversities among women. (Dan and Rosser 2003, 7)

Diversities among women serves as the theme uniting the essays on women's health selected for this anthology. Before women's health can reach phase V and be truly inclusive, much more attention must be de-voted to diversities among women. Demographic projections reveal that the majority of the U.S. population soon will come from the current ra-cial "minorities"; as the baby boom generation ages, the elderly popula-tion, predominantly female, will increase dramatically. Research on health of lesbians, women of color, women from non-U.S. cultures/coun-tries, and elderly women has remained underfunded, understudied, and overlooked (Rosser 1994). Disabled women remain largely invisible to both the U.S. population at large and the health research agenda in particular.

To rectify this dearth of research and avoid problems from failing to include the health of the majority of U.S. women, research and needs of diverse women must become a central focus of women's health education.

This volume provides a mechanism to center on diversity and bring the overlooked, understudied, and underfunded health issues of particular groups of women whose health issues have served neither as the center of women's health nor certainly as the attention of health issues for the over-all population to the fore. This selection includes essays from the *NWSA Journal* that focus on health issues for women of color, lesbians, and aging and disabled women, as well as those that use women's studies approaches to expand methods to study the health of women.

Women of Color

Racism intertwines with sexism and economics to move health care issues for women of color to the far margins or to move them entirely out of the national agenda for clinical research. Their gender and their color doubly remove them from the white male, from whose perspective the research agenda is formulated and whose body serves as the norm from which deviations are calculated. When included, women of color too often become misused as subjects in experiments that either lend credence to racial stereotypes or fail to distinguish true health problems among races.

Many of the health and disease concerns of women of color overlap with those of white women, which have only recently begun to be a focus of the national research agenda with the establishment of the Office of Research on Women's Health in 1990. Women of color also face many of the same problems with health and disease as do the men of their racial and ethnic groups. Men of color have not shared the central spotlight for research with white men. The Office for Minority Health Affairs was not established until 1991.

Racism and sexism have combined to severely limit advances in health care for women of color. The dearth of research in general and the often delimitative nature of this research have yielded only meager, and in many cases unreliable, data regarding frequency and cause of diseases, exacerbation of illness by environmental factors, and effective treatments for promoting health and preventing disease in women of color. Some complications of racism and sexism have effectively invalidated such research in the past. A major problem has been that the phrase "women of color" is too often taken to mean a coherent group when in fact it includes women of extremely diverse racial and ethnic backgrounds who are not closely related to each other genetically or culturally. They may, therefore, differ more from each other than they do from white women. Another controversy focuses on the appropriateness and reliability of undertaking race-based research, diagnosis, and treatment, since race is not a biological category. In this anthology, Zobeida Bonilla, in chapter 5, describes ways in which the editors and authors of the new *Our Bodies, Ourselves* attempted to include the overlapping, yet distinct issues faced by women of color of diverse races/ethnicities.

Considerable diversity exists within each group. For example, Asians and Pacific Islanders in the United States include more than twenty-five subgroups, such as Chinese, Filipinos, Japanese, Indians, Koreans, Vietnamese, Hawaiians, Samoans, Guamanians, Burmese, Cambodians, Laotians, Thais, and others (Manley et al. 1985). Although they share an origin in Asia and the Pacific Islands, they have different cultures, languages, and probably gene pools. Since many of the Asians and Pacific Islanders in the United States today are first-generation immigrants, virtually no baseline data exist on the health of these women. Less explicable is the fact that even for those whose ancestors immigrated to this country more than a century ago, only limited baseline data exist.

The Hispanic population also does not represent a homogeneous ethnic group. Mexican Americans, Puerto Ricans, Cubans, and individuals from sixteen other Latin American countries and Spain speak Spanish but have their origins in very different cultures and countries. Since many Chicanas and those from other Latin American cultures are also first-generation Americans, there is little history of research and few baseline data for Hispanic women either.

For American Indian and Alaska Native women, the first female Americans, predating not only white women but also white men, short tenure in the United States cannot be used to explain the absence of research (and their poor health). Similarly, the African American population, originally transported to the United States against its will, is the oldest and most stable non-indigenous minority group. Yet little good research has explored black women's health, despite the fact that, in many ways, black women are the most vulnerable of all minority women (Kasper 2000).

In the rare cases where women of color have been the focus of research, at best the results have yielded little or inadequate information about health and disease processes. At worst the women have served as guinea pigs for clinical trials of unsafe drugs or for experiments to document possible biological bases for social ills. In chapter 1, Lynn Roberts, Loretta Ross, and M. Bahati Kuumba explore how the legacy of forced sterilization, use of Puerto Rican women for testing birth control pills without informed consent, and general exploitation of women of color have complicated their reproductive rights and decisions. Andrea Smith, in chapter 3, builds on the arguments made by Roberts, Ross, and Kuumba, discussing how even the terminology used by white women remains complicating and inappropriate for women facing racial injustice on a daily basis.

Many studies (White 1990; Avery 1992; others) have defined access to health care as the controlling factor for health and disease in the lives of minority women. Researchers have also produced a considerable body of work that examines the relationship among poverty, access, and health care for minority women (Alcena 1992; Braithwaite and Taylor 1992; Kasper 2000). Jennifer Nelson, in chapter 2, documents the problem of access to health care complicated by poverty and location for African American women in rural Mississippi.

Lesbians

As women and as non-heterosexuals, lesbians are doubly distanced from the heterosexual male norm focus of health research and care. As I describe in chapter 7, usually lesbianism is ignored or overlooked, even when being a lesbian has implications for the issue under study. When lesbians are recognized, they are often subsumed as a subset of women or homosexuals, where heterosexual females (Bernhard and Dan 1986; Stevens and Hall 1988) or homosexual males (Trippet and Bain 1992) become the respective norms against which lesbians are measured. The implicit assumption underlying this failure to recognize the health care issues for lesbians is either that lesbians do not exist, that they have precisely the same health care issues as heterosexual females, or in rare cases that they share the same health care issues as male homosexuals (Trippet and Bain 1992).

This ignoring or lumping together of lesbian health care issues becomes exacerbated by homophobia on the part of health care professionals, as described by Elizabeth Sarah Lindsey in chapter 6. Not only does homophobia discourage lesbians from seeking necessary health care, but it also prevents health care workers from tying appropriate diagnoses and treatments to risk behaviors.

Aging Women

Until the Women's Health Initiative, very little research on women's menopausal experience existed. As the baby boom generation ages, the pharmaceutical companies developed an extreme interest in capturing the market of consuming women approaching menopause. These companies redefined menopause as a disease that required hormones to cure it and made large amounts of money by selling hormone replacement therapy (HRT) to women before, during, and after menopause. Indeed, Nancy Worcester, in chapter 10, documents the outrage that most women expressed against the pharmaceutical companies and health care industry after the announcement that HRT increased the risk of stroke, breast cancer, and blood clots and did not prevent heart attacks or Alzheimer's. They asked why they had been given HRT before such research had been completed.

Until the Women's Health Initiative, very little research compared the health of menopausal women who took HRT with those who did not take HRT. A primary reason was the general dearth of research on menopausal women. Feminists established the Society for Menstrual Cycle Research to fill that dearth, as Alice Dan documents in chapter 9. Heather Dillaway, in chapter 8, provides additional qualitative data to supplement the growing quantitative data documenting the wide variance of women's age and experience of menopause.

For elderly women, a recognized clinical specialty, gerontology, should address some of their health needs. Gerontology remains a relatively new, emerging field without a clear research agenda. It has already demonstrated androcentrism by excluding women from its most comprehensive longitudinal study. The Baltimore Longitudinal Study on Aging, the largest longitudinal study to assess the geriatric population, which was begun in 1958, included no women subjects for the first twenty years (Johnson 1992). This omission delayed the discovery of the link among osteoporosis, calcium, estrogen, and progesterone.

Recent census data projections completed by the Administration on Aging underscore the dramatic increase in the elderly population in the United States. In 2030, one-fifth of the total population will be 65 or older; the number of women 85 and older was 2.3 million in 2000 and is expected to reach 6.3 million by 2030, since women reaching 65 have an average additional life expectancy of 19.5 years (www.aaoa.govpop/statistics.asp). Elderly women outnumber elderly men by a ratio of 2:1. Because women die later in life than men, they accumulate more acute, chronic diseases, which tends to result in greater disability before death (Lewis 1985) and greater out-of-pocket expenses than do the acute illnesses suffered more commonly by men (Sofaer and Abel 1990). Their greater longevity also means that most women who serve as caretakers for a spouse when his health fails must rely on the support of health services, extended family, and friends during their own health care crises. Sondra Brandler, in chapter 11, describes the impact on the daughters who care for aging mothers as they themselves age.

This information strongly suggests that elderly women will become an increasingly significant proportion of the population who will need a disproportionately large amount of health care. Research on diseases, maintenance of health and well-being, and successful, cost-efficient health care practices appropriate for elderly women should be accorded high priority on the national health care agenda.

Women with Disabilities

Although women with disabilities typically differ from their able-bodied sisters because of mental or physical health issues that may lead them to frequent encounters with the health care system, in many ways they remain the most marginalized and invisible of women. In the newest version of *Our Bodies, Ourselves*, the authors/editors attempted to make disabled women more visible by integrating information through all of the chapters rather than having a separate chapter devoted to women with disabilities. In most ways, the issues of disabled women overlap with those of non-disabled women. *Excluded as research subjects, absent from clinical trials of drugs, compared with male norms*, and *out of central focus for research agendas* serve as descriptors that overlap health issues for both disabled and non-disabled women. Many women with disabilities are also women of color, and/or lesbians, and/or elderly. Christine Overall, in chapter 12, examines the striking similarities and connections between ableism and ageism as socially constructed systems of oppressions.

For many disabled women, issues of access, poverty, and environment become especially significant. Because of the relatively small numbers of women experiencing a particular disability, coupled with different manifestations of the disability, garnering research attention and funding may be especially difficult and acute.

In addition to the bias, ignoring, overlooking, and understudy of health issues faced by all women, disabled women experience additional, different issues. Disabled women are compared not only to the male norm, but also to the non-disabled female norm. One of the many facets of the disabled lived experience brought out by Ann Fox and Joan Lipkin in chapter 13 is the constant comparison of disabled women to non-disabled women in appearance, sexuality, and functioning.

Women's Studies Methods to Transform Health Research and Care

Large numbers of feminists are involved in various aspects of health care reform, ranging from policy formation through access and delivery. A considerable body of research evolved by women's studies scholars working through the traditional disciplines such as political science, public health, nursing, medicine, and social work provide feminist frameworks through which to suggest and evaluate health agendas and reforms. Sufficient numbers of scholars representing a variety of theoretical perspectives, including liberal, socialist, African American, and radical feminist, exist to provide some insights into possible advantages and disadvantages of various changes from the standpoints of different groups of women. Adriana Cavalcanti de Aguilar, in chapter 15, explores how women's studies approaches useful in Brazilian medicine might be brought to the U.S. health system.

Policy formation, widening access, and improving delivery represent crucial issues that must be resolved in order to improve health care in the United States. It is particularly important that feminist perspectives be voiced on those issues as changes are made. As outlined by Marianne McPherson in chapter 14, the editors tried very hard to include a broad variety of feminist voices in the 2005 edition of *Our Bodies, Ourselves.*

Basic scientific and clinical research constitutes an equally significant area for health care reform. Often the priorities for research, the topics chosen for study, the subpopulations of individuals included in and excluded from research protocols, and the theories and conclusions drawn from the data set the parameters for policy, access, and delivery. Women and feminist voices have been largely absent from the discussions of research agendas. Karen Messing provides a counter-example of how the subjects of research can help to set the agenda and approaches in chapter 16.

The connection between women's health and women's studies has never been more important. As women's health has experienced many successes over the last three decades, it has become a major component of the public agenda. Every week we see new women's health research reported in major newspapers. At the tenth anniversary symposium in September 2000 celebrating the Office of Research on Women's Health at NIH, Robert Bazell of NBC News described an endless demand for stories on women's health. Resources for research in women's health have multiplied, and with these successes have come increased competition and co-optation by those who are primarily interested in controlling women's health in their own interests. For example, in the wake of the revelation that hormone replacement therapy did not prevent heart disease or Alzheimer's, but increased the risk of stroke, blood clots, breast cancer, and incontinence, over six million women stopped taking hormone therapy and demanded to know more about the research and policies that had encouraged them to take it (Pearson 2006).

Rather than merely congratulating ourselves on how effectively we have established women's health as a priority for society, we must continue to insist that the vision of the women's health movement be the model of women's health research, teaching, and practice. As Carol Weisman documents in her 1998 book, health care could be viewed as a key social arena in which gender issues surface and are contested (Weisman 1998). Despite our accomplishments in raising awareness of the importance of women's health, feminist and woman-centered views are not well represented in the biomedical disciplines in which many of the new resources are being used; elderly women, disabled women, women of color, and lesbians are either barely represented or ignored. There is an urgent need to continue building on the strength of the women's health movement, with a strong collaborative link to women's studies to include the diversity of all women. This anthology takes another step in nurturing that relationship.

References

Alcena, Valiere. 1992. *The Status of Health of Blacks in the United States of America.* Dubuque, IA: Kendall/Hunt Publishing Co.

Avery, Byllye. 1992. The health status of Black women. In *Health Issues in the Black Community,* edited by Ronald Braithwaite and Sandra Taylor, 3–5. San Francisco: Jossey-Bass.

Ayanian, J.Z., and A.M. Epstein. 1991. Differences in the use of procedures between women and men hospitalized for coronary heart disease. *New England Journal of Medicine 325*: 221–25.

Bernhard, Linda, and Alice Dan. 1986. Redefining sexuality from women's own experiences. *Nursing Clinics of North America 21:* 123–36.

Braithwaite, Ronald, and Sandra Taylor, eds. 1992. *Health Issues in the Black Community.* San Francisco: Jossey-Bass.

Centers for Disease Control. 1987. Antibody to human immunodeficiency virus in female prostitutes. *Morbidity and Mortality Weekly Report 36:* 157–61.

Dan, Alice, and Sue V. Rosser. (2003) Editorial. *Women's Studies Quarterly 31*(1–2): 1–24.

Grobbee, D.E., E.B. Rimm, E. Giovannucci, G. Colditz, M. Stampfer, and W. Willett. 1990. Coffee, caffeine, and cardiovascular disease in men. *New England Journal of Medicine 321*: 1026–32.

Healy, Bernadine. 1991. The Yentl syndrome. *The New England Journal of Medicine 325*(4): 274–76.

———. 1992. Women's health, public welfare. *Journal of the American Medical Association, 264*(4): 566–68.

Johnson, Karen. 1992. Pro: Women's health: Developing a new interdisciplinary specialty. *Journal of Women's Health 1*(2): 95–100.

Kahn, S.S., S. Nessin, A. Gray, L.S. Czer, A. Chaux, and J. Martly. 1990. Increased mortality of women in coronary bypass surgery: Evidence for referral basis. *Journal of Women's Health 1*: 95–99.

Kasper, Anne. (2000). Barriers and burdens: Poor women face breast cancer. In *Breast Cancer: Society Shapes an Epidemic,* edited by Anne Kasper and Susan Ferguson. New York: St. Martin's Press.

Kelsey, Sheryl F., et al., and Investigators from the National Heart, Lung, and Blood Institute Percutaneous Transluminal Coronary Angioplasty Registry. 1993. Results of percutaneous transluminal coronary angioplasty in women: 1985–1986. National Heart, Lung, and Blood Institutes Coronary Angioplasty Registry. *Circulation* 87(3): 720–27.

Lewin, T. 2008. Doctors consider a specialty focusing on women's health. *New York Times*, September 16.

Lewis, M. 1985. Older women and health: An overview. *Women and Health* 10(2–3): 1–16.

Manley, Audrey, Jane Lin-Fu, Magdalena Maranda, Alan Noonan, and Tanya Parker. 1985. Special health concerns of ethnic minority women in women's health. *Report of the Public Health Service Task Force on Women's Health Issues.* Washington, DC: U.S. Department of Health and Human Services.

McIntosh, Peggy. 1984. The study of women: Processes of personal and curricular re-vision. *The Forum for Liberal Education* 5: 2.

Multiple Risk Factor Intervention Trial Research Group (MRFIT). 1990. Mortality rates after 10.5 years for participants in the multiple risk factor intervention trial: Findings related to a prior hypothesis of the trial. *Journal of the American Medical Association* 263: 1795.

Office of Women's Health. 1998. Directory of residencies and fellowship programs in women's health.

Pearson, Cynthia. 2006 (March–April). Menopause hormone therapy and age of initiation: Reasonable theory or marketing hoax?? *The Women's Health Activist.* Washington, DC: National Women's Health Network.

Pinn, Vivian, and Judith LaRosa. 1992. *Overview: Office of Research on Women's Health.* Bethesda, MD: National Institutes of Health.

Rosser, Sue V. 1994. *Women's Health: Missing from U.S. Medicine.* Bloomington: Indiana University Press.

Soafer, S., and E. Abel. 1990. Older women's health and financial vulnerability: Implications of the Medicare benefit structure. *Women's Health* 16: 47–67.

Steering Committee of the Physician's Health Study Group. 1989. Final report on the aspirin component of the ongoing physician's health study. *New England Journal of Medicine* 321: 129–35.

Steingart, R.M., M. Packes, P. Hamm, et al. 1991. Sex differences in the management of coronary artery disease. *New England Journal of Medicine* 321: 129–35.

Stevens, P.E., and J.M. Hall. 1988. Stigma, health beliefs, and experiences with health care in lesbian women. *Image: Journal of Nursing Scholarship* 10(2): 69–73.

Trippet, Susan E., and Joyce Bain. 1992. Reasons American lesbians fail to see traditional health care. *Health Care for Women International* 13(2): 145–54.

Weisman, Carol S. 1998. *Women's Health Care: Activist Traditions and Institutional Change.* Baltimore: Johns Hopkins University Press.

White, Evelyn (ed.) 1990. *The Black Women's Health Book.* Seattle, WA: The Seal Press.

PART ONE   **Women of Color**

CHAPTER ONE

The Reproductive Health and Sexual Rights of Women of Color: Still Building a Movement

LYNN ROBERTS, LORETTA ROSS, AND M. BAHATI KUUMBA

> *This cluster of articles is dedicated to the honor and memory of two of our beloved sister warriors and to all other sister warriors who have gone before them, as well as to the hope and promise of all those who will follow in their footsteps:*

GLORIA EVANGELINA ANZALDÚA[1]

1942–2004

PANDORA SINGLETON[2]

1955–2004

More than 600 activists gathered in Atlanta, Georgia, November 13–16, 2003, to participate in the first *SisterSong* Reproductive Health and Sexual Rights National Conference. The Collective was formed in 1997 with the shared recognition that as women of color we have the right and responsibility to represent ourselves and our communities. *SisterSong* is committed to educating women of color on reproductive and sexual health and rights and to working toward culturally and linguistically appropriate access to health services, information, and resources through the integration of the disciplines of community organizing, self-help, and human rights education. The *SisterSong* Women of Color Reproductive Health Collective is composed of more than 30 local, regional, and national grassroots member organizations and affiliates. Its nearly 300 individual members in the United States represent four primary ethnic populations/indigenous nations in the United States: Native American/Indigenous, Black/African American, Latina/Puerto Rican, and Asian/Pacific Islander.

The *SisterSong* conference was the largest gathering of women of color working on reproductive health issues in U.S. history, attracting many new voices to the reproductive justice movement.[3] More than half of the participants said that this was the first conference for and by women of color that they had ever attended. For four days, conference participants celebrated this historic and exceptional opportunity for women of color activists to lay the groundwork for a national women of color reproductive health and sexual rights movement in the United States. Both seasoned and emerging activists were able to reflect upon their work, expand their knowledge, celebrate their accomplishments, and develop and refine

Originally published in the spring 2005 issue (vol. 17, no. 1).

their strategies. They acknowledged the power of individual activism, the power of diversity among women of color, and the power of collective organizing.

In this issue, *SisterSong* offers a cluster of three articles by speakers at the conference. These articles are not just another form of historical evidence and opinion but a means of undermining the hegemonic narrative of the women's movement that continues to exclude our voices and neglect our needs. White, middle class, mainstream—these are the monikers that are often used to describe the women's movement—but through the *SisterSong* conference and these articles, we are identifying the silences and raising the voices of those whose experiences have not been documented.[4] There is no one story we are trying to tell, but rather these articles represent a harmony of our mixed voices. By attending to some of the silences, we seek to reveal what is not being talked about in the women's movement and, just as important, to mobilize us toward action.

Raising Our Voices

The three articles selected for this cluster of articles do not reflect the multiple and divergent thoughts, feelings, and experiences of all the conference attendees nor all the voices that should be heard. Yet, each piece resonates with the vision of *SisterSong* to build and sustain our women of color movement for reproductive justice.

The primary reasons for the existence of *SisterSong* are twofold: first, many women of color reproductive health organizations are small, fragile, and understaffed, yet they deliver valuable reproductive health services to communities of color and lead in advocating for reproductive justice in their communities. By uniting as a national collective, we are able to provide support for each other, train new leadership, develop financial and organizational stability, and help develop new women of color reproductive health organizations where needed. We are able to identify the particular reproductive health needs of women of color and promote culturally appropriate strategies for addressing these concerns. This commitment to capacity building is evident in the first article, Jennifer Nelson's documentation of women of color in the reproductive rights movement. Nelson's historical account of a community activist health center in the Mississippi Delta illustrates how women of color have the capacity to heal their own communities and, in turn, heal themselves.

The second motivating force of *SisterSong* is our belief that the mainstream reproductive rights movement marginalizes the voices of women of color. The neglect of women of color has weakened the pro-choice movement and, in fact, contributes to the incessant attacks on reproductive rights that largely target the most vulnerable women. As Andrea Smith points out in the second article in this issue, "The pro-choice and pro-life camps on the abortion debate are often articulated as polar opposites; [however], they both depend on similar operating assumptions that do nothing to support either life or real choice for women of color." According to Smith, the prison-industrial complex manifests the perverse connections between the current "choice" rhetoric, capitalism, the "pro-life" position, and oppressive intersecting forces of sexism, racism, and capitalism. Women of color also bear the brunt of punitive legislation such as the Hyde Amendment (that restricts government funding for abortions for poor women, women in the military, and women on Native American reservations) and welfare reform (that imposes limitations on family size, college education, and financial assistance).

In the third paper, Ester Shapiro shares her personal journey across and within many borders as coordinating editor of *Nuestros Cuerpos, Nuestras Vidas*, the Spanish cultural adaptation of *Our Bodies, Ourselves*, which brings into sharp relief some of the creative ways in which women of color are forging "new tools" for dismantling the master's house. The predominantly white movement has also failed to include or sufficiently address issues substantively affecting women of color, such as sterilization abuse, the lack of access to quality health care, infant mortality, immigration abuses, and population control strategies.

Making a Difference

Following the conference, *SisterSong* was part of the more than 1.15 million people who marched together for reproductive justice in Washington, D.C., on April 25, 2004, in support of women's rights. Despite the media's limited coverage, this March for Women's Lives was the largest women's protest march ever in U.S. history. It was remarkable because it represented a potentially pivotal point in our social justice movements by bringing together women's rights, civil rights, antiwar, and human rights activists to create a quilt of undivided rights that address the intersection of gender, race, and class that women—especially women of color—experience.[5]

SisterSong's participation in the march represents the fact that in the United States reproductive rights work among women of color parallels, yet at the same time is distinct from, that done by predominantly white, mainstream pro-choice organizations. The primary difference is that many women of color in the movement are moving away from or have never adopted the liberalist "choice" language as a defining framework and instead are embracing the global human rights framework.[6] The global human rights framework gives us the power of making global connections and the power of building a united human rights movement in which we defend not only our reproductive autonomy but also the right of our communities to self-determination.

As this volume goes to press, we anxiously await what many believe is the most crucial presidential election for women in many decades. Members of *SisterSong* are actively engaged in mobilizing women of color in their local communities to exercise their rights by educating them about the multiple issues and policies that affect their health and their communities. Whatever the outcome of the election, we recognize the urgent need to build a movement that will ensure the reproductive health of women of color. In this issue, we are honored to share just a few of the voices that are a part of this movement at this critical moment in history.

Notes

1. Gloria Evangelina Anzaldúa was an internationally recognized cultural theorist, creative writer, and independent scholar best known for her works *Borderlands/LaFrontera: The New Mestiza* and *This Bridge Called My Back: Writings of Radical Women of Color.* Anzaldúa was instrumental in developing a more inclusive feminist movement.

2. Pandora Singleton was the founding executive director of Project Azuka, an HIV/AIDS empowerment and support program for African American women and girls located in Savannah, Georgia. Project Azuka was one of the original member organizations of *SisterSong.*

3. In 1987 the Women of Color Program of the National Organization for Women (NOW) organized the first national conference for 400 women of color on reproductive rights, and in 1990 the National Black Women's Health Project (NBWHP) organized the first national conference on reproductive health for African American women.

4. While the historical contributions of women of color to the advancement of reproductive rights have been acknowledged in feminist literature, it is also recognized that there is insufficient documentation of our unique strategies for building and sustaining a movement that will address the multiple root causes of poor health in communities of color (Gilkes 1980; Gutierrez and Lewis 1997).

5. *SisterSong* was instrumental in broadening the agenda of the March for Women's Lives. Indeed, the very name of the march was changed due to the collective action of *SisterSong* and other women of color organizations. At the November conference, *SisterSong* issued a statement in support of the march as long as specific demands were met. These demands included the inclusion of

women of color in decision-making and assurance that the march be relevant to the lived realities of women of color. During the conference one plenary and a forum were held to allow attendees to voice their support of and opposition to the march. *SisterSong* coordinator Loretta Ross and National Black Women's Health Project founder Byllye Avery also convened several conference call dialogues with 40 women of color activists throughout the country to weigh in on issues surrounding the march. Ross was subsequently hired as co-coordinator of the march, although her role went virtually unrecognized by the media.

6. In actuality, black women may have been among the first feminists to fully embrace the concept of "choice." As welfare rights activist Johnnie Tillmon points out, "[n]obody realizes more than poor women that all women have the right to control their own reproduction" (1972, 111).

References

Gilkes, Cheryl Townsend. 1980. "Holding Back the Ocean with a Broom: Black Women and Community Work." In *The Black Woman*, ed. La Frances R. Rose. Beverly Hills: Sage Publications.

Gutierrez, Lorraine M., and Edith A. Lewis. 1997. "Education, Participation, and Capacity Building in Community Organizing with Women of Color." In *Community Organizing and Community Building for Health*, ed. Meredith Minkler, 216–29. New Brunswick, NJ: Rutgers University Press.

Nelson, Jennifer. 2003. *Women of Color and the Reproductive Rights Movement*. New York: New York University Press.

Tillmon, Johnnie. 1972. "Welfare Is a Women's Issue." *Ms.* (spring): 111.

CHAPTER TWO

"Hold your head up and stick out your chin":
Community Health and Women's Health in Mound Bayou, Mississippi

JENNIFER NELSON

Women's health activists of the late 1960s and 1970s radically transformed women's and reproductive health care by demanding that women,
rather than doctors, make fundamental decisions about their own health
care. They put the female patient at the center of the medical decision-
making process by demanding that doctors take seriously women's understandings of their own bodies. The fundamental definition, however,
of what constituted reproductive health care or women's health care did
not change. Women's health care and reproductive health care remained
within the traditional purview of OB/GYN services: Pap tests for cervical cancer, breast exams for breast cancer detection, birth control, prenatal care, birthing, and postpartum care for the mother. Yet when we shift
the perspective of the women's health movement to some of the poorest
women in the United States, those who lived in the counties surrounding the town of Mound Bayou in the Mississippi Delta region, we find
that this definition of women's/reproductive health care was far too narrow. Rather, women's and reproductive health care could only be understood within a broad context of health care needs that improved the life
quality of the entire community.

In the context of the Mississippi Delta in the 1960s, a narrow view of
women's health issues did not serve black women or their families as
long as basic economic and community development issues were neglected. Problems like sanitation, housing, clothing, transportation, and
food were all basic economic necessities that had to be provided to make
women's reproductive health a real possibility. The founders and staff
of the Delta Health Center in Mound Bayou, Mississippi, the first rural
community health center in the United States serving 14,000 people in
Bolivar, Coahoma, Sunflower, and Washington counties, realized that
achieving health for very poor rural women required that fundamental
development problems be addressed in conjunction with basic reproductive health care provision (Geiger 1974).[1] As a result of this redefinition of
what constituted health care, Delta Health Center nurse-midwives,
nurses, physicians, outreach workers, and other staff members linked
traditional OB/GYN care to broader community development issues.
They also focused on empowering poor women (and men) by involving

---

Originally published in the spring 2005 issue (vol. 17, no. 1).

them in their own health care delivery. In fact, most of those working with the health center were community members who also utilized the center as patients.[2]

The first two community health centers in the nation opened simultaneously in 1965 in Mound Bayou, Mississippi, and at Columbia Point (a 6,000-person housing project built on what used to be a city dump on an isolated peninsula jutting out into Boston harbor) in Massachusetts. Soon after, clinics opened in the South Bronx in New York City, in the Watts neighborhood of Los Angeles, California, in Chicago, Illinois, and in Denver, Colorado. By 1971 President Johnson's Office for Economic Opportunity (OEO) had provided $308 million and the federal Health, Education, and Welfare (HEW) Department had made available $110 million for the creation of new neighborhood health centers.[3] By 1974, there were more than 800 health centers across the country that served 4.2 million people. More than 70 percent of these people were poor (almost half had no employed family members), and over 40 percent were minors under the age of eighteen, groups that traditionally lack access to quality health care (Byrd and Clayton 2002, 336).

Delta Health Center patients found opportunities to complete their educations and become employed in the health profession at the center and elsewhere. (Some left the state to pursue careers as medical providers.) They trained and worked as social workers, medical doctors, outreach workers, registered nurses, nurses' aides, sanitarians, and technicians (Dorsey 2003). In 1969, Cynthia Kelly reported in the *American Journal of Nursing* that "of the 26 members of the nursing staff, 21 are long-time residents of the center's 500-square-mile 'district'" (Kelly 1969). Women involved in the health centers as both workers and patients argued that health care needed to embrace health education, GED and college prep courses, job placement, transportation, a clean environment, sanitation, legal services, a farm cooperative, nutrition counseling, child care, and, perhaps most important, empowerment fostered through participation in community building. Through their involvement, local black women ensured that the Delta Health Center conformed to values about health and health care held by the black community—not those imposed by white medical practitioners on blacks (Geiger 2003).

This broad notion of health care as a tool for community development and individual empowerment continued to be embraced and promulgated by African American women as they became active in the reproductive rights and the black women's health movements, which put a great emphasis on both community development and personal empowerment through self-help in the 1970s and 1980s. African American activists involved in black power and community development in the 1970s also embraced the link between empowerment, self-help, and community development; the roots of that perspective can be traced, in part, to the community health center experiment initiated in Mound Bayou (National Black Women's Health Project 1990, 291–92; Nelson 2003).

This essay begins to fill a wide gap in the existing historical literature documenting black women's relationship to health care by focusing on black women's experiences in the mid-1960s rural South. Most of the recent scholarship on rural black women and medicine has focused on the pre–World War II period and examined African American women's marginalization from mainstream medical care and their dependence on lay, or "granny," midwives (midwives with no formal medical training). Gertrude Fraser, Susan Smith, Holly Matthews, and Sharla Fett have all done important research that falls into this category (Fett 2002, 111–41; Fraser 1998, 25–106; Matthews 1992; Smith 1995, 118–48). Another avenue of research that has been pursued in recent years has focused on the postwar period, yet emphasized the reproductive abuses experienced by black women at the hands of physicians and the mainstream health care establishment. Dorothy Roberts has done some of the best work in this area in her book *Killing the Black Body* (Roberts 1997, 56–103).

In beginning to fill the gap between the two predominant areas of scholarship investigating black women's relationships to health care, my research offers a third course that includes important lessons learned from both prewar and postwar investigations, but also begins to break new ground by exploring how southern African American women became actively involved in creating and managing their own health care institutions that offered mainstream medical care provided by physicians, nurses, nurses' aides, and nurse-midwives in the post–World War II period. While these women were not always the principal providers of their own medical care, as is emphasized in the pre–World War II research on lay midwives, neither were they merely the victims of a racist medical system that was at its best negligent and at worst abusive. African American women in Mound Bayou, Mississippi, shaped health care to suit their community and individual needs by becoming centrally involved in the creation and maintenance of a community health center that served them.

The Delta Health Center in Mound Bayou also serves as a cogent example of community-based health care that will hopefully inspire a closer look at the health care system currently in place for the poor in the United States. A revival of neighborhood-based community clinics could help solve problems presently grappled with in attempting to provide quality health care to the poor. In particular, this innovative model brings poor people into the health care system as more than passive recipients of care. As providers of their own health care and decision-makers about what health care needs are most important, poor people would be able to better ensure that health care served them, their families, and their communities. Also, a closer look at the community health center model could broaden discussions about health to include the wider problems confronted by poor members of communities. It is my hope that this essay will inspire further discussion of how we might link public health to a broad set of community needs and demands defined by the people who use those services. This innovative model deserves reexamination given the current crisis in health care in this nation.

Historical Background

Black women in the South have a long history of providing health care to their communities that stretches from the first years of slavery into the first decades of the twentieth century. In the early part of the twentieth century, although nominally free, southern African American women and men were excluded from mainstream (white Jim Crow) medical facilities. At the same time, they expressed a strong personal preference for local black midwives over white physicians. This preference can be traced to the legacy of African American health care practices under slavery, which included traditions of lay midwifery among African American women. These traditions continued into the Jim Crow period as black lay midwives still provided the greater part of health care for their communities. The preference for midwifery eroded, however, in the first half of the twentieth century through a complex interaction between public health policymakers and physicians who barred local black midwives from medical practice through a system of regulation and forced "retirement." In the post–World War II period, as lay midwives all but disappeared from the rural South, there was a growing acceptance of physician-based medical care by black women (Fett 2002, 111–41; Fraser 1998, 25–106; Matthews 1992; Smith 1995, 118–48).

Yet, the increasing acceptance of physician- and hospital-based medical care by blacks continued to be hampered by the persistence of the Jim Crow medical system, which sorely underserved black patients and left little to fill the gap in rural reproductive health services left by the eradication of lay midwife practices. Few white physicians worked in rural black areas, and those who did often neglected poor blacks. Hospitals that did serve African Americans often turned poor patients away if they could not pay. Health insurance was largely unavailable to blacks because of discrimination by national insurance companies like Metropolitan Life (Wailoo 2001, 100).

There were hospitals created by black fraternal organizations to serve blacks, such as the International Order of Twelve Knights and Daughters of Tabor, which founded Taborian, a black hospital in Mound Bayou, Mississippi ("Mound Bayou's Crisis" 1974; Kelly 1969). Unfortunately, it was totally inadequate to meet community health care needs—it only had a 50-bed capacity. Members of the fraternal organization who founded the hospital paid dues for care; dues also covered burial as well as health services. This facility was the only hospital for blacks in the region. Like Taborian, black hospitals remained woefully underfunded and inadequate to meet most black community health needs.

By the 1950s and 1960s, as the cotton harvest became mechanized and white plantation owners saw no economic incentive to provide medical care to blacks who lived on their land, many rural African Americans went completely without health services. Often they were also without basic transportation to get to a hospital even if one existed in their area (" 'To be, or not to be': Mound Bayou" 1973; "Mound Bayou's Crisis" 1974). As Dr. L.C. Dorsey, social activist and former director of the Delta Health Center, explained in a telephone interview, "Doctors on plantations found conditions so unpleasant they didn't want to treat African Americans. Health care for poor people and poor black people was dependent on home remedies" (Dorsey 2003). Richard Hall, a reporter writing about the Delta Health Center for *Life Magazine,* observed that "blacks in the farm country outside Mound Bayou were accustomed to suffering the pain of their illnesses until it became unbearable. Only then would they seek out a doctor. Even if the doctor was black, he would frequently demand payment on the spot; and if he was white, he would often only talk to them across a desk, asking questions" (Hall 1969).

There were other social barriers stemming from within black communities that also prevented Delta residents from accessing mainstream health care even when it was available. African Americans in the Delta were frequently distrustful of white health care providers because of medical abuses—particularly the Tuskegee (Alabama) experiment (1932–1972) and the high incidence of involuntary sterilization—that had targeted blacks. This attitude needed to be addressed before African Americans would use mainstream health services, or even community health centers, in large numbers. As Dorsey explained, "Black people were suffering from the aftershocks of the Tuskegee experiment . . . I thought it would be real easy to tell people, 'you got free health care,' but many of them were suspicious. Many had known people who had gone to Tuskegee and not come back or died there" (Dorsey 2003).

The Delta Health Center case suggests that African Americans needed to become agents in the provision of their own health care in order for health care institutions serving poor blacks in the South to succeed. Community control over the Delta Health Center fostered a strong sense of personal and community empowerment by providing the opportunity for blacks to command the expansion of an entire nexus of interrelated health care services that included reproductive health but also embraced sanitation, housing, education, and jobs. Empowerment was linked to the creation of services by and for the community, rather than the imposition of services on the community by outsiders.

Dorsey's interaction with the Delta Health Center characterizes how community involvement in medical services could help transform black women's lives in the Delta beyond simple health care provision. Dorsey was born on a plantation to sharecropper parents (just a generation removed from slavery) in Washington County, Mississippi. She grew up in neighboring LeFleur County without access to education or job experience beyond farming. As a teenager, Dorsey was a social activist (a self-described fieldworker) with the Council of Federated Organizations (COFO), the Student Non-Violent Coordinating Committee (SNCC), and the Southern Christian Leadership Conference (SCLC). From her involvement in the civil rights movement, Dorsey heard about the Delta Health Center and was intrigued because she wanted to become engaged with a project that would be sustainable in a community over a long period of time. She explained that she was hired to be a part of community health outreach with the center although she had no other experience except her activism. Dorsey said Dr. John Hatch, director of community health action at the health center and one of the center's founders, wanted to give young people the chance to grow in the organization, so he hired people with little or no work experience. After a stint as an outreach worker, Dorsey applied to direct the community farm associated with the clinic. Again, she noted she had no direct experience but was given an opportunity to develop her skills on the job. Dorsey made clear that her work with the Delta Health Center helped build her confidence to the point that she eventually completed her Ph.D. at SUNY Stony Brook in New York state and returned to the center to become its executive director in the 1980s (Dorsey 2003).

The Mound Bayou Community Health Center: Foundations of Community Medicine

There were three important theoretical foundations underlying the creation of the Delta Health Center that made it both unique and successful. First, there was a vision of medicine as not only a tool for individual health care but as a tool for community transformation. As Dr. H. Jack Geiger, a white physician who co-founded the Delta Health Center, expressed, the architects of the center wanted to "use health care as a . . . point of entry for social change" (2003). Second, the founders of the Delta Health Center believed that fundamentally medicine was a right, not a class or race privilege. Finally, the Delta Health Center promoted personal empowerment by giving members of the community an "assured role in the design and control of their own health services" (Geiger 1984, 12–14).

Dr. Geiger imported the seeds for the community medical center from South Africa when he traveled there in the 1950s to investigate one of the only successful international examples of community medicine serving a poor population. In South Africa he worked at a health center in Pholela created in 1940 by the physician Dr. Sydney Kark. Pholela was a Zulu "tribal reserve" that suffered from desperate poverty. The emphasis at the clinic was not merely on individual health but on the health of the entire community. Kark and other health care providers at the Pholela Health Center were principally attentive to environmental factors, including sanitation, as major contributors to ill health. Kark believed that this model was so effective he exported it to other South African health centers, including one at Lamontville, an African housing project outside of the city of Durban. Kark and his colleagues targeted communities with "high birth rates, high death rates, a heavy burden of both infections and chronic disease, low levels of employment, low literacy, substandard housing and nutrition, and limited medical care resources" (Geiger 1984, 17).

In June 1964, during the Student Non-Violent Coordinating Committee's "Freedom Summer," Geiger connected his experiences with the health centers in South Africa to the desperate poverty he found in the southern United States. Geiger traveled to Mississippi in 1964 as cofounder of the Medical Committee for Human Rights (MCHR). MCHR consisted of a group of New York physicians who contributed to the stepped-up civil rights activity of Freedom Summer by providing health care to civil rights volunteers, as well as to local poor black people who were not involved in the movement. In that capacity Geiger journeyed to the Deep South with "hundreds of other physicians, nurses, and health worker volunteers . . . to help provide medical care, support, and protection for civil rights workers." Geiger and other MCHR activists remained in Mississippi after Freedom Summer and dedicated their services to building long-term community-based institutions that could help address both the economic and social oppression experienced by African Americans in the South (Geiger 1996, 15; Dittmer 1995, 335).

During his stint as a doctor-activist in Mississippi during Freedom Summer, Geiger found that African Americans lived in communities that were as poor and unhealthful as those he had seen in the tribal reserves of South Africa. He wrote that he "took a long, close look at the poverty, misery, and deprivation—and, inevitably, illness—in the sharecropper shacks and small-town black slums of the Deep South." He recognized he didn't have to go to Africa to find poverty; "there was a third world in the United States" (Geiger 1996, 15).

The mid-1960s were a pivotal time in the civil rights movement. Freedom Summer was a formidable effort that brought new energy into the movement. SNCC organizers believed that by bringing northern college students to Mississippi, national attention would be focused on the fight for voting rights and racial justice. It was also a summer of severe violence, including lynchings, beatings, bombings, and the burning of buildings. Yet, activists also began to see a transformation in the political orientation of the movement. With the passage of the Civil Rights Act of 1964 and the Voting Rights Act of 1965, many people around the nation believed the movement had achieved its goals. Of course, blacks in Mississippi knew that racial justice was still not a reality as resistance to both acts by white Mississippians was strong. Organizations like SNCC became increasingly frustrated with the idea of integration and nonviolence and, as a result, began to focus on black power and black nationalism. As an interracial and nonviolent effort focused on local community development and empowerment, the Delta Health Center stands out as a continuation of earlier civil rights movement goals. At the same time, it also embraced some of the new ideas put forth by black nationalists, primarily the creation of majority black-run institutions to foster both community building and empowerment of the individuals involved in the institutions (Dittmer 1995, 242–49; Curry 1996, 58–65).

Together, in Greenville, Mississippi, with other civil rights and SNCC activists, Geiger decided that a community health center was perhaps the best way to make a long-term commitment to improving comprehensive health problems associated with poverty among African American Delta residents (Geiger 2003). He also believed that the health center should be controlled by local blacks who would use it. Fellow activists Dr. Count Gibson, chairman of Preventive Medicine at Tufts University Medical School, and Dr. John Hatch, civil rights volunteer, offered to partner with Geiger. Dr. Hatch was the only African American of the three. He was born in Kentucky and, as he explained in an interview, had grown up in Arkansas on "the banks of the Mississippi River" and often earned money "working in the fields picking cotton" (Hatch 2003). Dr. Hatch trained as a social worker at Atlanta University and joined the faculty as an assistant professor of preventive medicine at Tufts Medical School (Hall 1969). Geiger and the other founders of the project received support from the Office of Economic Opportunity (OEO), which was part of President Johnson's "War on Poverty," and later, after the Nixon administration dismantled OEO, from the Department of Health, Education, and Welfare (HEW). Gibson, Geiger, and Hatch believed that "community health centers [could] be used as a route to social, economic, and political change." They argued further that "a new model for primary care . . . would draw on the resources of the people themselves, making them active rather than passive participants" (Geiger 1996, 16).

As in South Africa, the first health centers were created in two locations, one urban and one rural. The urban site was in Boston and the rural one in Mound Bayou in northern Bolivar County, Mississippi. In 1965, founders of the Delta Health Center carefully chose to locate the

center in the Delta community of Mound Bayou, an all-black community of 12,000 residents, because it was an historically all-black town.
Freedman Isaiah T. Montgomery had founded the town in 1887. Since its
founding, Mound Bayou had been unique in the Mississippi Delta. Em-
mett J. Stringer, a leader in the National Association of Colored People
(NAACP) at the time of the 1954 *Brown v. Board of Education* Supreme
Court decision, recalled that growing up in Mound Bayou had a very
positive influence on his development as a "race man." He said, "Having
seen black mayors and bankers and policemen and superintendents
of schools, I knew what was possible, probable, and desirable" (Dittmer
1995, 42).

Yet, Bolivar County had long been one of the poorest counties in the
nation. The infant mortality rate of the county was astoundingly high in
the 1960s; about 60 per 1,000 infants died before their first year. (As a
point of comparison, that is about the same rate as Burundi, Uzbekistan,
and Nepal; the U.S. rate is currently 6.8 per 1,000.) The residents of Mound
Bayou lived on a median annual income of less than $1,000 per family
per year and suffered from lack of health care as well as poor sanitation,
including unprotected water supplies, because 70 percent of the population was without a clean water supply. Mound Bayou residents suffered
from a lack of adequate shelter as well, because approximately 90 percent
of dwellings were unfit for human habitation (Geiger 2003; Geiger 1984,
25; Geiger 1974, 139).

Before the health center in Mound Bayou even opened its doors, project
staff began to drum up grassroots community support. The project immediately incorporated local people into the organization by recruiting
residents of Mound Bayou and Bolivar County to go door to door to community homes, churches, and schools to discuss community health needs.
Ten local health associations were formed from these efforts. These community health associations defined priority health needs to be addressed
by the neighborhood health center. Priority health requirements ranged
from drinking water in a community where people had to walk three
miles for clean water to health care for children and the elderly.

Members of the community health associations expanded the traditional idea of health care by pointing out that food, jobs, and housing were
fundamental requirements for good health. For Geiger and other organizers of the project, it was essential to the success of the clinic that local
people defined health needs for themselves. That these were not always
traditionally defined health care needs was not a problem. The clinic
founders believed that they needed to respond to health priorities set by
the people themselves. Geiger believed that the clinic could not be sustained if a group of outsiders imposed health care services on the community without giving the community a fundamental role in identifying

and prioritizing what those services should look like. By 1969, 7,000 black residents of Bolivar County were involved in implementing the services sponsored by the health center; these were services the community members had created for themselves (Geiger 1974, 139–40).

By attending to what local people needed and wanted, the community clinic improved upon more traditional medical provision in the rural South. Geiger wrote that the Mound Bayou clinic provided "the essentials of community-oriented primary care: family health care teams; community organization and health education; the training of local workers as family health aides, environmental sanitarians and health [educators]" (Geiger 1996, 16; Geiger 1974, 139). The ten local health associations formed into the larger Mound Bayou Health Council, which became the community governing board for the health center. The health council was comprised entirely of African American community residents, all of whom were also patients at the health center. The creation of the health council allowed the health center to file as a Community Development Corporation (with OEO), helping them to institutionalize their broad point of view on health, which encompassed much that was outside of the traditional health care rubric, such as "early childcare, nutritional and social programs for the isolated rural elderly, a bus transportation system, legal services, and housing rehabilitation" (Geiger 1996, 17). Health care was much more than seeing a doctor for these community activists. It meant building a strong economic and social base for the community as a whole (Geiger 1974, 139). A community vegetable garden became a 500-acre farm cooperative founded by 1,200 families in the region. "The first farm co-op of people who don't own farms," Geiger commented (2003). In just over seven months the co-op grew more than one million pounds of food and effectively ended hunger in the area. As Geiger explained, the most important lesson to impart from the Mound Bayou experiment to health care providers is that "your [health care providers] priorities may not be those of the people you are concerned with . . . People who are concerned with survival are going to be worried about that before they are concerned with tuberculosis. They are going to be concerned with housing, jobs, food, their kids, and some other things" (Geiger 1974, 141–42).

Women in the Community Health Center: Providers and Patients

According to Geiger, most of the Delta Health Center patients were women, children, and elderly men. Because there was so little paid labor in the region (at its height unemployment reached 75 percent), many young men migrated north to find jobs. As a result of out-migration, the average age of Mound Bayou residents was only about 15 years old, and the average age of men in the community was about 50 years old. Thus, women and their children were very much at the center of the Delta Health Center as both patients and workers (Geiger 2003).

As in other rural and primarily African American communities in the South, there were few practicing physicians in the area and even fewer who would treat blacks. Black physicians were even scarcer (Wailoo 2001, 101). The Delta Health Center filled that gap with two white nurse-midwives, Sister Mary Stella Simpson and Asa Johansen, both of whom joined the clinic when it opened its doors. Other medical staff at the Delta Health Center included a black female obstetrician/gynecologist, Dr. Helen Barnes, who joined the health center in 1968, and local women trained as nurses and nurses' aides. Dr. Barnes set up a program for pre-natal care, delivery, and contraceptive services, which was supported in the 1970s with federal Title X money, a program created by President Nixon to promote family planning among poor Americans. Born in Mississippi, Barnes left the state to earn her medical degree from Howard University in Washington, D.C. Completing her degree in 1958, she returned to the Mississippi Delta to serve as one of the few black general practitioners in Greenwood, Mississippi. After returning north to finish a residency in OB/GYN at Kings County Hospital in Brooklyn, New York, she joined the Delta Health Center (Barnes 2003).

Clementine Murray, a local resident of Bolivar County and the mother of nine children, trained as a nurse's aide at the Delta Health Center in 1966. When she trained for her position the health center was still in its first temporary residence, which was an abandoned movie theater (Kelly 1969). Murray expressed the strong sense of personal empowerment she garnered from her work with the health center by testifying that she managed to juggle both her full-time work at the center and the arduous work in her own home raising her children because she was so fully committed to the center as a community resource. Her pride in the health center gave her energy to "hold your head up and stick out your chin and say, 'I can if I want to' " (1969).

Women's Health as Community Health

Both Dr. Barnes and Dr. Dorsey explained that there was no such thing as "women's health care" among African American women in rural Mississippi in the 1960s. Health care was not discussed in terms of its specific relevance to women beyond providing basic OB/GYN services in conjunction with other health services. Like Geiger, Barnes discovered that she could not address OB/GYN or infant health without addressing the larger environmental and economic problems that faced the community. She recalled that "we had pediatrics and surgery, but I also found out that it's all right to practice medicine and deal with sanitation and feed people—write a prescription for evaporated milk." Like general health, women's health could not be limited to a narrow conception of medical practice. The practice of medicine necessarily expanded to embrace the environmental and economic problems of the Mississippi Delta community. Dr. Barnes continued, "I delivered babies every day and night and the nurse-midwives would go out to do home visits—take care of the babies. [They would] look and see if they had screens and if they didn't have running water they would dig a well" (Barnes 2003). Thelma Walker, another local woman who became the nursing administrator of the center, added:

> If a nurse in the field finds a home without a water supply—out go the sanitarians and engineers with the well digger invented right here at the center and they dig a well in half a day. If there are rats coming through the floor, we exterminate them. A leaking roof? A privy falling down? Out go workers from the center—and these are local people—to patch the roof, build a new privy or take healthy adults tools from the tool bank we've scrounged together so they can make their own repairs. (Kelly 1969)

Although the ideas of "women's health" and "reproductive health" need to be reconceived in the context of the Mississippi Delta in the mid-1960s, there is evidence that African American women responded positively to contraceptives when they were made available. Dr. Barnes distributed large numbers of contraceptives as part of a "community health improvement program" created by federal Title X money in 1970. Barnes explained that for many poor black women this was the first time they had been introduced to any kind of family planning. For the most part, she said, black women responded positively to the idea that they could limit their fertility using contraceptive measures. She recalled that women also came to her to be sterilized when they felt they no longer wanted to bear children. Her experience confirms other evidence that African American women wanted to control their fertility as long as they could do so voluntarily (Barnes 2003; Rodrique 1999, 293–305).

At the same time, in the early 1970s, many African Americans, including black nationalists but also other women of color involved in the burgeoning feminist movement, viewed federally sponsored birth control programs as genocidal. The African American reaction against birth control was very much linked to the way that federal programs provided contraceptive services. These programs were associated with ideas of population reduction rather than with notions of creating healthy communities. Black women were particularly adamant that birth control and abortion services needed to be accompanied by other health services that allowed black families to bear and raise the healthy children they wanted.

The emphasis on population reduction as a solution to black poverty made many African Americans very suspicious (Nelson 2003, 55–84). As Barnes noted when I asked her why blacks were suspicious of white health care providers, "You can get kicked in the shins only so many times before you decide that you won't trust people anymore" (Barnes 2003). To gain the trust of the populations she worked with, Barnes explained, we "set up a clinic in a community and found more people came to the clinic year after year after year because we were proving to the community that we were going to stay and do what we said" (Barnes 2003).

A collection of letters written by Sister Mary Stella Simpson, one of the nurse-midwives at the center, serves as a particularly cogent example of how women's health, in particular, needed to be understood in conjunction with larger community development needs. Simpson arrived in Mississippi in 1966 from Evansville, Indiana, to work at the newly opened Delta Health Center. As a native of rural Arkansas Simpson said she "was very familiar with the kind of poverty . . . found in Mound Bayou." Her letters paint a vivid picture of health conditions in the Mississippi Delta during this decade (Simpson 1978, 5).

One letter reveals the extent to which African Americans in the Mississippi Delta lacked even basic necessities such as adequate shelter, food, and clothing, as well as health care and access to education. Simpson recognized these as fundamental problems that could not be separated from her primary task of providing OB/GYN care to poor women:

> Today was my first day for [obstetrical/gynecological] home visits . . . On the very first one I had to come back to town to get milk for a baby. He had finished his last bottle. It had gotten really cold, and the 14 people in that family all congregate in one room around a small wood burning stove . . . The children were all barefoot, therefore could not go to school. The parents have no way of getting shoes for them since they have no income . . . A year old baby was very ill with diarrhea—had it for a week. So I had to drive the mother with all [her] six children to the clinic. The baby had to be hospitalized. (Simpson 1978, 20)

Another letter addresses the extraordinarily poor housing occupied by Delta blacks. Again, adequate housing could not be separated from this particular woman's need for prenatal health care: "I went into a shack out in the country on one [prenatal] visit today and found the ceiling was made of cardboard boxes and the roof leaked badly. What a sight! I did the prenatal exam as if this situation was a daily occurrence. 'We'll fix it when it stops raining,' says the husband as he sweeps the water through the cracks in the floor" (Simpson 1978, 39).

Through her letters written home to her convent sisters, Mary Stella Simpson provided a detailed overview of the persistent and basic health problems confronted by poor African American women who were served by the Delta Health Center. Within days of her arrival in the Mississippi Delta, Simpson learned that OB/GYN care was not enough to improve the lives of the women and children she treated. As Geiger, Barnes, and Dorsey already noted, Simpson found that OB/GYN care also needed to be accompanied by a nexus of health-related provisions such as sanitation, screens on windows to keep out mosquitoes, housing, clothing, nutritional information, and food. Without these basic necessities, the provision of women's reproductive health care was virtually pointless.

Persistent problems recorded by Simpson were lack of food and inadequate housing and clothing. In one letter she wrote, "The last place I visited was the worst ever. The dogs and cats go and come through the walls. It has a high front porch and an old washtub turned upside down for a step. I was scared stiff to put my weight on it, but it held. The mother and daughter were wearing rags held together by safety pins and had bare feet" (Simpson 1978, 20). The lack of basic necessities was so profound that health center doctors, nurses, and nurse-midwives spent much of their time helping to find food and clothing, repairing screens on windows, pressuring landowners to provide better housing, and connecting patients with welfare entitlements such as food stamps.

Women also lacked basic health education, which compromised the health of their children. Although the health center midwives and physicians, including Sister Simpson, encouraged breast-feeding, few women practiced it at first. The local Mound Bayou hospital, Taborian, actually discouraged women from breast-feeding their children because it was viewed as inconvenient (for the hospital, of course, not the mothers). This left women with no option but to use formula, which required sterilizing bottles and finding clean water. Many homes on the white-owned plantations and farms in the region were without running water or a well. Some families used water from the bayou until it dried up in the summer. Some families were also without the means to boil water, and women often didn't know that a bottle could not be rinsed and reused. Because of the unsanitary conditions, diarrhea was a constant problem with small children and a major cause of high infant mortality (Simpson 1978, 19, 82).

The women in Mound Bayou and Bolivar County were very enthusiastic about breast-feeding when they were given some coaching as to how to get started. Because good mothering is something that is learned and neither instinctual nor natural, new mothers often need to be shown how to breast-feed their babies (Tardy 2000; Boston Women's Health Book Collective 1998, 507). In the past it had been grandmothers and granny-midwives who passed on this knowledge. Without an indigenous group of health care providers, however, women in Mound Bayou and surrounding areas were often reliant on indifferent physicians and hospital staff until the community Delta Health Center was founded. Sister

Simpson recorded the enthusiasm for breast-feeding she witnessed among the new mothers:

> We are starting to see results! Breast-feeding is beginning to catch on. We hope to have 100 percent of our mothers feeding this way before the year ends. The mothers enjoy our classes, too . . . We seem never to get away from the sessions . . . They ask questions for hours! One of the mothers delivered her baby only a few days before the next class. She didn't want to miss it, so we went to her home and had class there! (Simpson 1978, 82)

For many of these patients, a home visit by a nurse-midwife was their first ever encounter with a health care practitioner. Many women had received no prenatal care, had never had any sort of medical care as children, and bore their children without any medical support. Simpson also confirmed reports that some doctors and hospitals in the area that did provide care for poor African Americans were neglectful or inadequate for the population. In one case a mother took her 11-month-old baby who would not eat to two different doctors before Simpson helped her to get her child into a hospital that would feed the child intravenously. Another 18-year-old patient was due to deliver her baby any day and was experiencing pre-eclampsia. She had extremely high blood pressure and protein in her urine but had never been seen by a doctor (Simpson 1978, 40). Simpson also cared for a child whose hand had been badly burned and had healed into a fist—the child would remain handicapped for the rest of his life—because a neighborhood doctor had neglected to treat him properly (Simpson 1978, 32).

With basic health care problems unmet it was extremely difficult to carve out a separate OB/GYN practice or define an area of health care as "women's health care" or "reproductive health care." Improving the general health of the entire community was a "women's issue" as it bolstered the health of the women in the community tremendously. Sister Simpson noted that prenatal care was seldom the only care given on a home visit: "If the prenatal exam was the only thing we did on such visits, they wouldn't take so long. But when you see a little one with impetigo all over his face, you doctor him, which often takes a couple of hours" (Simpson 1978, 29). As Barnes pointed out, "Medicine may be the way we got in the door, but medicine is not the number one priority. There are other priorities; food is number one and then a way to make a living" (Barnes 2003).

The clinic quickly transformed women's health and general health in the four-county area served by the Delta Health Center. When the health center was first established, clinic services and training for community staff occurred in an abandoned church parsonage and in an old movie theater in town. After about a year, a new building was built for the health center. By 1969, the clinic was able to provide hospital equipment to patients in their homes when there was not enough space to accommodate patient needs at Taborian. Prenatal and antenatal care both improved dramatically over the first three years of the clinic's existence. Thelma Walker reported that OB/GYN care had grown from almost nothing in the community to a majority of pregnant patients attending the clinic before the fifth month of their pregnancies. Many of these women gave birth at the hospital or at home with a midwife in attendance and were then followed up postpartum at the health center. Their infants received care from birth onward. Walker explained that it was "quite a change . . . from the days when Sister Mary Stella and Aase [sic] Johansen saw many mothers for the first time when they were ready to deliver—or had delivered—and from the time when little children never saw a doctor or nurse until they were so ill with diarrhea or pneumonia that it was touch and go to save them." She added that the "two nurse midwives have helped in prenatal care or delivery of over 100 babies, all living, many at home, but now most mothers have their babies in the hospital" (Kelly 1969).

Ultimately, the Delta Health Center brought poor black women in the Delta the mainstream health services that were available to most other populations in the United States by 1966. But, unlike most other health centers or hospitals serving poor women in America, poor women provided and managed much of their own health care in Mound Bayou. The health center workers, including the physicians, nurses, nurse-midwives, nurses' aides, sanitarians, and health outreach educators, were black women and men who understood that African Americans had been neglected and even abused by mainstream (white Jim Crow) health provision in the past. Clinic staff also addressed fundamental factors contributing to ill health that few people had defined previously as legitimate to a medical practice. As Dorsey explained, Dr. John Hatch, director of health outreach, decided to create a farm collective because he believed that the only antidote to hunger was food (Dorsey 2003). Lack of food was a medical issue, and, I would add, a women's health issue and a reproductive health issue. Women could not bear healthy children without adequate nutrition. Dr. Geiger pointed to the success of the cooperative farm: "In one spring and summer, they have grown one million pounds of food, enough to end hunger in Northern Bolivar County—sweet potatoes, Irish potatoes, snap beans, butter beans, black-eyed peas, collard greens and the like" (Kelly 1969).

Unfortunately, the national neighborhood health center project initiated by Jack Geiger and John Hatch lost federal government support in the 1970s. With the decline in commitment to the "War on Poverty," the OEO and HEW handed the centers over to state public health departments and drastically reduced their funding by shifting over to the Medicaid and Medicare reimbursement system (Byrd and Clayton 2002, 337). The Delta Health Center was sustained through the efforts of the community; however, due to federal government cutbacks, they also suffered funding shortfalls that made their service to the community more difficult. Yet, the notion that overall community health was fundamental to women's reproductive health would continue to resonate and develop as black women defined reproductive health and reproductive rights for themselves in the next decade.

Conclusion

It is imperative to my larger project on the women's health movement of the 1960s and 1970s, which this essay is a part of, to know how effective the community clinics were beyond the more anecdotal evidence provided by those who created and used them. Of course, local voices are essential to a history of community health centers, but without concrete statistical evidence linking improvements in women's health to the neighborhood health centers and their provision of a broad nexus of community services, it is more difficult to make the case that this innovative system of health care should be revived to better serve poor rural women in the South. We do know that infant and maternal mortality rates declined steadily nationwide throughout the twentieth century, but we still don't know the root cause of this decline. In the state of Mississippi infant mortality rates fell from nearly 70 per 1,000 black infants who died before the age of one year in the 1960s to 10.7 per 1,000 for white children and 15.3 per 1,000 for black children in 2000. Although this is still very high compared to national rates, the second highest rate in the country, it is a vast improvement over a 40-year period. We need to find out to what extent these reductions can be solidly attributed to local community efforts to link traditional medicine to broader community development. Anecdotal and subjective evidence point toward a convincing correlation between community involvement, community development, and improved health care and health, but we need to find stronger links if we want to make the case that medicine in this century should be more broadly defined and community based.

Substantiating the correlation between improved health care and community-based and inclusive medicine is also important to providing more equitable reproductive health care to poor African American women in this century. By all the indicators of inadequate reproductive health it is plain that black women in the South are disproportionately disadvantaged: they consistently have higher infant and maternal death

rates than either white or Hispanic women; they disproportionately deliver low birth weight babies; they have some of the highest teenage pregnancy rates; and they are less likely than their wealthier counterparts to
be screened for breast or cervical cancer. Black women also have a disproportionate number of abortions nationwide, and by many accounts,
they still suffer from forced and coerced sterilization and population
control (Roberts 1997, 97, 101). In the area of general health, African
American women in the South also suffer more often from heart disease,
cancer, diabetes, and other diseases related to obesity. These problems
are even more pronounced in rural southern states like Mississippi (Mississippi State Department of Health 2001; Sarah Isom Center 2004, 47–
50, 54–56).

In order to solve these problems, we need to better understand the recent historical contours of African American women's intervention in
the creation of public health policy and then ask why the medical establishment is still under-serving them (and sometimes even abusing them).
We need to understand what critiques of gynecological and obstetrical
medical care African American women have offered in order to begin to
transform our public health structures into equitable health systems. As
in the community health center example in Mound Bayou, we need to
listen to black women in their communities in order to figure out how
best to solve dire health problems that still strike black women down
before their time.

Notes

1. The Mississippi Delta is a diamond-shaped region of western Mississippi
    bordering the Mississippi River and stretching from Memphis, Tennessee,
    all the way south to Natchez, Mississippi. Since the Civil War it has pro-
    duced huge quantities of cotton through a sharecropping system that kept
    African Americans financially dependent on white plantation owners.

2. I use the term *empowerment* to capture the important black feminist con-
    cept of moving masses of people ("critical mass") to political action in their
    everyday lives, as discussed by Patricia Hill Collins (Collins 1998, 229–51). I
    also found useful Barbara Ransby's discussion of the radicalism of participa-
    tory democracy in her biography of Ella Baker. I believe that Baker's demo-
    cratic ideal as demonstrated by her commitment to attaining political power
    for "the many" was also very much a part of the strategy of those who
    founded and ran the Delta Health Center (Ransby 2003).

3. Between 1965 and 1971, OEO funded more than 100 health centers. HEW
    funded more than 50 (Geiger 1984, 13, 19).

References

Barnes, Helen. 2003. Phone interview with author, 23 January.

Boston Women's Health Book Collective. 1998. *Our Bodies Ourselves for the New Century.* New York: Simon & Schuster.

Byrd, Michael, and Linda Clayton. 2002. *An American Health Dilemma.* Vol. 2. New York: Routledge.

Collins, Patricia Hill. 1998. *Fighting Words: Black Women and the Search for Justice.* Minneapolis: University of Minnesota Press.

Curry, Constance. 1996. *Silver Rights.* New York: Harvest Books.

Dittmer, John. 1995. *Local People: The Struggle for Civil Rights in Mississippi.* Urbana: University of Illinois Press.

Dorsey, L.C. 2003. Phone interview with author, 17 January.

Fett, Sharla. 2002. *Working Cures: Healing, Health, and Power on Southern Slave Plantations.* Chapel Hill: University of North Carolina Press.

Fraser, Gertrude Jacinta. 1998. *African American Midwifery in the South: Dialogues of Birth, Race, and Memory.* Cambridge, MA: Harvard University Press.

Geiger, H. Jack. 2003. Phone interview with author, 7 October.

———. 1996. "A Life in Social Medicine." In *The Doctor-Activist: Physicians Fighting for Social Change,* ed. Ellen L. Bassuk. New York: Plenum Press.

———. 1984. "Community Health Centers: Health Care as an Instrument of Social Change." In *Reforming Medicine: Lessons of the Last Quarter Century,* ed. Ruth and Victor Sidel, 11–32. New York: Pantheon.

———. 1974. "Community Control—or Community Conflict?" In *Neighborhood Health Centers,* ed. Robert M. Hollister, Bernard M. Kramer, and Seymour S. Bellin, 133–41. Lexington: Lexington Books.

Hall, Richard. 1969. "A Stir of Hope in Mound Bayou." *Life Magazine.* Delta Health Center Records, Box 12, Folder: "Articles on Mound Bayou/Bolivar County Health Needs." Southern Historical Collection, University of North Carolina, Chapel Hill.

Hatch, John. 2003. Phone interview with author, 13 October.

Kelly, Cynthia. 1969. "Health Care in the Mississippi Delta." *American Journal of Nursing* 69(4). Delta Health Center Records, Box 12, Folder: "Articles on Mound Bayou/Bolivar County Health Needs." Southern Historical Collection, University of North Carolina, Chapel Hill.

Matthews, Holly F. 1992. "Killing the Medical Self-Help Tradition Among African Americans: The Case of Lay Midwifery in North Carolina, 1912–1983." In *African Americans in the South: Issues of Race, Class, and Gender,* ed. Hans Baer and Yvonne Jones, 60–78. Athens: University of Georgia Press.

Mississippi State Department of Health. 2001. Vital Statistics Mississippi.

"Mound Bayou's Crisis." 1974. *Time Magazine,* 25 November, n.p. Delta Health Center Records, Box 12, Folder: "Articles on Mound Bayou/Bolivar County Health Needs." Southern Historical Collection, University of North Carolina, Chapel Hill.

National Black Women's Health Project. 1990. "Reproductive Rights Position Paper." In *From Abortion to Reproductive Freedom: Transforming a Movement*, ed. Marlene Gerber Fried. Boston: South End Press.

Nelson, Jennifer. 2003. *Women of Color and the Reproductive Rights Movement*. New York: New York University Press.

Ransby, Barbara. 2003. *Ella Baker and the Black Freedom Movement: A Radical Democratic Vision*. Chapel Hill: University of North Carolina Press.

Roberts, Dorothy. 1997. *Killing the Black Body: Race, Reproduction, and the Meaning of Liberty*. New York: Pantheon Books.

Rodrique, Jessie. 1999. "The Black Community and the Birth Control Movement." In *Women and Health in America*, 2nd ed., ed. Judith Walzer Leavitt, 293–305. Madison: University of Wisconsin Press.

Sarah Isom Center. 2004. *A Weave of Women: The Sarah Isom Report on the Status of Women in Mississippi*.

Simpson, Mary Stella. 1978. *Sister Stella's Babies: Days in the Practice of a Nurse Midwife*. New York: American Journal of Nursing Company.

Smith, Susan L. 1995. *Sick and Tired of Being Sick and Tired: Black Women's Health Activism in America, 1890–1950*. Philadelphia: University of Pennsylvania Press.

Tardy, Rebecca W. 2000. "'But I Am a Good Mom': The Social Construction of Motherhood Through Healthcare Conversations." *Journal of Contemporary Ethnography* 29(4): 433–73.

"'To be, or not to be': Mound Bayou." 1973. *Medical World News*, 16 March, 55. Delta Health Center Records, Box 12, Folder: "Articles on Mound Bayou/Bolivar County Health Needs." Southern Historical Collection, University of North Carolina, Chapel Hill.

Wailoo, Keith. 2001. *Dying in the City of the Blues: Sickle Cell Anemia and the Politics of Race and Health*. Chapel Hill: University of North Carolina Press.

CHAPTER THREE

Beyond Pro-Choice versus Pro-Life: Women
of Color and Reproductive Justice

ANDREA SMITH

Once, while taking an informal survey of Native women in Chicago about their position on abortion—were they "pro-life" or "pro-choice"—I quickly found that their responses did not neatly match up with these media-mandated categories.

EXAMPLE 1:
> *Me:* Are you pro-choice or pro-life?
> *Respondent 1:* Oh, I am definitely pro-life.
> *Me:* So you think abortion should be illegal?
> *Respondent 1:* No, definitely not. People should be able to have an abortion if they want.
> *Me:* Do you think then that there should not be federal funding for abortion services?
> *Respondent 1:* No, there should be funding available so that anyone can afford to have one.

EXAMPLE 2:
> *Me:* Would you say you are pro-choice or pro-life?
> *Respondent 2:* Well, I would say that I am pro-choice, but the most important thing to me is promoting life in Native communities.

These responses make it difficult to categorize the Native women queried neatly into "pro-life" or "pro-choice" camps. Is Respondent #1 pro-life because she says she is pro-life? Or is she pro-choice because she supports the decriminalization of and public funding for abortion? I would argue that, rather than attempt to situate these respondents in pro-life or pro-choice camps, it is more useful to recognize the limitations of the pro-life/pro-choice dichotomy for understanding the politics around reproductive justice. Unlike pro-life versus pro-choice advocates who make their overall political goal either the criminalization or decriminalization of abortion, the reproductive frameworks these Native women are implicitly articulating are based on fighting for life and self-determination of their communities. The criminalization of abortion may or may not be a strategy for pursuing that goal.

In previous works, I have focused more specifically on Native women and reproductive justice (A. Smith 2001). Here, I am using these Native women's responses to questions about abortion to argue that the pro-life

Originally published in the spring 2005 issue (vol. 17, no. 1).

versus pro-choice paradigm is a model that marginalizes women of color, poor women, and women with disabilities. The pro-life versus pro-choice paradigm reifies and masks the structures of white supremacy and capitalism that undergird the reproductive choices that women make, and it also narrows the focus of our political goals to the question of criminalization of abortion. Ironically, I will contend, while the pro-choice and pro-life camps on the abortion debate are often articulated as polar opposites, both depend on similar operating assumptions that do nothing to support either life or real choice for women of color. In developing this analysis, I seek to build on previous scholarship that centers women of color as well as reflect on my fifteen years as an activist in the reproductive justice movement through such organizations as the Illinois National Abortion and Reproductive Rights Action League (NARAL), the Chicago Abortion Fund, Women of All Red Nations, Incite! Women of Color Against Violence, and the Committee on Women, Population and the Environment. I begin by examining the limitations of the pro-life position. I then explore the problems with the pro-choice position. The essay concludes with suggestions for moving beyond this binary stalemate between "pro-life" and "pro-choice."

Pro-Life Politics, Criminalization of Abortion, and the Prison Industrial Complex

The fetus is a life—but sometimes that life must be ended.
—Jeanette Bushnell, Seattle-based Native health activist (2004)

The pro-life position maintains that the fetus is a life; hence abortion should be criminalized. Consequently, the pro-life camp situates its position around moral claims regarding the sanctity of life. In a published debate on pro-life versus pro-choice positions on the issue of abortion, Gary Crum (former vice-president of South Carolina Citizens for Life) argues that the pro-life position is "ethically pure" (Crum and McCormack 1992, 54). Because of the moral weight he grants to the protection of the life of the fetus, Crum contends that abortion must be criminalized. Any immoral actions that impact others should be a "serious crime under the law" (1992, 28). The pro-choice position counters this argument by asserting that the fetus is not a life, and hence policy must be directed toward protecting a woman's ability to control her own body. To quote sociologist Thelma McCormack's response to Crum: "Life truly begins in the . . . hospital room, not in the womb" (Crum and McCormack 1992, 121). Gloria Feldt, president of Planned Parenthood, similarly asserts that if the fetus is established as a life, the principles of *Roe v. Wade* must necessarily be discarded (Feldt 2004, 90).

Jeanette Bushnell's statement that *"the fetus is a life—but sometimes that life must be ended"* suggests, however, a critical intervention in the pro-life argument. That is, the major flaw in the pro-life position is NOT the claim that the fetus is a life, but the conclusion it draws from this assertion: that because the fetus is a life, abortion should be criminalized. In this regard, reproductive rights activists and scholars could benefit from the analysis of the anti-prison movement, which questions criminalization as an appropriate response to social issues. As I shall demonstrate, assuming a criminal justice regime fails to address social problems or to adjudicate reproductive issues and results in further marginalization of poor women and women of color. To make this connection, I must first provide a critical history of the failures of the prison system to deal effectively with social problems.

The anti–prison industrial complex movement has highlighted the complete failure of the prison system to address social concerns. In fact, not only do prisons not solve social problems, such as "crime," they are more likely to increase rather than decrease crime rates (Currie 1998; Donziger 1996; Walker 1998). Most people in prison are there for drug- or poverty-related crimes. Prisons do not provide treatment for drug addiction, and it is often easier to access drugs in prison than on the outside. For people who are in prison because of poverty-related crimes, a prison record ensures that it will be much more difficult for them to secure employment once they are released. Consistently, study after study indicates that prisons do not have an impact on decreasing crime rates. For instance, the Rand Corporation found that California's three strikes legislation, which requires life sentences for three-time convicted felons, did not reduce the rate of "murders, rapes, and robberies that many people believe to be the law's principal targets" (Walker 1998, 139). In fact, changes in crime rates often have more to do with fluctuations in employment rates than with increased police surveillance or increased incarceration rates (Box and Hale 1982; Jankovic 1977). In addition, as documented by prison activist groups such as the Prison Activist Resource Center, government monies are siphoned away from education and social services into prisons, thus destabilizing communities of color and increasing their vulnerability to incarceration (Prison Activist Resource Center 2004).

The failure of prisons is well known to policymakers. In fact, John Dilulio, prominent right-wing analyst who was one of the major advocates for the buildup of the prison industrial complex, later renounced his position and came out in support of a prison moratorium (Dilulio 1999). Given that this failure is well known, it then becomes apparent that the purpose of prisons has never been to stop crime. Rather, as a variety of scholars and activists have argued, the purpose has been in large part to control the population of communities of color. As Michael Mancini (1991) and Angela Davis (2003) point out, the racial background of the prison population prior to the Civil War was white. After the Civil War, the Thirteenth Amendment was passed, which prohibits slavery—except for prisoners. The slavery system was then essentially replaced by the convict leasing system, which was often even more brutal than the former. Under slavery, slave-owners at least had a financial incentive to keep slaves alive. In the convict leasing system, no such incentive existed—if a prisoner died, she or he could simply be replaced by another prisoner (Davis 2003; Mancini 1991). The regime of the prison was originally designed to "reform" the prisoner by creating conditions for penitence (hence the term penitentiary) (Ignatieff 1978). After the Civil War, however, the prison adopted similar regimes of punishment found in the slavery system that coincided with the re-enslavement of black communities into the convict leasing system (Davis 2003). As Davis argues, "racisms . . . congeal and combine in prisons"; they exist to maintain the capitalist and white supremacist underpinnings of U.S. society (Davis 2003, 26). The continuing racism of the prison system is evidenced by who is in prison. In 1994, for instance, one out of every three African American men between the ages of 20 and 29 was under some form of criminal justice supervision (Mauer 1999). Two-thirds of men of color in California between the ages of 18 and 30 have been arrested (Donziger 1996, 102–4). Six of every ten juveniles in federal custody are American Indian and two-thirds of women in prison are women of color (Prison Activist Resource Center 2004).

In a statement that also applies to the criminalization of abortion, Davis further argues that it is critical to disarticulate the equation between crime and punishment because the primary purpose is not to solve the problem of crime.

> "Punishment" does not follow from "crime" in the neat and logical sequence offered by discourses that insist on the justice of imprisonment, but rather punishment—primarily through imprisonment (and sometimes death)—is linked to the agendas of politicians, the profit drive of corporations, and media representations of crime. Imprisonment is associated with the racialization of those most likely to be punished . . . If we . . . strive to disarticulate crime and punishment . . . then our focus must not rest only on the prison system as an isolated institution but must also be directed at all the social relations that support the permanence of the prison. (2003, 112)

Prisons simply are not only ineffective institutions for addressing social concerns, they drain resources from institutions that could be more effective. They also mark certain peoples, particularly people of color, as inherently "criminal," undeserving of civil and political rights—thus increasing their vulnerability to poverty and further criminalization.

Davis's principle of disarticulation is critical in reassessing the prolife position. That is, whether or not one perceives abortion to be a crime, it does not therefore follow that punishment in the form of imprisonment is a necessary response. Criminalization individualizes solutions to problems that are the result of larger economic, social, and political conditions. Consequently, it is inherently incapable of solving social problems or addressing crime. Alternative social formations and institutions that can speak to these large-scale political and economic conditions are the appropriate place to address social issues, such as reproductive justice. As Davis argues: "Prison needs to be abolished as the dominant mode of addressing social problems that are better solved by other institutions and other means. The call for prison abolition urges us to imagine and strive for a very different social landscape" (cited in Rodriguez 2000, 215). Thus, even if we hold that a top social priority is to reduce the number of abortions, there is no evidence to suggest that involving the criminal justice system will accomplish that goal, given that it has not been effective in reducing crime rates or addressing social problems. In addition, increased criminalization disproportionately affects people of color—and in the case of abortion, women of color and poor women. An interrogation of the assumptions behind the pro-life movement suggests that what distinguishes the pro-life position is not so much a commitment to life (since criminalization promotes death rather than life, particularly in communities of color and poor communities), but rather a commitment to criminal justice interventions in reproductive justice issues.

An assessment of recent debates within the anti-domestic/sexual assault movements further illustrates this argument. As I, and others, have argued, the anti-violence movement, as it became increasingly funded by the state, began to rely on criminal justice interventions (A. Smith 2005). Domestic violence and sexual assault agencies formed their strategy around the slogan that sexual and domestic violence is a crime. The response then of activists was to push for increased criminalization of sexual and domestic violence through mandatory arrest policies, no-drop prosecution policies, and longer sentencing. Sadly, the result of this approach was that not only did it not reduce violence rates, it often contributed further to women's victimization. For instance, under mandatory arrest laws, the police often arrest the women who are being battered. In fact, the *New York Times* recently reported that the impact of strengthened anti-domestic violence legislation is that battered women kill their abusive partners less frequently; however, batterers do not kill their partners less frequently, and this is more true in black than white communities (Butterfield 2000). Thus, ironically, laws passed to protect battered women are actually protecting their batterers! While prisons currently are not filled with batterers and rapists, this approach contributed to the growth of the prison industrial complex by implicitly buying into a criminal justice regime on which the prison system depends. Legislators attach violence against women provisions (such as the Violence Against Women Act) to repressive anti-crime bills, and by so doing legislators can then rely on anti-violence activists to support the legislation as a whole.

Similarly, the pro-life position implicitly supports the prison industrial complex by unquestioningly supporting a criminal justice approach that legitimizes rather than challenges the prison system. As Davis (2003) argues, it is not sufficient to challenge the criminal justice system; we must build alternatives to it. Just as the women of color anti-violence movement is currently developing strategies for ending violence (A. Smith 2005), a consistent pro-life position would require activists to develop responses to abortion that do not rely on the prison industrial complex. Otherwise, these pro-life activists will continue to support policies that are brutally oppressive, particularly to communities of color and poor communities.

Interestingly, this critique of the prison system is prevalent even within conservative evangelical circles. For example, Charles Colson, a prominent Christian Right activist, founder of Prison Fellowship, and former attorney with the Nixon administration, served time in prison for his role in the Watergate break-in. Following his imprisonment, Colson began to work on prison reform, organizing the Prison Fellowship and its associated lobbying arm, Justice Fellowship. Many platforms implicitly or explicitly supported by Prison Fellowship and Justice Fellowship could be used to question the wisdom of the criminalization of abortion: decarceration for drug offenders (Colson 1977, 17; Colson 1980, 52); minimum wage compensation for prison labor (Lawton 1988, 38); decarceration of all nonviolent offenders ("The first thing we have to do with prisons today is to get the nonviolent people out") (Forbes 1982, 33: Smarto 1993; 46); prison construction moratoriums (Colson 1985, 29; Mill 1999; Van Ness 1985); eradication of mandatory sentencing (Forbes 1982, 33); suffrage for convicted felons (Colson 1985, 34); and expansion of community sentencing programs (Colson 1985, 29; Pulliam 1987; Van Ness 1985). In fact, Colson argues that 50 percent of people in prison today should be released immediately (Fager 1982, 23). To quote Colson:

> The whole system of punishment today is geared toward taking away people's dignity, putting them in an institution, and locking them up in a cage. Prisons are overcrowded, understaffed, dirty places. Eighty percent of American prisons are barbaric—not just brutal, but barbaric . . . Prison as a punishment is a failure. Mandatory sentences and longer sentences are counterproductive . . . the tougher the laws, I'm convinced, the more lawless and violent we will become. As for public safety, it can hardly be said that prisons contribute to public safety . . . Prisons obviously are not deterring criminal conduct. The evidence is overwhelming that the more people we put in prison, the more crime we have. All prisons do is warehouse human beings and at exorbitant cost. (Colson 1983, 15; Fager 1982, 23; Forbes 1982, 34)[1]

Yet, despite his sustained critique of the failure of the prison system, Colson never critiques the wisdom of criminalization as the appropriate response to abortion. In the name of promoting life, the pro-life movement supports one of the biggest institutions of violence and death in this society. But given that this critique of criminalization is not inaccessible to large sectors of the pro-life movement, there should be opportunities to make anti-criminalization interventions into pro-life discourse. Thus, the major flaw in the pro-life position is not so much its claim that the fetus is a life, but its assumption that because the fetus is a life, abortion should be criminalized. A commitment to criminalization of social issues necessarily contributes to the growth of the prison system because it reinforces the notion that prisons are appropriate institutions for addressing social problems rather than causes of the problems. Given the disproportionate impact of criminalization on communities of color, support for criminalization as public policy also implicitly supports racism.

In addition, I am suggesting that those committed to pro-choice positions will be more effective and politically consistent if they contest the pro-life position from an anti-prison perspective. For instance, increasingly, poor women and women of color are finding their pregnancies criminalized. As Dorothy Roberts (1997) and others have noted, women of color are more likely to be arrested and imprisoned for drug use because, as a result of greater rates of poverty in communities of color, they are more likely to be in contact with government agencies where their drug use can be detected. While white pregnant women are slightly more likely to engage in substance abuse than black women, public health facilities and private doctors are more likely to report black women than white women to criminal justice authorities (Maher 1990; Roberts 1997, 175). Meanwhile, pregnant women who would like treatment for their addiction can seldom get it because treatment centers do not meet the needs of pregnant women. One study found that two-thirds of drug treatment centers would not treat pregnant women (Roberts 1997, 189). Furthermore, the criminalization approach is more likely to drive pregnant women who are substance abusers from seeking prenatal or other forms of health care for fear of being reported to the authorities (Roberts 1997, 190). Roberts critiques communities of color for often supporting the criminalization of women of color who have addictions and for failing to understand this criminalization as another strategy of white supremacy that blames women for the effects of poverty and racism. Lisa Maher (1990) and Rickie Solinger (2001, 148) note that a simple choice perspective is not effective for addressing this problem because certain women become marked as women who make "bad choices" and hence deserve imprisonment.

Similarly, Elizabeth Cook-Lynn (1998) argues in "The Big Pipe Case" that at the same time Native peoples were rallying around Leonard Peltier, no one stood beside Marie Big Pipe when she was incarcerated on a felony charge of "assault with intent to commit serious bodily harm" because she breast fed her child while under the influence of alcohol. She was denied services to treat her substance abuse problem and access to abortion services when she became pregnant. But not only did her community not support her, it supported her incarceration. Cook-Lynn argues that in doing so, the community supported the encroachment of U.S. federal jurisdiction on tribal lands for an issue that would normally be under tribal jurisdiction (1998, 110–25). Cook-Lynn recounts how this demonization of Native women was assisted by the publication of Michael Dorris's (1989) *The Broken Cord*, which narrates his adoption of a Native child who suffered from fetal alcohol syndrome. While this book has been crucial in sensitizing many communities to the realities of fetal alcohol syndrome, it also portrays the mother of the child unsympathetically and advocates repressive legislative solutions targeted against women substance abusers. Thus, within Native communities, the growing demonization of Native women substance abusers has prompted tribes to collude with the federal government in whittling away their own sovereignty.

In the larger society, Barbara Harris started an organization called CRACK (Children Requiring a Caring Kommunity) in Anaheim, California, which gives women $200 to have sterilizations. Their mission is to " 'save our welfare system' and the world from the exorbitant cost to the taxpayer for each 'drug addicted birth' by offering 'effective preventive measures to reduce the tragedy of numerous drug-affected pregnancies' " (Kigvamasud'Vashi 2001). Some of CRACK's initial billboards read, "Don't let a pregnancy ruin your drug habit" (Kigvamasud'Vashi 2001). The organization has since opened chapters in several cities around the country, and has changed its name to Positive Prevention to present a less inflammatory image. Nonetheless, its basic message is the same—that poor women who are substance abusers are the cause of social ills and that the conditions that give rise to poor women becoming substance abusers do not need to be addressed.

Unfortunately, as both Roberts (1997) and Cook-Lynn (1998) point out, even communities of color, including those who identify as both pro-life and pro-choice, have supported the criminalization of women of color who have addiction issues. The reason they support this strategy is because they focus on what they perceive to be the moral culpability of women of color for not protecting the life of their children. If we adopt an anti-prison perspective, however, it becomes clear that even on the terms of moral culpability (which I am not defending) it does not follow that

the criminal justice approach is the appropriate way to address this social concern.[2] In fact, criminal justice responses to unwanted pregnancies and/or pregnant women who have addiction issues demonstrate an
inherent contradiction in the pro-life position. Many pro-life organizations have been ardent opponents of population control programs and
policies—advocating against the promotion of dangerous contraceptives
or the promotion of sterilization in third-world countries. Yet, their position depends on the prison industrial complex that is an institution of
population control for communities of color in the United States.

Meanwhile, many pro-choice organizations, such as Planned Parenthood, have supported financial incentives for poor and criminalized women
to be sterilized or to take long-acting hormonal contraceptives (Saletan
2003).[3] As I will discuss later, part of this political inconsistency is inherent in the articulation of the pro-choice position. But another reason is that
many in the pro-choice camp have also not questioned criminalization as
the appropriate response for addressing reproductive health concerns. The
pro-choice camp may differ from pro-life groups regarding which acts
should be criminalized, but it does not necessarily question the criminalization regime itself.

The Pro-Choice Position and Capitalism

The pro-choice camp claims a position that offers more choices for women
making decisions about their reproductive lives. A variety of scholars and
activists have critiqued the choice paradigm because it rests on essentially individualist, consumerist notions of "free" choice that do not take
into consideration all the social, economic, and political conditions that
frame the so-called choices that women are forced to make (Patchesky
1990; J. Smith 1999; Solinger 2001). Solinger further contends that in the
1960s and 1970s, abortion rights advocates initially used the term *rights*
rather than *choice*; rights are understood as those benefits owed to all
those who are human regardless of access to special resources. By contrast, argues Solinger, the concept of choice is connected to possession of
resources, thus creating a hierarchy among women based on who is capable of making legitimate choices (2001, 6). Consequently, since under a
capitalist system, those with resources are granted more choices, it is not
inconsistent to withdraw reproductive rights choices from poor women
through legislation such as the Hyde Amendment (which restricts federal
funding for abortion) or family caps for TANF (Temporary Assistance for
Needy Families) recipients.[4] Solinger's argument can be demonstrated in
the writings of Planned Parenthood. In 1960, Planned Parenthood commissioned a study that concluded that poor and working-class families

lacked the rationality to do family planning, and that this lack of "rationality and early family planning as middle-class couples" was "embodied
in the particular personalities, world views, and ways of life" of the poor
themselves (Rainwater 1960, 5, 167). As Solinger states:

> "Choice" also became a symbol of middle-class women's arrival as indepen-
> dent consumers. Middle-class women could afford to choose. They had earned
> the right to choose motherhood, if they liked. According to many Americans,
> however, when choice was associated with poor women, it became a symbol of
> illegitimacy. Poor women had not earned the right to choose. (2001, 199–200)

What Solinger's analysis suggests is that, ironically, while the pro-choice
camp contends that the pro-life position diminishes the rights of women
in favor of "fetal" rights, the pro-choice position actually does not as-
cribe inherent rights to women either. Rather, women are viewed as having reproductive choices if they can afford them or if they are deemed
legitimate choice-makers.

William Saletan's (1998) history of the evolution of the pro-choice paradigm illustrates the extent to which this paradigm is a conservative one.
Saletan contends that pro-choice strategists, generally affiliated with the
National Abortion and Reproductive Rights Action League (NARAL), in-
tentionally rejected a rights-based framework in favor of one that focused
on privacy from *big government*. That is, government should not inter-
vene in the woman's right to decide if she wants to have children. This
approach appealed to those with libertarian sensibilities who otherwise
might have had no sympathy with feminist causes. The impact of this
strategy was that it enabled the pro-choice side to keep *Roe v. Wade*
intact—but only in the most narrow sense. This strategy undermined any
attempt to achieve a broader pro-choice agenda because the strategy could
be used against a broader agenda. For instance, the argument that government should not be involved in reproductive rights decisions could also be
used by pro-life advocates against federal funding for abortions (Saletan
2003). Consequently, Saletan argues, "Liberals have not won the struggle
for abortion rights. Conservatives have" (1998, 114).

Furthermore, this narrow approach has contributed to some pro-choice
organizations, such as Planned Parenthood and NARAL, often developing strategies that marginalize women of color. Both supported the Freedom of Choice Act in the early 1990s that retained the Hyde Amendment
(Saletan 2003). The Hyde Amendment, besides discriminating against
poor women by denying federal funding for abortion services, discrimi-
nates against American Indian women who largely obtain healthcare
through Indian Health Services, a federal agency. One of NARAL's petitions stated: "The Freedom of Choice Act (FOCA) will secure the original vision of *Roe v. Wade*, giving *all* women reproductive freedom and

securing that right for future generations [emphasis mine]."[5] Apparently, poor women and indigenous women do not qualify as "women."[6]

Building on this analysis, I would argue that while there is certainly a sustained critique of the choice paradigm, particularly among women of color reproductive rights groups, the choice paradigm continues to govern much of the policies of mainstream groups in a manner that sustains the marginalization of women of color, poor women, and women with disabilities. One example is the extent to which pro-choice advocates narrow their advocacy around legislation that affects the one choice of whether or not to have an abortion without addressing all the conditions that gave rise to a woman having to make this decision in the first place. Consequently, politicians, such as former President Bill Clinton, will be heralded as "pro-choice" as long as they do not support legislative restrictions on abortion regardless of their stance on other issues that may equally impact the reproductive choices women make. Clinton's approval of federal welfare reform that places poor women in the position of possibly being forced to have an abortion because of cuts in social services, while often critiqued, is not viewed as an "anti-choice" position. On Planned Parenthood's and NARAL's websites (www.plannedparenthood.org; www.naral.org) there is generally no mention of welfare policies in these organizations' pro-choice legislation alerts.

A consequence of the choice paradigm is that its advocates frequently take positions that are oppressive to women from marginalized communities. For instance, this paradigm often makes it difficult to develop nuanced positions on the use of abortion when the fetus is determined to have abnormalities. Focusing solely on the woman's choice to have or not have the child does not address the larger context of a society that sees children with disabilities as having worthless lives and that provides inadequate resources to women who may otherwise want to have them. As Martha Saxton notes: "Our society profoundly limits the 'choice' to love and care for a baby with a disability" (1998, 375). If our response to disability is to simply facilitate the process by which women can abort fetuses that may have disabilities, we never actually focus on changing economic policies that make raising children with disabilities difficult. Rashmi Luthra (1993) notes, by contrast, that reproductive advocates from other countries such as India, who do not operate from this same choice paradigm, are often able to develop more complicated political positions on issues such as this one.

Another example is the difficulty pro-choice groups have in maintaining a critical perspective on dangerous or potentially dangerous contraceptives, arguing that women should have the "choice" of contraceptives. Many scholars and activists have documented the dubious safety record of Norplant and Depo-Provera, two long-acting hormonal contraceptives (Krust and Assetoyer 1993; Masterson and Guthrie 1986; Rob-

erts 1997; A. Smith 2001). In fact, lawsuits against Norplant have forced
an end to its distribution (although Norplant that remains on the shelves
can be sold to women). In 1978, the Food and Drug Administration (FDA)
denied approval for Depo-Provera on the grounds that: (1) dog studies
confirmed an elevated rate of breast cancer; (2) there appeared to be an
increased risk of birth defects in human fetuses exposed to the drug; and
(3) there was no pressing need shown for use of the drug as a contraceptive (Masterson and Guthrie 1986). In 1987, the FDA changed its regulations and began to require cancer testing in rats and mice instead of dogs
and monkeys; Depo-Provera did not cause cancer in these animals, but
major concerns regarding its safety persist (Feminist Women's Health
Centers 1997). Also problematic is the manner in which these contraceptives are frequently promoted in communities of color and often without
informed consent (Krust and Assetoyer 1993; Masterson and Guthrie
1986; A. Smith 2001).[7] Yet none of the mainstream pro-choice organizations have ever seriously taken a position on the issue of informed consent as part of their agenda.[8] Indeed, Gloria Feldt, president of Planned
Parenthood, equates opposition to Norplant and Depo-Provera as opposition to "choice" in her book *The War on Choice* (Feldt 2004, 34, 37).
Planned Parenthood and NARAL opposed restrictions against sterilization abuse, despite the thousands of women of color who were being
sterilized without their consent, because they saw such policies as interfering with a woman's "right to choose" (Nelson 2003, 144; Patchesky
1990, 8).

Particularly disturbing has been some of the support given by these
organizations to the Center for Research on Population and Security,
headed by Stephen Mumford and Elton Kessel, which distributes globally
a form of sterilization, Quinacrine. Quinacrine is a drug that is used to
treat malaria. It is inserted into the uterus, where it dissolves, causing the
fallopian tubes to scar and rendering the woman irreversibly sterile. Family Health International conducted four *in vitro* studies and found Quinacrine to be mutagenic in three of them (Controversy Over Sterilization
Pellet 1994; Norsigian 1996). It, as well as the World Health Organization,
recommended against further trials for female sterilization, and no regulatory body supports Quinacrine. However, the North Carolina–based
Center for Research on Population and Security has circumvented these
bodies through private funding from such organizations as the Turner
Foundation and the Leland Fykes organization (which, incidentally, funds
pro-choice and anti-immigrant groups). The Center for Research on Population and Security has been distributing Quinacrine for free to researchers and government health agencies. There are field trials in eleven countries, with more than 70,000 women sterilized. In Vietnam, a hundred
female rubber plant workers were given routine pelvic exams during
which the doctor inserted the Quinacrine without their consent. Thus

far, the side effects linked to Quinacrine include ectopic pregnancy, puncturing of the uterus during insertion, pelvic inflammatory disease, and severe abdominal pain. Other possible concerns include heart and liver damage and exacerbation of pre-existing viral conditions. In one of the trials in Vietnam, a large number of cases that had serious side effects were excluded from the data (Controversy Over Sterilization Pellet 1994; Norsigian 1996).

Despite the threat to reproductive justice that this group represents, the Feminist Majority Foundation featured the Center for Research on Population and Security at its 1996 Feminist Expo because, I was informed by the organizers, they promoted choice for women. Then in 1999, Planned Parenthood almost agreed to sponsor a Quinacrine trial in the United States until outside pressure forced it to change its position (Committee on Women, Population and the Environment 1999). A prevalent ideology within the mainstream pro-choice movement is that women should have the choice to use whatever contraception they want. This position does not consider: (1) that a choice among dangerous contraceptives is not much of a choice; (2) that pharmaceutical companies and the medical industry have millions of dollars to promote certain contraceptives, compared to the few resources women's advocacy groups have to provide alternative information on these same contraceptives; and (3) that the social, political, and economic conditions in which women may find themselves are such that using dangerous contraceptives may be the best of even worse options.

One reason that such groups have not taken a position on informed consent in the case of potentially dangerous contraceptives is due to their investment in population control. As Betsy Hartmann (1995) has argued, while contraceptives are often articulated as an issue of choice for white women in the first world, they are articulated as an instrument of population control for women of color and women in the third world (Hartmann 1995). The historical origins of Planned Parenthood are inextricably tied to the eugenics movement. Its founder, Margaret Sanger, increasingly collaborated with eugenics organizations during her career and framed the need for birth control in terms of the need to reduce the number of those in the "lower classes" (Roberts 1997, 73). In a study commissioned in 1960, Planned Parenthood concluded that poor people "have too many children" (Rainwater 1960, 2); yet something must be done to stop this trend in order to "disarm the population bomb" (Rainwater 1960, 178). Today, Planned Parenthood is particularly implicated in this movement as can be seen clearly by the groups it lists as allies on its website (www.plannedparenthood.org): Population Action International, the Population Institute, Zero Population Growth, and the Population Council. A central campaign of Planned Parenthood is to restore U.S. funding to the United Nations Population Fund. In addition, it asserts its commitment to addressing *rapid population growth* on this same website. I will not repeat the problematic analysis, critiqued elsewhere, of this population paradigm that essentially blames third-world women for poverty, war, environmental damage, and social unrest, without looking at the root causes of all these phenomena (including population growth)—colonialism, corporate policies, militarism, and economic disparities between poor and rich countries (Bandarage 1997; Hartmann 1995: Silliman and King 1999).

As Hartmann (1995) documents, the United Nations Population Fund has long been involved in coercive contraceptive policies throughout the world. The Population Council produced Norplant and assisted in Norplant trials in Bangladesh and other countries without the informed consent of the trial participants (Hartmann 1995). In fact, trial administrators often refused to remove Norplant when requested (Cadbury 1995). All of these population organizations intersect to promote generally long-acting hormonal contraceptives of dubious safety around the world (Hartmann 1995). Of course, Planned Parenthood provides valuable family planning resources to women around the world as well, but it does so through a population framework that inevitably shifts the focus from family planning as a right in and of itself to family planning as an instrument of population control. While population control advocates, such as Planned Parenthood, are increasingly more sophisticated in their rhetoric and often talk about ensuring social, political, and economic opportunity, the *population* focus of this model still results in its advocates working to reduce population rather than to provide social, political, and economic opportunity.

Another unfortunate consequence of uncritically adopting the choice paradigm is the tendency of reproductive rights advocates to make simplistic analyses of who our political friends and enemies are in the area of reproductive rights. That is, all those who call themselves pro-choice are our political allies while all those who call themselves pro-life are our political enemies. An example of this rhetoric is Gloria Feldt's description of anyone who is pro-life as a "right-wing extremist" (Feldt 2004, 5). As I have argued elsewhere, this simplistic analysis of who is politically progressive versus conservative does not actually do justice to the complex political positions people inhabit (A. Smith 2002). As a result, we often engage uncritically in coalitions with groups that, as anti-violence activist Beth Richie states, "do not pay us back" (2000, 31). Meanwhile, we often lose opportunities to work with people with whom we may have sharp disagreements, but who may, with different political framings and organizing strategies, shift their positions.

To illustrate: Planned Parenthood is often championed as an organization that supports women's rights to choose with whom women of color should ally. Yet, as discussed previously, its roots are in the eugenics

movement and today it is heavily invested in the population establishment. It continues to support population control policies in the third
world, it almost supported the development of Quinacrine in the United
States, and it opposed strengthening sterilization regulations that would
protect women of color. Meanwhile, the North Baton Rouge Women's
Help Center in Louisiana is a crisis pregnancy center that articulates its
pro-life position from an anti-racist perspective. It argues that Planned
Parenthood has advocated population control, particularly in communities of color. It critiques the Black Church Initiative for the Religious
Coalition for Reproductive Choice for contending that charges of racism
against Sanger are *scare tactics* (Blunt 2003, 22). It also attempts to provide its services from a holistic perspective—it provides educational and
vocational training, GED classes, literacy programs, primary health care
and pregnancy services, and child placement services. Its position: "We
cannot encourage women to have babies and then continue their dependency on the system. We can't leave them without the resources to care
for their children and then say, 'Praise the Lord, we saved a baby'" (Blunt
2003, 23).

It would seem that while the two organizations support some positions that are beneficial to women of color, they both equally support
positions that are detrimental to them. If we are truly committed to reproductive justice, why should we presume that we should necessarily
work with Planned Parenthood and reject the Women's Help Center?
Why would we not instead position ourselves independently from both of
these approaches and work to shift their positions to a stance that is
truly liberatory for all women?

Beyond Pro-Life versus Pro-Choice

To develop an independent position, it is necessary to reject the pro-life
versus pro-choice model for understanding reproductive justice. Many reproductive advocates have attempted to expand the definitions of either
pro-life or pro-choice depending on which side of this divide they may rest.
Unfortunately, they are trying to expand concepts that are inherently designed to exclude the experiences of most women, especially poor women,
women of color, indigenous women, and women with disabilities.

If we critically assess the assumptions behind both positions, it is
clear that these camps are more similar than they are different. As I have
argued, they both assume a criminal justice regime for adjudicating reproductive issues (although they may differ as to which women should
be subjected to this regime). Neither position endows women with inherent rights to their body—the pro-life position pits fetal rights against
women's rights whereas the pro-choice position argues that women

should have freedom to make choices rather than possess inherent rights to their bodies regardless of their class standing. They both support positions that reinforce racial and gender hierarchies that marginalize women of color. The pro-life position supports a criminalization approach that depends on a racist political system that will necessarily impact poor women and women of color who are less likely to have alternative strategies for addressing unwanted pregnancies. Meanwhile, the pro-choice position often supports population control policies and the development of dangerous contraceptives that are generally targeted toward communities of color. And both positions do not question the capitalist system—they focus solely on the decision of whether or not a woman should have an abortion without addressing the economic, political, and social conditions that put women in this position in the first place.

Consequently, it is critical that reproductive advocates develop a framework that does not rest on the pro-choice versus pro-life framework. Such a strategy would enable us to fight for reproductive justice as a part of a larger social justice strategy. It would also free us to think more creatively about whom we could work in coalition with while simultaneously allowing us to hold those who claim to be our allies more accountable for the positions they take. To be successful in this venture, however, it is not sufficient to simply articulate a women of color reproductive justice agenda—we must focus on developing a nationally coordinated women of color movement. While there are many women of color reproductive organizations, relatively few actually focus on bringing new women of color into the movement and training them to organize on their own behalf. And to the extent that these groups do exist, they are not generally coordinated as national mobilization efforts. Rather, national work is generally done on an advocacy level with heads of women of color organizations advocating for policy changes, but often working without a solid base to back their demands (Silliman et al. 2005).

Consequently, women of color organizations are not always in a strong position to negotiate with power brokers and mainstream pro-choice organizations or to hold them accountable. As an example, many women of color groups mobilized to attend the 2004 March for Women's Lives in Washington, D.C., in order to expand the focus of the march from a narrow pro-choice abortion rights agenda to a broad-based reproductive rights agenda. While this broader agenda was reflected in the march, it became co-opted by the pro-choice paradigm in the media coverage of the event. My survey of the major newspaper coverage of the march indicates that virtually no newspaper described it as anything other than a pro-choice or abortion rights march.[9] To quote New Orleans health activist Barbara Major, "When you go to power without a base, your demand becomes a request" (2003). Base-building work, on which many women of color organizations are beginning to focus, is very slow work that may not show results for a long time. After all, the base-building of the Christian Right did not become publicly visible for 50 years (Diamond 1989). Perhaps one day, we will have a march for women's lives in which the main issues addressed and reported will include: (1) repealing the Hyde Amendment; (2) stopping the promotion of dangerous contraceptives; (3) decriminalizing women who are pregnant and who have addictions; and (4) ending welfare policies that punish women, in addition to other issues that speak to the intersections of gender, race, and class in reproductive rights policies.

At a meeting of the United Council of Tribes in Chicago, representatives from the Chicago Pro-Choice Alliance informed us that we should join the struggle to keep abortion legal or else we would lose our reproductive rights. A woman in the audience responded, "Who cares about reproductive rights; we don't have any rights, period." What her response suggests is that a reproductive justice agenda must make the dismantling of capitalism, white supremacy, and colonialism central to its agenda, and not just as principles added to organizations' promotional material designed to appeal to women of color, with no budget to support making these principles a reality. We must reject single-issue, pro-choice politics of the mainstream reproductive rights movement as an agenda that not only does not serve women of color, but actually promotes the structures of oppression that keep women of color from having real choices or healthy lives.

Notes

1. This block quote is a compilation of Colson quotes from three different sources (Colson 1983, 15; Fager 1982, 23; Forbes 1982, 34).

2. As Roberts (1997) and Maher (1990) note, addiction is itself a result of social and political conditions, such as racism and poverty, which the U.S. government does not take steps to alleviate, and then blames women who are victimized by these conditions. Furthermore, the government provides no resources for pregnant women to end their addictions; it simply penalizes them for continuing a pregnancy. Thus assigning moral culpability primarily to pregnant women with addiction problems is a dubious prospect.

3. Additionally, several reproductive rights advocates at the historic *SisterSong* Conference on Women of Color and Reproductive Justice held in Atlanta, November 13–16, 2003, noted that some local Planned Parenthood agencies were currently offering financial incentives for women who are addicted to accept long-acting contraceptives or were distributing literature from CRACK. This

policy was not uniform among Planned Parenthood chapters, however, and many Planned Parenthood chapters condemn this practice.

4. For further analysis of how welfare reform marks poor women and women of color as women who make "bad choices" and hence should have these choices restricted through marriage promotion, family caps (or cuts in payments if recipients have additional children), and incentives to use long-acting hormonal contraceptives, see Mink 1999.

5. The petition can be found on the Web at http://www.wanaral.org/s01take action/200307101.shtml.

6. During this period, I served on the board of the Illinois National Abortion and Reproductive Rights Action League (NARAL), which was constituted primarily of women of color. Illinois NARAL broke with National NARAL in opposing the Freedom of Choice Act (FOCA). Despite many heated discussions with NARAL president Kate Michelman, she refused to consider the perspective of women of color on this issue.

7. I was a co-organizer of a reproductive rights conference in Chicago in 1992. There, hotline workers from Chicago Planned Parenthood reported that they were told to tell women seeking contraception that Norplant had no side effects. In 2000, women from a class I was teaching at University of California, Santa Cruz, informed the class that when they asked Planned Parenthood workers what were the side effects of Depo-Provera, the workers said that they were not allowed to tell them the side effects because they were supposed to promote Depo-Provera. Similar problems in other Planned Parenthood offices were reported at the previously mentioned *SisterSong* conference. These problems around informed consent are not necessarily a national Planned Parenthood policy or uniform across all Planned Parenthood agencies.

8. In 1994 when NARAL changed its name from the National Association for the Repeal of Abortion Laws to the National Abortion and Reproductive Rights Action League, it held a strategy session for its state chapters that I attended. Michelman and her associates claimed that this name change was reflective of NARAL's interest in expanding its agenda to new communities, and informed consent around contraceptives would be included in this expanded agenda. I asked how much of NARAL's budget was going to be allocated to this new agenda. Their reply: none. They were going to release a report on these new issues, but they were going to work only on the issues NARAL had addressed traditionally.

9. Newspapers surveyed that focused solely on abortion rights include *The New York Times* (Toner 2004); *Connecticut Post* ("Abortion-Rights Marchers Crowd D.C." 2004); *New York Newsday* (Phelps 2004); *Syracuse Post Standard* (Gadoua 2004); *The Record* (Varoqua 2004); *The Baltimore Sun* (Gibson 2004); *The Commercial Appeal* (Wolfe 2004); *Richmond Times Dispatch*

(T. Smith 2004); *Marin Independent Journal* ("Marchers Say Bush Policies Harm Women" 2004); *Salt Lake Tribune* (Stephenson 2004); *The Capital Times* (Segars 2004); *Dayton Daily News* (Dart 2004); *Milwaukee Journal Sentinel* (Madigan 2004); *Cleveland Plains Dealer* (Diemer 2004); *Minneapolis Star Tribune* (O'Rourke 2004); *Chicago Daily Herald* (Ryan 2004); *Chicago Sun-Times* (Sweeney 2004); *The Columbus Dispatch* (Riskind 2004); *San Francisco Chronicle* (Marinucci 2004); and *Dayton Daily News* (Wynn 2004). There was coverage of "other" issues in a few papers: "The concerns they voiced extended beyond the issues of abortion to health care access, AIDS prevention, birth control and civil rights" in *San Francisco Chronicle* (Marinucci 2004); "Another group flashed signs calling for the government to recognize same-sex marriage" in the *Houston Chronicle* (Black 2004); "Various trends and vendors on the Mall also promoted other political causes, including welfare, the Falun Gong movement in China, homosexual 'marriage,' the socialist movement, environmentalism, and striking Utah coal miners" in the *Atlanta Journal-Constitution* (Dart and Pickel 2004); " 'This morning I was saying that I was mainly here for abortion,' said Gresh, reflecting on the march. 'But now, going through this, I realize that there are so many issues. Equal pay is a big issue. And globalization, and women's rights around the world' " in the *Pittsburgh Post-Gazette* (Belser 2004).

References

"Abortion-Rights Marchers Crowd D.C." 2004. *Connecticut Post*, April 26.

Bandarage, Asoka. 1997. *Women, Population and Global Crisis*. London: Zed.

Belser, Ann. 2004. "Local Marchers Have Many Issues." *Pittsburgh Post-Gazette*, April 26, A4.

Black, Joe. 2004. "Marchers Rally for Abortion Rights." *Houston Chronicle*, April 26, A1.

Blunt, Sheryl. 2003. "Saving Black Babies." *Christianity Today* 47 (February): 21–23.

Box, Steve, and Chris Hale. 1982. "Economic Crisis and the Rising Prisoner Population in England and Wales." *Crime and Social Justice* 17: 20–35.

Bushnell, Jeanette. 2004. Interview with author, May 21.

Butterfield, Fox. 2000. "Study Shows a Racial Divide in Domestic Violence Cases." *The New York Times*, May 18, A16.

Cadbury, Deborah. 1995. *Human Laboratory*. Video, BBC.

Colson, Charles. 1985. "God Behind Bars." *Christian Life* 47 (September): 28–32.

———. 1983. "Why Charles Colson's Heart is Still in Prison." *Christianity Today* 27 (September 16): 12–14.

———. 1980. "Prison Reform: Your Obligation as a Believer." *Christian Life* 41 (April): 23–24; 50–56.

———. 1977. "Who Will Help Penitents and Penitentiaries?" *Eternity* 28 (May): 12–17, 34.

Committee on Women, Population and the Environment. 1999. Internal Correspondence.

Controversy Over Sterilization Pellet. 1994. *Political Environments 1* (Spring): 9.

Cook-Lynn, Elizabeth. 1998. *Why I Can't Read Wallace Stegner and Other Essays.* Madison: University of Wisconsin Press.

Crum, Gary, and Thelma McCormack. 1992. *Abortion: Pro-Choice or Pro-Life?* Washington, DC: American University Press.

Currie, Elliott. 1998. *Crime and Punishment in America.* New York: Metropolitan Books.

Dart, Bob. 2004. "Abortion-Rights Backers March." *Dayton Daily News,* April 26, A1.

Dart, Bob, and Mary Lou Pickel. 2004. "Abortion Rights Supporters March." *Atlanta Journal-Constitution,* April 26, A1.

Davis, Angela. 2003. *Are Prisons Obsolete?* New York: Seven Stories Press.

Diamond, Sara. 1989. *Spiritual Warfare.* Boston: South End Press.

Diemer, Tom. 2004. "Thousands Rally for Choice 500,000 to 800,000 March in D.C. in Support of Abortion Rights." *Cleveland Plains Dealer,* April 26, A1.

Dilulio, John. 1999. Keynote Address, Justice Fellowship Conference. Washington, DC, February.

Donziger, Steven. 1996. *The Real War on Crime.* New York: HarperCollins.

Dorris, Michael. 1989. *The Broken Cord.* New York: Harper & Row.

Fager, Charles. 1982. "No Holds Barred." *Eternity 33* (April 1982): 20–24.

Feldt, Gloria. 2004. *The War on Choice.* New York: Bantam Books.

Feminist Women's Health Centers. 1997. "Depo-Provera (The Shot)," http://www.fwhc.org/bcdepo.html.

Forbes, Cheryl. 1982. "What Hope for America's Prisons." *Christian Herald 105* (April): 32–40.

Gadoua, Renee. 2004. "A Woman Should Decide." *Post-Standard,* April 26, B1.

Gibson, Gail. 2004. "Thousands Rally for Abortion Rights." *Baltimore Sun,* April 26, A1.

Hartmann, Betsy. 1995. *Reproductive Rights and Wrongs: The Global Politics of Population Control.* Boston: South End Press.

Ignatieff, Michael. 1978. *A Just Measure of Pain.* New York: Pantheon Books.

Jankovic, Ivan. 1977. "Labour Market and Imprisonment." *Crime and Social Justice 8*: 17–31.

Kigvamasud Vashi, Theryn. 2001. "Fact Sheet on Positive Prevention/CRACK (Children Requiring a Caring Kommunity)." Seattle: Communities Against Rape and Abuse.

Krust, Lin, and Charon Assetoyer. 1993. "A Study of the Use of Depo-Provera and Norplant by the Indian Health Services." Lake Andes: South Dakota: Native American Women's Health Education Resource Center.

Lawton, Kim. 1988. "So What Should We Do with Prisoners." *Christianity Today 32* (November 4): 38–39.

Luthra, Rashmi. 1993. "Toward a Reconceptualization of 'Choice': Challenges at the Margins." *Feminist Issues 13* (Spring): 41–54.

Madigan, Erin. 2004. "Hundreds of Thousands March for Abortion Rights." *Milwaukee Journal Sentinel,* April 26, A3.

Maher, Lisa. 1990. "Criminalizing Pregnancy—The Downside of a Kinder, Gentler Nation?" *Social Justice 17* (Fall): 111–35.

Major, Barbara. 2003. Keynote Address, National Women's Studies Association National Conference. New Orleans, June.

Mancini, Michael. 1991. *One Dies, One Gets Another.* Columbia: University of South Carolina Press.

"Marchers Say Bush Policies Harm Women." 2004. *Marin Independent Journal,* April 26, Nation/World.

Marinucci, Carla. 2004. "Hundreds of Thousands in D.C. Pledge to Take Fight to Polls." *San Francisco Chronicle,* April 26, A1.

Masterson, Mike, and Patricia Guthrie. 1986. "Taking the Shot." *Arizona Republic,* n.p.

Mauer, Marc. 1999. *Race to Incarcerate.* New York: New Press/WW Norton.

Mill, Manny. 1999. "No Prisons in Heaven." *New Man 8* (January/February): 74.

Mink, Gendolyn, ed. 1999. *Whose Welfare?* Ithaca: Cornell University Press.

Nelson, Jennifer. 2003. *Women of Color and the Reproductive Rights Movement.* New York: New York University Press.

Norsigian, Judy. 1996. "Quinacrine Update." *Political Environments 3* (Spring): 26–27.

O'Rourke, Lawrence. 2004. "Thousands Rally for Abortion Rights." *Star Tribune,* April 26, A1.

Patchesky, Rosalind. 1990. *Abortion and Woman's Choice.* Boston: Northeastern University Press.

Phelps, Timothy. 2004. "Demonstration in D.C." *New York Newsday,* April 26, A05.

Prison Activist Resource Center. 2004. http://www.prisonactivist.org.

Pulliam, Russ. 1987. "A Better Idea than Prison." *Christian Herald 110* (November): 28–31.

Rainwater, Lee. 1960. *And the Poor Get Children.* Chicago: Quadrangle Books.

Richie, Beth. 2000. "Plenary Presentation." In *The Color of Violence: Violence Against Women of Color,* ed. Incite! Women of Color Against Violence, 124. University of California, Santa Cruz: Incite! Women of Color Against Violence.

Riskind, Jonathan. 2004. "Supporters of Abortion Rights Seek Forefront." *The Columbus Dispatch,* April 25, A1.

Roberts, Dorothy. 1997. *Killing the Black Body.* New York: Pantheon Books.

Rodriguez, Dylan. 2000. "The Challenge of Prison Abolition." *Social Justice 27* (Fall): 212–18

Ryan, Joseph. 2004. "Abortion Rights Supporters Jump in to Rejuvenate Cause." *Chicago Daily Herald,* April 26, 15.

Saletan, William. 2003. *Bearing Right.* Berkeley: University of California Press.

———. 1998. "Electoral Politics and Abortion." In *The Abortion Wars,* ed. Rickie Solinger, 111–23. Berkeley: University of California Press.

Saxton, Martha. 1998. "Disability Rights." In *The Abortion Wars,* ed. Rickie Solinger, 374–93. Berkeley: University of California Press.

Segars, Melissa. 2004. "Rally For Women's Rights." *The Capital Times,* April 26, A1.

Silliman, Jael, Loretta Ross, Marlene Gerber Fried, and Elena Gutierrez. 2005. *Undivided Rights*. Boston: South End Press.

Silliman, Jael, and Ynestra King, eds. 1999. *Dangerous Intersections: Feminist Perspectives on Population, Environment and Development*. Boston: South End Press.

Smarto, Don, ed. 1993. *Setting the Captives Free*. Grand Rapids: Baker Book House.

Smith, Andrea. 2005. "Domestic Violence, the State, and Social Change." In *Domestic Violence at the Margins: A Reader at the Intersections of Race, Class, and Gender*, ed. Natalie Sokoloff. New Brunswick: Rutgers University Press.

———. 2002. "Bible, Gender and Nationalism in American Indian and Christian Right Activism." Santa Cruz: University of California.

———. 2001. "'Better Dead Than Pregnant' The Colonization of Native Women's Health." In *Policing the National Body*, ed. Anannya Bhattacharjee and Jael Silliman, 123–46. Boston: South End Press.

Smith, Justine. 1999. "Native Sovereignty and Social Justice: Moving Toward an Inclusive Social Justice Framework." In *Dangerous Intersections: Feminist Perspectives on Population, Environment and Development*, ed. Jael Silliman and Ynestra King, 202–13. Boston: South End Press.

Smith, Tammie. 2004. "Marchers Call for 'A Choice' About Reproductive Rights." *Richmond Times Dispatch*, April 26, A1.

Solinger, Rickie. 2001. *Beggers and Choosers*. New York: Hill and Wang.

Stephenson, Kathy. 2004. "Utahns Take Part in D.C. and at Home." *Salt Lake Tribune*, April 26, A6.

Sweeney, Annie. 2004. "Chicagoans Head to D.C. for Pro Choice March." *Chicago Sun-Times*, April 26, 18.

Toner, Robin. 2004. "Abortion Rights Marches Vow to Fight Another Bush Term." *The New York Times*, April 26, A1.

Van Ness, Daniel. 1985. "The Crisis of Crowded Prisons." *Eternity 36* (April): 33–73.

Varoqua, Eman. 2004. "N.J. Supporters Form Large Column for Rights." *The Record*, April 26, A01.

Walker, Samuel. 1998. *Sense and Nonsense about Crime*. Belmont: Wadsworth Publishing Company.

Wolfe, Elizabeth. 2004. "Rights March Packs Mall." *The Commercial Appeal*, April 26, A4.

Wynn, Kelli. 2004. "Hundreds Go to D.C. for March Today." *Dayton Daily News*, April 25, B1.

CHAPTER FOUR

Because Words Are Not Enough: Latina Re-Visionings of Transnational Collaborations Using Health Promotion for Gender Justice and Social Change

ESTER R. SHAPIRO

> *This chapter honors the memory of Helen Rodriguez Trias, Puerto Rican pediatrician and activist, whose leadership built bridges and inspired North/South collaborations toward a shared vision of women's health and rights throughout the Americas.*

Latinas Bridging Local and Global Gender Politics: Transnational Health Promotion as Activist Strategy

International movements working toward women's equality and empowerment have focused on gender and health, especially reproductive health and rights and freedom from violence, as fundamental to women's sovereignty and full participation as citizens (Keck and Sikkink 1998; Palomino 2002; Petchesky 2003; Petchesky and Judd 1998; Shepard 2002). These international movements have used recent World Health Organization paradigms of health promotion that define health as the presence of well-being and the resources for its actualization (Kickbusch 2003). These international movements contribute to emerging interdisciplinary, multisystemic, contextual definitions of women's empowerment emphasizing quantitative and qualitative measures of access to resources, agency in self-determination of strategic life choices, and well-being outcomes, while working to achieve equitable access to conditions promoting good health as a human right (Kabeer 1999; Kar, Pascual, and Chickering 1999; Kar et al. 2002; Malhotra 2002; Shapiro 2000). Recent decades have seen enormous growth in scholarship on transnational feminist activism, including recognition of transnational feminism's contribution of global strategies and debate of its value to local organizations (Alvarez 1998, 2000; Basu 1995, 2000; Mendoza 2002; Naples and Desai 2002). In this essay, I use concepts bridging U.S. Latina and transnational feminisms to analyze the contributions of a U.S. Latina perspective in creating *Nuestros Cuerpos, Nuestras Vidas* (*NCNV*), the Spanish cultural adaptation of *Our Bodies, Ourselves* (*OBOS*). I analyze how a U.S. Latina perspective

---

Originally published in the spring 2005 issue (vol. 17, no. 1).

contributed to the transformation of the text into a meaningful forum for conversations on feminist activism encompassing women's unique localized cultural experience and connecting that experience to transnational networks and strategies for achieving gender justice and social change.

A great deal of the literature on women's and feminists' transnational organizing emphasizes work centered in international settings rather than in U.S. communities of color (Alvarez 2000; Kaplan and Grewal 2002; Kaplan, Alarcon, and Moallem 1999; Mohanty 2003; Naples and Desai 2002; Yuval-Davis 1999). However, a growing literature on Latino communities emphasizes the impact of border-crossing and transnational migration experiences on U.S. Latinas (Zavella 2002; Conway, Bailey, and Ellis 2001). Frameworks exploring the transnational terrain from the standpoint of U.S. third-world communities argue for relational, process-oriented perspectives examining the historical unfolding of power relations as expressed in the practice of everyday life in local contexts (Bonilla et al. 1998; Naples and Desai 2002; Shohat 2002; Velez-lbanez and Sampaio 2002). Engendering these perspectives through the study of *everyday transnationalism and transnationalism from below*, we can better map pathways by which women's everyday survival strategies become a vehicle for personal and collective empowerment.[1] Transnational activism in women's health promotion offers important lessons for supporting linked processes of personal, organizational, and social change, creating "virtuous circles" that expand women's empowerment.[2] While bridging global and local perspectives on women's activism in debates on methods of transnational organizing, Latinas working in U.S. settings offer meaningful contributions to understanding the lived experience of transnationalism as it affects everyday survival. U.S. Latinas also offer meaningful contributions to the study of strategies supporting the formation of oppositional organizations and communities of solidarity (Acosta-Belen and Bose 2000; Mohanty 2003; Sanchez 2001; Zavella 2002).

U.S. Latinas come from all over Latin America and the Caribbean, representing diverse nationalities, political and economic circumstances of migration, and generations. In addition, U.S. Latinas settle in different parts of the United States. Immigrating Latinas each encounter existing or receiving communities and, in turn, create distinctive dynamics of language, race, culture, and educational and economic opportunities as ecologies of acculturation and potential transculturation.[3] Feminist scholarship on Latina political participation has documented women's frequent participation in highly localized community-based activism specific to sending and receiving communities (Hardy-Fanta 2002). A powerful foundation of Chicana feminist writing is increasingly being expanded by a diverse group of Latinas from Puerto Rico, Cuba, Central America, and Latin America (see Torres 1998; Latina Feminist Group 2002). Puerto Rican feminists on both the island and the U.S. mainland offer especially meaningful work bridging Latin American and Caribbean-based feminist activism and U.S. Latina perspectives (Warren and Colon 2003). Interdisciplinary, comparative perspectives highlighting the complexity of Latina experience in transnational settings can help us address intersections of gender, class, race, language, and ethnicity as sites of oppression and as powerful resources for resistance and transcendence. These approaches need to be multidimensional and place-based, capable of moving between the intimate politics of personal experience and the structural politics of social change while also recognizing their interdependence.

The Political Is Personal:
Transnationalism as Lived Experience and Activist Practice

While transnational feminist and cultural studies have become the focus of disciplinary debate, it is important to remember that the violent displacements of family lives as they collide with the forces of politics and history are deeply personal. I was born in Havana, Cuba, and grew up in Miami, Florida, as part of a tightly knit Eastern European Jewish extended family whose five generations of living memory included two world wars and two revolutions across three continents and five languages. In the United States, both Cuban and Jewish diaspora narratives begin with forced exile from a Promised Land and close with insistence on eventual return; both stories erase the complex interweaving of many cultures, languages, and generations as they evolve both at home and in diaspora. My family, too, created an official story of triumph over adversity, literally whitewashing the ethnic and racial solidarities and identities that characterized our multiracial, culturally complex diaspora sojourns as Jews in Europe, in Palestine, in Cuba, and in the United States. I was taught to fear politics and dedicate myself to family loyalty by means of a gender-stereotyped, materialistic strategy for preserving family security and unity. My apparent wholesale rebellion against these imposed values was revealed over the years as profound loyalty to a radically different set of values: the deeply ethical valuing of our human interdependence and dedication to uncovering the abuses of power that erode our abilities to sustain loving environments of healthy mutuality (Shapiro 1994b, 2002, 1994/2005).

With my own family as a starting point, I study the complex ecologies of time and space and of material and symbolic resources that make it possible for us to recognize difference while practicing solidarity in interdependent processes of everyday survival and change. Beginning with my own boundary-crossing life and work, I have struggled to confront the ethnocentrism, individualism, racism, and unacknowledged investments of my academic discipline, my work as a clinical psychologist, and my U.S. feminism (Shapiro 1996a, 2001). Seeking new words with which to honor our immigrant family struggles to survive and creatively adapt to new homes, I study how women explore this new territory and bear many of its burdens, finding ways to build bridges of continuity in a landscape of change (Shapiro 1996b). I also discovered how as immigrants we are encouraged to drink the U.S. *Milk of Amnesia* (Tropicana 2000) and forsake our collective responsibilities as engaged citizens fighting for justice; as immigrants this was the price of admission to a fragmenting, isolating consumer culture in which everything is for sale, including our intimate relationships. We know from the research literature on racial disparities in health, from feminist debates on gender and culture, and from many testimonials by U.S. women of color that border-crossing offers both burden and opportunity in the struggle to make the best of both worlds rather than simply experience the worst.

My own encounter with Latin American and Caribbean feminisms through the prism of a particular activist project provided the catalyst for new personal, intellectual, and political knowledge and practice. As coordinating editor of *Nuestros Cuerpos, Nuestras Vidas* (*NCNV*), I became inspired by the work of Latin American and Caribbean feminists to revisit my assumptions about gender, culture, and health promotion that were formed within my coming of age as a North American feminist and by my life and work in the United States. The process of adaptation, initially biased toward an overemphasis on the U.S. text, became transformed as the U.S. Latina editors discovered and negotiated differences by critically examining the connection of both *OBOS* and *NCNV* to the political movements each edition represented and exploring the place of U.S. Latinas in bridging the texts. Initially, the Latina editorial groups framed our explorations of Latin American and Caribbean feminist organizations and their work as part of gathering culturally meaningful materials and incorporating the work of these organizations to expand the predominantly U.S.-based resources included in every edition of *Our Bodies, Ourselves*. Yet, beginning with these textual explorations, we found that following their implications catalyzed a deeper consideration of the complex, highly specific encounters between individual lives in everyday practices, cultural meanings, and community connections inspiring personal change in solidarity with others toward creating a more just society. These encounters themselves illuminated new facets of border-crossing methods, infusing familiar words with new meanings, as *citizenship*, *self-help*, and *choice* became clarified, redefined, and transformed in their new locations, politics, poetics, and practice of gender and social justice.

From *Our Bodies, Ourselves* to *Nuestros Cuerpos, Nuestras Vidas* (*Our Bodies, Our Lives*): Creating a Transnational Trialogue

Our Bodies, Ourselves (*OBOS*), the groundbreaking women's health information resource book, highly influential in the 1970s, sold millions of copies in the United States and was translated or adapted into nineteen languages. Women all over the world see the book as a catalyst mobilizing the women's health movement in reproductive health and rights, social and domestic violence, and gender justice. However, the book remains embedded in models and methods of white North American feminism (Davis 2003; Thayer 2000). *Nuestros Cuerpos, Nuestras Vidas* (*NCNV*) (2000) was written collaboratively with more than 30 Latin American women's health groups and coordinated by a group of Boston-based Latinas, creating a transformational *trialogo* between the North American text, the concepts, materials, and methods of Latin American and Caribbean women's health activists, and U.S. Latinas working at the intersection of language, gender, culture, and health promotion for social change. The cultural adaptation project was initiated at a time of enormous transition for the partners involved in the trialogue: for the Boston Women's Health Book Collective (BWHBC) as an organization shifting from a founder's collective to a nonprofit organization with a racially and culturally diverse staff and board, for the Latin American and Caribbean feminist groups during the intensified organizing that preceded and followed the Cairo and Bejing meetings, and for Latinas working within the BWHBC.[4]

Constructing these collaborations as U.S. Latinas working within a legendary organization of second-wave feminism and adapting a movement's canonical text forced us to confront some of the text's North American assumptions in light of Zavella's (2002) *peripheral vision* and Sandoval's (2000) *differential consciousness*, strategies our Latina editorial committee used in solving problems presented by the original cultural adaptation plan.[5] We also learned from our Latin American and Caribbean collaborators as they grappled with their own struggles as a growing movement confronting the ways the region's feminist activisms had tilted toward institutionalization and professionalization. These transnational collaborations viewed through a Latina lens helped us create a text based on culturally meaningful images of healthy interdependence, mutuality, spirituality, and active citizenship for gender justice, clarifying pathways and processes linking our personal struggles and strengths, social inequities, and the transformative power of gender equality.

The original planning for the cultural adaptation, *Nuestros Cuerpos, Nuestras Vidas* (*NCNV*), was designed as a Latin American adaptation of the updated *Our Bodies, Ourselves* (*OBOS*). U.S. Latinas were not part of this updated planned adaptation. Rather, *NCNV* was initially conceptualized as a Latin American international edition that could document and include the nearly two decades of feminist activism in the region, which the 1973 edition of *OBOS* and an early direct translation had helped catalyze and inspire (Gomez 1993). Members of the Boston Women's Health Book Collective (BWHBC) attended the Fifth Feminist Encuentro in Puerto Plata, Argentina, in 1990 to arrange a cultural adaptation to be conducted in the region. However, no single group had the resources to coordinate the complex cultural adaptation process without overburdening their local and regional work. Feminists in the region were confronting enormous challenges and opportunities in the aftermath of brutal dictatorships and transitions to democracy. Instead, participants from the region requested that the translation and cultural adaptation be coordinated from Boston, with individual groups adapting specific chapters most closely connected to their own areas of activism. At that stage a group of U.S. Latinas from different backgrounds but predominantly from the Caribbean, with our own complex migration histories, race and class backgrounds, and Spanish-language competence, became the intermediaries between the U.S. text and the models, methods, and materials being generated by the Latin American and Caribbean organizations involved in adapting the text.

Initially, the editorial group of Latinas began our work following the agreed-upon framework that regional feminist groups would receive translated chapters that they would adapt and that Latinas would serve as coordinators for what was fundamentally a conversation between the English-speaking U.S. text and the Latin American and Caribbean groups working on adaptations. Very quickly, we confronted flaws in the project, including an extremely poor initial translation, an inadequate time-line for the Latin American groups to make their contribution, and no funding for the dialogues and face-to-face meetings required to transform the text to transcend the basic structure of the U.S.-based chapters. These errors required an extended phase for reediting the text to restore the companionable, accessible voice so critical to *OBOS*'s success. This extended editing phase supported a longer process of reflection and reorganization of the project, generating a transformative transnational trialogue that more centrally incorporated U.S.-based Latina contributions to a transformed text.

Early in this process, our *NCNV* editorial group was told that publishers were interested in an *NCNV* edition for U.S. Latinas. Although reluctant to circulate two editions in Spanish, we considered the possibilities of creating a U.S. Latina edition as an independent project. Struggling with the complexity of a text that was already seeking ways to incorporate the enormous national and regional differences characterizing the Latin American and Caribbean edition, we despaired that neither our timeframe nor our resources would permit us the ambitious undertaking of incorporating a U.S. Latina perspective. Rosie Muñoz Lopez proposed the solution that was elegantly simple by deploying a differential consciousness to reframe a concept in order to use it in a new setting. Muñoz Lopez noted that *OBOS* itself incorporated the voices of a shifting "we" that was textually interpreted in context as sometimes referring to all U.S. women and at other times to specific women. Through the participation of Latinas in the organization the U.S. Latina perspective had been expanded beginning with the 1984 edition.[6] Why not use a similar strategy in the Spanish cultural adaptation, letting the "we" who speaks be defined in context while further expanding the sections referring to U.S. Latinas? After all, U.S. Latinas had our own ties to national origin, and the book could address us as women of Latin America and the Caribbean wherever in the world we were living. With this reframe of the text as a transnational edition for the Americas, our work group of Latinas became more active in reflecting on our relationship to the U.S. text and to Latin American and Caribbean feminist movements as Latinas with our own standpoint and migration circumstances. Looking back on this moment with the perspective of the book's completion, this decision reflected the recognition that our roles as Latinas translating two movements to unknown readers required the creation of a textual voice inviting readers to complete the text as they applied it to their own very specific circumstances and contexts. From this moment onward, the Latina editorial committee began to travel beyond the original work plan for *NCNV*. We restructured a methodology for adaptation as we discovered the fundamental ways the original adaptation plan contradicted the methods that had made *OBOS* a compelling voice for women's health as a vehicle for social change.

Transnationalism and Textual Transformations: *OBOS* and *NCNV* as Evolving Tools for Social Change

Considering *OBOS*'s importance in U.S. and global feminist and women's health movements, it has been remarkably little studied in scholarly literature (Davis 2003). Yet, as Latinas working between the U.S. text and the Latin American and Caribbean adaptations, we were forced to study the fundamental structure of *OBOS* as a way of exploring its culturally based, textual and political strategies and assumptions. I was the only member of the editorial team to also be on the first nonprofit board of the organization, and throughout my work with the organization these dual roles were a source of rich learning and tremendous conflict.[7] In untangling my subjectivity and responsibilities within both roles, I found it essential to begin to study the history of *OBOS* as text and its relationship to the founding members within a changing organization and a changing U.S. feminist movement. This comparative, border-crossing approach mirrored the strategic methodologies of U.S. feminists of color, whose surviving and thriving at intersecting spaces of oppression and opportunity requires interpreting very specific situations. These strategic methodologies are undertaken to discern the play of power and privilege, achieving a critical perspective on power and difference that helps generate a flexible, strategic third path.[8] Over the course of the project, this implicit border-crossing methodology became more explicitly a perspective deliberately embodied in the text. In the spirit of Aida Hurtado's method in *The Color of Privilege: Three Blasphemies on Race and Feminism* (1996), we questioned sources of race-and class-based subjectivities rarely spoken of in interracial feminist conversations. The following sections articulate the three necessary and forbidden questions posed within our editorial working group of Latinas that helped us identify points of difference and connection and transform their embodiment in the text.

Is It a Book, or Is It a Movement? Questioning *OBOS* as Text and Its Relationship to Changing U.S. Feminisms

The first irreverent question in confronting a canonical text within an idealized organization was to ask how *OBOS* as text had changed during its 25-year history. We explored how *OBOS* had expanded in size along with the U.S. women's health movement it helped create while declining in readership and political influence. *OBOS* emerged in 1969 as a mutual education course entitled "Women and Their Bodies," as a group of young Boston feminists prepared materials that would permit them to challenge a patriarchal health care system. The fundamental "bone structure" of *OBOS* emerged from the founders' methods of engagement with each other and with the thriving feminist movement of the early 1970s. These powerful participatory methods for social change embodied in the text began with women's testimonials describing their struggles with reproductive and other women's health issues, as well as their coming to consciousness of their own strengths. The text then offered accessible health information, especially in the important and tightly regulated areas of reproductive health, contraception, and abortion rights during a period when the right to a legal abortion was still being won. The text also offered a socialist feminist analysis of patriarchy and capitalism as forces in the health care system. Finally, the text included descriptions of emerging women-centered health centers and political organizations, with their names, addresses, and contact information. Initially distributed in mimeograph form, then published by the local, nonprofit New England Press, *OBOS* reached its widest distribution when it was commercially published by Simon & Schuster in 1973 and remained on the bestseller list for most of the 1970s. Because *OBOS*'s publication coincided with the first international women's health meetings, the book also circulated throughout the world and was deeply influential to emerging global feminist networks.

In subsequent editions, *OBOS* expanded in size along with its own growing feminist and women's health organizations (Norsigian et al. 1999; Ruzeck and Becker 1999). The fundamental textual elements remained the same, but they shifted significantly in their proportion and in their political framework and connections. Textually, the book grew enormously in the content of information and in the links to bibliographic and organizational resources, becoming much more like an encyclopedia than like a friend and guide. Politically, the book became allied more with consumer education movements and with the growing number of professionalized women's health care and advocacy organizations with their investments in the systems' status quo. As one of the founders tellingly described the evolution of the text, "The first edition blamed 'Capitalism, capitalism, capitalism' and later editions blamed 'Stress, stress, stress.'" Our Latina work group argued that in creating the cultural adaptation, we needed to restore more of the original balance of political analysis to content while recognizing that politically, times had changed and few of the world's women were inspired by imposed political ideologies, whether feminist or socialist.

In creating an alternative framework for this rebalancing, we turned to Paolo Freire's participatory education as a tool widely used in both Latin American and U.S. Latino communities (Darder 2002; P. Freire 1994; A. Freire and Macedo 2000; Nieto 2003). We saw participatory education, with its use of testimonials on lived experience, emergent critical analysis of the politics of personal experience, accessible women's health information, and connection to activist resources as a tool that would preserve the fundamental structure of *OBOS*. However, participatory education formulates the connection between text and action with a greater emphasis on methodologies linking motivations, knowledge, and action. In participatory education, testimonial creates the groundwork for affirming experientially based knowledge. The power of the learner's experiential knowledge is expanded with egalitarian application of the teacher's tools for creating knowledge, which include both information and critical analysis of how what appear to be unique individual problems are fundamentally socially structured. More important, the *conscientization*, or awareness and critique of unjust circumstances, is accompanied by *annunciation* of what can be, in highlighting the successes of women working in many activist spheres (P. Freire 1994; A. Freire and Macedo 2000). In proposing to use participatory education as a culturally meaningful method of adaptation, we turned to a generative tool that continued to yield new learning as we used it to shift the book's center of gravity symbolically and pragmatically.

Why Were Latinas Left Out of the Conversation?
Expanding Latina Contributions to the Trialogue

The shift to an explicit participatory education methodology as the foundation for updating and culturally adapting the text also helped us achieve a new understanding of the role of Latinas and other women of color in the Boston Women's Health Book Collective (BWHBC)'s struggle to become a more diverse, inclusive organization.[9] The first edition of *OBOS* (1973) was translated into Spanish by Leonora Taboada and Raquel Salgado, and circulated widely in U.S. Latina communities and throughout Latin America. At that time, Elizabeth McMahon Herrera, a Colombian immigrant to the United States, joined the BWHBC and founded Amigas Latinas en Acción Pro-Salud (ALAS) as a working Latina collective that would generate a cultural adaptation of *OBOS* for use with U.S. Latinas. The working group very quickly changed their focus from generating an alternative culturally adapted text to generating culturally meaningful participatory methods for active education and community engagement. Within both BWHBC and ALAS, this shift to an emphasis on participatory methodology and use of culturally meaningful accessible media in addition to text was interpreted as necessary for low-literacy Latinas who lacked the educational skills to make use of a text whose increasingly scientific information required a college education. For more than a decade, ALAS continued to work within BWHBC at the margins of the organization, with a very limited part-time staff member creating multimedia materials or conducting community-based theater workshops that were seen as only needed for U.S. Latinas and not for the organization's "traditional constituencies."[10]

As we clarified differences between BWHBC's priorities and perspectives embodied in *OBOS* as text and carried over into the *NCNV* work plan, our Latina work group revisited the structure of the adaptation with this fundamental question: what would happen if we privileged the Latin American and Latina point of view? We began to see ALAS as the medium for participatory community education and local organizing that would revitalize the link between text and action. As we began to directly contact our Latin American and Caribbean collaborators, we began to see new points of connection between our work and theirs, discovering ways we understood each other's culturally informed textual and political strategies. We had an opportunity to further develop these points of connection (Puntos de Encuentro) because the lengthened editorial process necessary to improve the initial poor translation coincided with new funding for the use of NCNV in community education settings.[11] Making the most of the opportunity presented by this new funding, we shifted the definition and organizational positioning of ALAS from remediation for low-literacy Latinas to embodiment of the inspiring tools of translating words into action.[12] Using this reframing of the ALAS work, we revisited our library of Latin American and Caribbean materials in participatory health promotion and reproductive health, seeing more clearly the common threads connecting our Latina work in health promotion with the emphasis on methodology and media characterizing visions of learning and changing in our communities.

As we proceeded, we identified key organizations from different regions as consultants, using the BWHBC's links as part of a worldwide feminist network of activist groups and regional documentation centers.[13] Initially, these collaborations were hampered by lack of Latina participation in international meetings. The adaptation plan had not included any opportunities for Latina project directors and editors to visit key groups and their documentation centers, building on the relationships with these groups established by BWHBC founders through their long history of movement participation. However, several of us were able to visit Taller Salud in Puerto Rico and its documentation center while visiting family on the island. Nirvana Gonzalez, who founded and directed Taller Salud's documentation center and was active in the regional movement from the first feminist Encuentros, became a crucial guide to key historical, conceptual, and methodological materials. Gonzalez had participated in every regional Feminist Encuentro and proved to be an essential guide to its key texts and their living history in the work of activist organizations throughout the region. She was especially aware of the lack of Caribbean representation on the board of the Latin American and Caribbean women's health network and the regional imbalances and biases that resulted from this lack of representation. Because of Puerto Rico's unique location as a U.S. colony, yet with its own independent ties to Caribbean and Latin American feminist and political movements, we came to see Puerto Rican feminists as uniquely positioned to reflect on and inform the cultural adaptation's transnational perspective. Most Latinas on the editorial team were Puerto Rican– or Caribbean-born and -identified, and we began to examine regional tensions between more theoretically oriented feminist writings and writings emphasizing participation.

Although we didn't recognize the implications of our affinities and selections at the time, we kept returning to the writings of Latin American and Caribbean feminist organizations generated through processes involving both local grassroots community organizations and national/ transnational policy and advocacy. These organizations provided community-based services while using community practice–based knowledge to nurture and inform their strategic policy and advocacy work in national, regional, and international forums. For example, Flora Tristan, a feminist organization based in Peru, sent us their publication in holistic health care, *De Salvia y Toronjil* (*Of Sage and Lemon Balm*), which included an eloquent yet accessible analysis of the consequences of medicalized, fragmented health services in interfering with holistic healing by silencing the wise voice of the healer within. Flora Tristan developed their feminist health center's guide to holistic health as part of delivering direct services to women in both urban and rural settings. At the same time, their organization has been centrally involved in global meetings, and Virginia Vargas, a Flora Tristan founder, was selected by regional activists as their representative for the 1995 United Nations meeting on the status of women in Bejing. When we received *De Salvia y Toronjil*, we were in the process of restructuring the order of chapters to better convey a progression from critique of the health care system to proposals for what might be possible. We had decided to move rewritten chapters on International Feminisms, Health Care Systems, and Organizing for Change to the beginning of the book from their location at the back of *OBOS* to be followed by the section Taking Care of Ourselves, which opens the book in English. We felt that a chapter on Holistic Health provided a clearer bridge to an alternative vision for health, and we substantially rewrote the chapter to include indigenous healing practices and forms of prayer as dimensions of integral or holistic health. Maria Marmo Skinner, production editor for *NCNV*, was a gifted artist and holistic health practitioner whose work resonated with the spirituality and poetics of the holistic health practice materials created by members of Flora Tristan. We located and incorporated materials by other regional groups linking a sacred aesthetics of healing to their political organizing in health. As we re-visioned the Holistic Health chapter to emphasize the sacred healing arts, we learned that *OBOS* editors had chosen to omit all references to religion and spirituality to avoid association either with anti-abortion politics or with nonscientific health care methods. Enhancing the connection between culturally based spiritual practices and feminist politics in health permitted us to introduce a woman-centered indigenous approach to spirituality in this and other chapters as an indispensable dimension of health for women in the region. For U.S. Latinas and other U.S. women of color, spirituality remains a critical resource for health.

Our selection of a culturally meaningful document denoting patient's rights offers another example of a document we selected for its content and only later came to appreciate for the participatory processes that achieved its accessible, inclusive tone and its empowering message of citizen participation and advocacy. The *OBOS* chapter on Health Systems includes an excellent but very detailed legalistic definition of patient's rights, written for a legal and medical audience and requiring a high level of education. We replaced this with a document titled *Declaration of Rights: Rights and Responsibilities of Users of Reproductive Health Services* written by Consorcio Mujer, a consortium of feminist organizations in Peru. We learned much later that the document had been generated by an extensive participatory process involving both users and providers of reproductive health services (Shepard 2002) and based on Consorcio Mujer's application of the concept of citizen participation and reproductive health and rights to quality care in reproductive services.

Although in working with Latin American and Caribbean women's health groups we were hampered by costly communications and limited opportunities for face-to-face collaboration, documenting the work of U.S. Latinas in reproductive health was hampered by lack of national organizations or regional networks with this focus. At the time, the National Latina Health Organization, based in Oakland, had remained active primarily in California. As we called groups around the country, conducting the outreach that would help us create a database of U.S. Latina activists, organizations, and resources, we found that most major U.S. Latino organizations maintained profoundly traditional views of gender roles and reproductive decision-making. At this phase of conceptualizing our goals and methods, we did not see our role as proactively generating organizational capacity, either within BWHBC or in building networks among existing Latina organizations. The National Latina Institute for Reproductive Health, developing a U.S. Latina agenda in reproductive health and rights, was beginning regional organizing in 1995 and invited our adaptation team to attend a New England meeting. Due to other work obligations, none of us was able to attend. Upon reflection, I would now characterize our absence as a failure to give this collaboration and capacity-building meeting a high enough priority. Our work plan failed to recognize the significance of these collaborative networks in nurturing, as well as reflecting, a U.S. Latina feminist movement to be embodied within *NCNV.* Three years later, at a different phase in the development of our methodology, we had a new appreciation of the links between the text and participation in building activist networks and began to work more closely with the National Latina Institute for Reproductive Health in connection with our local Latina organizing.[14]

Are Latinas U.S. or Third-World Feminists? Questioning the Inclusiveness of Latin American Feminisms

Our third irreverent question emerged as we immersed ourselves in the texts of the Latin American and Caribbean women's health movement and confronted an enormous range of texts from different regions and branches of the feminist movement. Our editorial team of Latinas changed participants over time, and the group of seven co-editors coordinating the project differed in our nationalities, migration status, and level of Spanish-language literacy. Within our work group, Puerto Rican women who had lived their own border-crossing experience of island and mainland were the best equipped to understand the Latin American and Caribbean feminist movement. Puerto Rican feminists had a long history of struggle with the issues of political and language sovereignty at stake in the translation adaptation project, and appreciated issues of dominance from both sides of the Americas. Puerto Rican feminists experienced discrimination from a Southern Cone–dominated Latin American movement as well as from U.S. feminist groups. For example, we were surprised to discover that many global health databases, such as the World Health Organization's Pan American Health Organization (PAHO), did not tabulate separate data for Puerto Rico because of its status as a U.S. territory. I, and other members of the editorial team who had immigrated to the United States as children, struggled with Spanish-language literacy, finding some texts to be difficult in their use of intellectual, theoretical language and others to be lyrical and accessible. Over time, we realized that the Latin American feminist movement had its own historical and contemporary rifts, and we began to map the history and location of points of collaboration and divergence.

One especially useful resource for understanding this evolving, living feminist history in the region was the "Memorias/Memories," documenting regional feminist Encuentros/Encounters, several of which were published and distributed to regional documentation centers. The first Encuentro was held in 1981 in Bogota, Colombia, the second in 1983 in Lima, Peru, the third in 1985 in Brazil, with subsequent Encuentros held every two to three years in rotation throughout the region (Alvarez et al. 2003). The tenth feminist Encuentro is currently being planned for October 2005, in Sao Paulo, Brazil. The fourth Encuentro, held in Taxco, Mexico, in 1987, documented its extraordinary diversity and plurality through a collection of individual and group participant testimonials, images, policy reports, and poetry. Starting in 1996, with the seventh Encuentro in Chile, members of the Latina editorial team began to participate in these regional Encuentros, expanding our opportunity to join with and learn from these extraordinarily vibrant meetings and to incorporate these perspectives into our vision for the text as an expression of that movement. At the same time, we were struck by significant rifts representing struggles within the movement as well as evolving regional politics. In the Chile Encuentro in 1996, the organizers were strongly committed to financial autonomy from government and foundation sources, and issued a controversial mandate that no participants could attend who received funds from these sources. The receipt of government or foundation funds was seen as compromising to the integrity of their feminist projects. The subsequent discussion, carried on in early electronic forums and documented in a special issue of the Uruguayan feminist magazine *Cotidiano Mujer*, brought forward an important critique of the risks involved in the institutionalization of regional feminism, a critique that became destructively acrimonious.

A grant supporting connections between U.S. Latina and Latin American feminist organizations permitted our Latina work group's attendance at the Dominican Republic Encuentro of 1999 to identify opportunities for collaboration using *NCNV* as a tool for shared activism in women's health and rights. The Dominican Encuentro followed our ALAS/*NCNV* gatherings of Latinas working in feminist health promotion in San Juan, Puerto Rico, and Brooklyn, New York, and I felt fortunate to have Nirvana Gonzalez and Eugenia Acuña, a founder of Taller Salud now living and working in New York City, and collaborators in those meetings, as guides at the Encuentro. Steeped in their own long trajectory as border-crossing feminists within the movement, they helped me navigate the Encuentro, identify women whom I had come to "know" from reading their texts, select significant workshops, and interpret critical events in light of the Encuentro's history. After the painfully divisive 1996 Encuentro in Chile, the organizing committee worked to create a forum for healing and unity by incorporating participatory methodologies into all the workshops as a way of encouraging full involvement by women from different sectors, communities of feminist work, and levels of education.

In previous Encuentros, U.S. Latinas had been registered as "foreign" participants, but the more than 100 Dominican women residing in the United States and attending the Encuentro refused to accept that designation, insisting that they were Dominican women wherever in the world they lived. As the first Encuentro held in the Caribbean, the meeting drew a substantial delegation of Francophone women, especially Haitian, and women from the English-speaking Caribbean. However, the organizing committee failed to organize translation for these participants and did not consider the political dynamics of exclusion in light of Dominican policies of discrimination against Haitians. During the introductory plenary at which all participants were gathered, the Haitian women seized the microphone, confronted the organizing committee on their failure to consider this linguistic exclusion and its political and racial dimensions, and threatened to walk out of the Encuentro. Their statement was supported by nearly every participant, who noisily supported their declarations and threatened to leave the plenary in solidarity. Initially defensive, members of the organizing committee quickly acknowledged the ways the failure to provide translation was a failure of political vision rather than a lack of resources.

An additional point of contention in the Dominican Encuentro grew out of the emphasis on participatory methods at the workshops, which led a group of participants interested in discussing political movement strategy more directly to convene a workshop in the hotel's discotheque. Attended by 100 women of many backgrounds and ages, this meeting offered an unexpected opportunity to voice my concerns as a U.S. Latina to the creators of many of the texts that had informed, enriched, and transformed our work. The meeting, organized as a dialogue on next steps in the movement, was opened to all who wished to speak with the goal of articulating points of agreement and controversy concerning next steps. Speaking from my position as an *NCNV* editor, I thanked participants for their contributions to our work while pleading with them to consider the accessibility of their political texts, many of which remained theoretically abstract and difficult to read with our U.S. border-crossing Spanish. I felt the greatest resonance with the statements from the network of women in feminist communications, who similarly pleaded for the need to more systematically include media strategies as part of their political work. The Dominican Encuentro lacked communications access for representatives of the media, which feminist communications specialists from the region felt was emblematic of the low priority given to this critical movement strategy. I was also struck by the recurrent theme of missed opportunities to engage intergenerational relationships and the need to pass the torch of activism, a theme I was especially attuned to because of the difficulties encountered by so many feminist organizations in involving the next generation.

One particularly poignant series of exchanges occurred as parallel concerns that never became an engaged dialogue. A group of young feminists posed their concern that a new generation was learning about the movement through academic and nongovernmental organizations (NGOs) settings without feeling the vital engagement with the lived experience of activism and longed-for mentorship in those roles to the senior, established women in the movement. A well-known figure in the movement responded jokingly, "Don't worry, youth is a temporary condition," an intervention that unfortunately only served to confirm young feminists' worry that their concerns would not be taken seriously. Another well-known participant in the movement spoke of her fears as one among many single women confronting old age and finding that their nontraditional lives dedicated to building a movement left them alone, without the traditional resources of husbands and extended family. The work of incorporating diverse women, young women, and women from the U.S. diasporas was greatly advanced at the Dominican Encuentro but remained a work in progress.

In the Costa Rica Encuentro of 2002, a strong representation of Feminist Radio and a sophisticated communications strategy emphasized a balance of theory, methods of political development, communications and learning, self-care, and the healing arts. The conference focused on globalization, with a careful balance of plenaries offering sophisticated analysis on globalization by established scholars and activists in the field and participatory workshops addressing very diverse issues. I was drawn to a workshop on transnationalism, whose description in the catalogue offered a forum to talk about how Latin American and Caribbean women living and working in diaspora could contribute to the work of the movement. I sat in a circle under an open-air tent on the beach with twenty other women, all of us waiting for the facilitator. When we learned that because the facilitator's flight had been delayed she would not be arriving, the group began to disband. Suggesting that we not leave but instead stay and explore the questions bringing us together to see whether we could build a dialogue based on those questions, I became the group's facilitator and recorder. Our group included women from Colombia, Nicaragua, Mexico, and Argentina living in Europe; European women living and working in Latin America; Latin American academics working on transnational migration; and me, as a Cuban American living in the United States and redefining my life and work within a transnational feminist movment in the region. We titled our session "Las Ventajas de ser Desarraigadas/The Advantages of Being Uprooted," appreciating our multiple perspectives on the lived experience of globalization in contributing to the Encuentro's themes. Although the session included our complicated subjectivities on transnationalism, we used these to discuss the role of transnational organizing strategies in furthering feminism at a newly dangerous intersection. Participants were divided on the value of the great investment in the Bejing meeting and in other international forums.

Our dialogue affirmed the importance of communications and organizational networks that helped us maintain our connections to one another. We noted the great diversity of our positions at the margins or at the centers of power, and wondered how we could make use of these different positions constructively. A Colombian woman living in Belgium who worked for an NGO that provided funding to transnational organizing worked to create a bridge to Colombia throughout her private life and professional work. One participant, originally from Spain and living in Guatemala, joined with others to comment that we were using old paradigms of North/South while confronting new conditions of discrimination and injustice under new political economies. One participant who had been to Bejing and worked in rural Brazil used a forum of monthly meetings to sustain momentum and participation in women's issues in her community. Some workshop participants expressed great frustration with the location of the conference at a costly resort, and the ways costs limited the participation of many women's organizations at a time when funders were carefully selecting priorities for funding. A Honduran participant offered an optimistic example of the ways her Center for Women's Studies had succeeded in involving rural women in advocacy by using the Global Women's March as a vehicle for working locally on women's employment and labor rights. Their center organized a campaign event that helped them identify participants who could work from their own rural areas, decentering their networks, which had previously been centered in the capital of Tegucigalpa. She noted that in Honduras, banana plantations, mining, and *maquiladoras* had long ago "transnationalized" and "globalized" women's lives and work by creating the split between wealthy far-away owners and desperately poor local workers. In their labor advocacy work, they could not turn to the neoliberal state, as it worked in collusion with global capital. However, feminist activists found a helpful community of solidarity in first-world consumers who did not want to purchase *ropa sucia*, or tainted clothing, made through the labor of exploited workers. We closed with the affirmation that each of us may place only so many bricks, and some of the bricks may fall, but together we can build something massive and enduring.

By attending the Encuentros, I began to appreciate in new ways the longstanding debates concerning the role of broader women's organizations within a dedicated feminist movement and how different approaches to political organizing generated debates about political inclusiveness, social class, and race. As our ALAS/*NCNV* team came to appreciate these cultural and political complexities and histories, we were better able to engage them and strategically select textual materials and political voices. In engaging these activists and movements as living, evolving individuals and organizations rather than as information and text, we began to experience the text itself as a transnational border-crosser that held within its bound pages the representation of our participation in that movement. Our words in the text began to embody and invoke that movement. Together we recognized the many pathways by which diverse women might encounter the text and use it to learn about themselves in solidarity with their communities by sharing their stories and struggling together for their rights.

Puerto Rico as Bridge to Transnational Feminism in the Americas

Throughout our work of cultural adaptation, we kept returning to the critical role of Puerto Rican feminists as bridging U.S. Latina and Latin American and Caribbean feminisms in expanding the potential for transnational collaborations. During nearly twenty years of participation in local, regional, and global feminist movements, Nirvana Gonzalez had advocated for the development of a documentation center with key texts from organizations all over the region. In the chapter on Health Systems in *NCNV*, we reprinted a political analysis written by Gonzalez to address how Taller Salud's founders had selected women's health as the political medium for a feminist transformation of gender justice and social change (see *NCNV* 2000, 45–46). Recognizing the importance of locally based feminist organizations in Puerto Rico as links both to U.S. Latina and to regional and global women's health movements, we used the funding opportunity offered by an organizing grant from the Open Society Institute's U.S. reproductive health initiative to expand our learning about programs and their health promotion methodologies linked to political activism. In July 1999, as we were writing the final introductions to *NCNV*, we visited San Juan and held meetings with feminist activists and organizations working throughout the island. Taller Salud founding director Laura Colon drove us to two small rural towns where we experienced a dramatic highlighting of the relational and political differences between a grassroots empowerment approach and a professionalized social services approach to work with women experiencing domestic violence.

I have two enduring images from that visit, as the contrast between the two settings. In the self-organized group, called Cimarronas/Run-Away Slaves, we were ushered into an open communal dining room where the women offered us a lunch they had prepared in honor of our visit. As we sat around the table, they described the near closing of their domestic violence center and their determination to contribute volunteer time and resources to keeping it open so they could share the sense of safety and learning they experienced with other women. In the professionalized domestic violence center, we were brought into a traditional human services waiting room while we waited for the director. While we waited, we made friendly eye contact with a woman sitting across from us. A few minutes later, her counselor entered hurriedly and approached the waiting woman with no apology. The employee's demeanor conveyed the self-important posture and formality of a trained professional. As they walked away into a private room for a counseling session, the counselor loudly stated, "Now let's get started to see if we can do something about your problems." Although our colleagues in Taller Salud had deliberately selected these two centers for their contrasting approaches, we did not expect to see the consequences of empowerment versus a clinical approach exposed so starkly. Our conversations with participants and staff at both these sites emphasized the dangers of drifting toward professionalization in providing social services rather than promoting social justice. These two visits reinforced the vital importance of protecting community participation as a means of sustaining the integrity of feminist emancipatory projects as organizations engage funders, influence governments, and become involved in transnational advocacy networks and strategies (see Alvarez 2000; Minkler and Wallerstein 2004; Torres and

Cernada 2003). These visits with Puerto Rican feminists and their organizations, at a time when we were finalizing the final introductions in the text, inspired us to build "an altar of words" invoking connections between *NCNV* as a text, the ALAS approach to methodology, and the work of Taller Salud and other Puerto Rican feminists using health promotion as a feminist tool.

Lessons Learned:
Latina Organizing—Linking Local and Global Strategies

The Latina re-visionings and lessons learned in this final section are more of a work in progress than a finished product. Our Latina ALAS/*NCNV* work group's vision of a transnational collaborative process, emphasizing participatory methodologies, was successful in transforming *NCNV* as text. However, we were not as successful in helping to shift the organizational priorities of the Boston Women's Health Book Collective or their approach to the book in English.[15] At the time of the organization's 1999 strategic planning, I organized a panel on women of color's vision of participation in community organizing to articulate a vision of the book's potential not just as a mirror but as a tool for movement building, applicable not only for Latinas but for diverse women working in cross-racial coalitions. We suggested that an updating of *Our Bodies, Ourselves* consistent with the work of *NCNV* required deemphasizing the text as an encyclopedic resource and emphasizing participatory methodologies, systematic community outreach, and coalition building, along with the use of multiple media and new technologies. Significantly, the South African Women's Health Project, whose visually beautiful and pedagogically accessible women's health book based on *OBOS* provided our editorial work group with an inspiring example, chose not to publish a second edition of their book, emphasizing instead the creation of adaptable materials for use in their community health promotion workshops. Without a shift in the organization's priorities, the work on *NCNV* within Our Bodies, Ourselves as an organization has rested on the shoulders of a single Latina, and has emphasized development of a public health curriculum for use by *promotoras*. While this is an extremely valuable first step, it falls far short of actualizing our vision of transnational organizing by using *NCNV* as a tool, which remains a work in progress.

The following summary reflects our ALAS/*NCNV* work group's re-visioning of work in women's health promotion for personal and social change. Consistent with new work in culturally based community health promotion (Minkler and Wallerstein 2004; Torres and Cernada 2003), these re-visionings emphasize leadership development (Shapiro and Leigh

2005) and active health citizenship (Shepard 2002) as methodologies that shift the emphasis from health information as content to health as a human right and a matter of gender and social justice.

Latina Leadership Development in Gender, Culture, and Reproductive Health and Rights: Vision/Mission of Health Promotion for Leadership Development and Social Change

- Health promotion education, to be culturally meaningful, relevant to women's own lives, and effective in mobilizing personal and community change, needs to start with women's own stated needs and concerns; speak our language using culturally meaningful images and sacred healing arts; and use these as a pathway for identifying strengths and resources with which to solve our own problems in solidarity with others.
- Culturally meaningful health promotion connects body with mind, spirit, and community; promotes active engagement in a shared vision of change; and supports women making connections and building relationships to other women and to their communities to create the conditions promoting health.
- The first priority of health promotion education is to offer women the support and sense of self-efficacy that will help use available resources and advocate for new culturally and community-based resources to address sources of distress and ill-health while promoting vibrant well-being.
- Access to health care is redefined as, first and foremost, women's access to resources within their own communities that contribute to improved health, and only secondarily as access to the existing health care system with its many barriers for diverse women users.
- Collaboration requires that we work across professional and community boundaries, get to know other groups' strengths and resources, and participate in an "exchange of gifts."
- Women educators, outreach workers, and administrators first need to connect with ourselves and each other to become aware of the implications of injustices as burdens and barriers to wellness in our own lives and begin a process of mutual healing.
- The international and third-world women's health movements can help invigorate and inspire Latinas and other women from U.S. communities of color who have not felt a connection to the North American feminist movement.
- Latin American and Caribbean women's health activists offer U.S. Latinas working in health promotion for gender justice and social change a culturally compatible approach to building activist networks and methods for

designing culturally meaningful materials for health promotion education grounded in participatory education principles and linked to the women, communities, and movements creating them.

Expanding the Borderlands: Transnational Opportunities for U.S. Latinas in Gender, Culture, and Health

As a faculty member in psychology and Latino studies at an urban public university, I have returned to this public university as a home base for developing the next steps in transnational collaborations emphasizing campus and community collaborations. Learning from my transnational community to make the best of both worlds, I have come to appreciate the advantages of my privileged location at a third-world university, remembering the words of Leopoldina Rendon, director of the documentation center at the Mexican feminist organization Comunicación, Intercambio y Desarrollo Humano en América Latina/Communication, Interchange and Human Development in Latin Amé3rica (CIDHAL): "We are poor in material resources, but rich in human resources." Among the states initiating the most significant cuts in public higher education, Massachusetts was one of only two states to have increased the gap between rich and poor during the boom years, and it is home to one of the poorest and one of the youngest Latino populations in the United States. The University of Massachusetts at Boston is also the most racially diverse four-year college in New England and home to an inspiring array of ethnic minority and public policy institutes with significant community partnerships. Among these friends, I have initiated a home for my transnational work in Latina health promotion within a project in gender, culture, and health at the Mauricio Gaston Institute for Latino Public Policy, which is part of an inter-university program in Latino research, a network of Latino research institutes linked to community constituencies.[16] The project emphasizes participatory health promotion methodologies; a view of gender justice as good for both men and women; inclusion of a spiritual perspective in reproductive health and rights; and *ciudadanía*/citizenship concepts of political participation. The project aims to create strategic partnerships locally, nationally, and internationally, emphasizing development of multimedia materials, outreach campaigns, and participatory action research in gender justice, health promotion, and social change. The project supports initiatives and programs in leadership development, network organizing, and capacity building using Latin American models and methods of *ciudadanía*/citizenship and health promotion in reproductive health and rights (Palomino 2002; Shepard 2002, 2003; Thayer 2000); definitions of reproductive justice and human rights meaningful in local Latino/a communities; family-friendly and spiritually based feminisms; and health promotion approaches to family health using cultural strengths.

I am currently working as participatory program evaluator with Entre Nosotras. This program is a culturally meaningful Spanish-language HIV prevention program for Latinas, using community *promotoras* to conduct workshops on healthy sexuality and empowerment. Entre Nosotras operates in partnership with Mujeres Unidas, a community-based Latina adult education and empowerment center, and with Iris Rivera, founder of Casa Iris, who opened Boston's conversation for Latinas living with AIDS and striving to transform their communities. In the spirit of creating communities in which economic hardship and family violence do not blight the possibilities for love given and received in women's lives and for generations to come, Entre Nosotras uses lessons learned the hard way but shared generously with other women. I had the honor of traveling to the March for Women's Lives with the Boston Latina delegation organized by Maridena Rojas, project director for Entre Nosotras. I served as their translator when Rojas and community activist Jacqueline Peña presented their work at the Latina Summit organized by the National Latina Institute for Reproductive Health.

As a university-based Latina and academic activist, my vision of what is possible has been nourished by the extraordinary women I met through my travels with *Nuestros Cuerpos, Nuestras Vidas*, and the projects they introduced me to. I take example and inspiration from the Latin American Women's Health Network's Universidad Itinerante/Itinerant University, envisioned and until recently directed by Maria Isabel Matamala, a Chilean feminist who co-directed the Latin American Women's Health Network (RSMLAC) and currently works at the Pan American Health Organization on monitoring the impact of health sector privatization on women's health. Itinerant University is an educational and capacity-building campus/community collaboration held throughout the region, which brings together a local women's organization, a local activist university, and the Latin American Women's Health Network to design workshops that will offer training in gender justice and health while establishing and strengthening collaborative networks. I also look to the Regional Training Program in Politics and Public Policy (PRIGEPP), a virtual educational program in capacity building and leadership development for women's participation in governance and policy founded by Gloria Bonder. Conducted virtually, it is physically located at Facultad Latino-americana de Ciencias Sociales/Latin American Faculty in Social Sciences (FLACSO), the regional social sciences faculty at its Buenos Aires, Argentina campus (http://www.prigepp .org/site/home.asp). Finally, we are inspired by a world of work in Latin American and Caribbean activism in women's health and rights (see Chant and Craske 2003; Shepard 2003; Stephen 1997; Thayer 2000). Our inspiration extends also to global feminism, to which we bring our unique local perspectives and our solidarity.

Acknowledgments

Nuestros Cuerpos, Nuestras Vidas represents the loving labor of many hands and passionate activism of many communities; I want to thank my colleagues on the Latina editorial committee, in ALAS throughout the years, the founders, staff, and board of the Boston Women's Health Book Collective/*Our Bodies, Ourselves*, our Latin American and Caribbean collaborators (listed at http://www.ourbodiesourselves.org/ncnv_eng.htm), and the Entre Nosotras community at Action for Boston Community Development.

Notes

1. Zavella (2002) describes the "peripheral vision" of everyday transnationalism as women working in canneries and food industries at the U.S./Mexico border evaluate shifting economic and political contingencies to determine where they will move in pursuit of their family's economic survival; Naples and Desai (2002) review vocabularies, definitions, and strategies for connecting global transnational movements with local strategies of "transnationalism from below"; Thayer (2001) describes how women's organizations in the Brazilian *sertao* (backlands) appropriated and transformed concepts from an urban Brazilian feminist organization, themselves translating and transforming U.S. feminist concepts.

2. Complex systems theory approaches to women's empowerment through health promotion use concepts from ecologies of human development in living systems to describe "virtuous circles" in which resource-rich environments protect and promote positive development, in contrast to "vicious circles" in which depriving, violent, and unjust circumstances increase exposure to risks and stressors undermining capacities for development; see Kar, Pascual, and Chickering (1999); Kar et al. (2002); Shapiro (1994/2005); Shapiro and Leigh (2005).

3. Cuban anthropologist Fernando Ortiz (1940/1995) proposed the construct of transculturation as an alternative to Malinowski's acculturation in describing new forms created by cultural encounters in Cuba and the Caribbean.

4. For detailed discussion of these organizational transitions, see Main (1997); for detailed description of the organizational strategies permitting the transformation of the NCNV adaptation, see Shapiro (2005).

5. Similarly, I describe "strategic reflection" as a method for assessing barriers and leveraging resources in achieving desired goals under circumstances of

oppression, changing the contexts for one's own contingent development (Shapiro 2005; Shapiro and Leigh 2005).

6. A group of U.S. Latinas formed Amigas Latinas en Acción (ALAS) in 1979, initially to generate a cultural adaptation of the 1976 Spanish translation for use by U.S. Latinas, but continued their work with an emphasis on participatory education using media; see later discussion of the changing role of ALAS in the organization.

7. For detailed discussion of these organizational transitions, see Main (1997); for detailed description of the organizational strategies permitting the transformation of the NCNV adaptation, see Shapiro (2005).

8. In addition to Sandoval (2000), see Zavella (2002) on peripheral vision; Moya argues that U.S. women of color have contributed to a collective project of social change by developing a distinctive border-crossing critical consciousness characterized by the capacity to learn from difference and demonstrating "the viability of, and methods involved in, creating coalitions across difference" (2002, 97).

9. The December 1997 issue of *Sojourner* includes an open letter from Boston Women's Health Book Collective women of color who had resigned from the organization after highly contentious battles over its racial inclusiveness, transparency, and accountability; a response from the board of directors (which I co-signed as a member of the new diverse board); and an analysis of the organizational processes involved by Shelly Main, based on interviews with former and current staff, founders, and board.

10. As a board member involved in the organization's strategic planning, I was part of an intense debate on who constituted the organization's constituencies and whether they overlapped with the purchasers of current *OBOS* editions.

11. Puntos de Encuentro is the name of a Nicaraguan feminist organization specializing in young women's political participation and popular education methods (http://www.puntos.org.ni/).

12. This re-visioning of ALAS and its vital relationship to *NCNV* was supported by funding from the Boston Foundation, which subsidized local community workshops and local development of a Latina health network, and by funding from the Open Society Institute supporting U.S. Latina organizing nationally and transnationally, using *NCNV* and its activist networks.

13. Colleagues at regional documentation centers included Nirvana Gonzalez at Taller Salud in Puerto Rico; Isabel Duques and colleagues at ISIS international in Chile, who run the Latin American Women's Health Information Center, making activist databases and documents available regionally;

Leonora Rendon and colleagues Communicacion, Intercambio y Desarrollo Humano en America Latina/Communication, Interchange and Human Development in Latin America (CIDHAL) in Cuernavaca, Mexico, with its own women's health programs and a thriving regional documentation center; Adrianna Gomez and colleagues at the Latin American and Caribbean Women's Health Network/RSMLAC in Chile, publishing a quarterly women's health magazine, coordinating regional activist campaigns, and maintaining a database of women's health organizations in the region; Cecilia Olivares and colleagues at Centro de Informacion y Desarrollo de la Mujer/ Center for Women's Information and Development (CIDEM) in Bolivia, at that time coordinating the Latin American regional campaign to legalize abortion; and Elsa Gomez Gomez, director of the Pan American Health Organization's Women and Development Section.

14. After a period of reorganization, the National Latina Institute for Reproductive Health has relocated from Washington, D.C., to Brooklyn, New York, and changed its methods of work to emphasize grassroots leadership development, community organizing, and coalition building that supports their national policy work in Latina reproductive health and rights, described at http://www.latinainstitute.org/mission.html.

15. The organization changed its name from Boston Women's Health Book Collective (BWHBC) to Our Bodies, Ourselves to emphasize the centrality of the text in their public recognition and their organizational priorities.

16. The Inter University Program in Latino Research is housed at Notre Dame University, http://www.nd.edu/~iuplr/.

Resource References

Nuestros Cuerpos, Nuestras Vidas: *NCNV* is available for bulk ordering of clinic discount copies, and the webpage has a free, downloadable guide for its use in health promotion workshops, information, and contact person at http://www.ourbodiesourselves.org.
Entre Nosotras: a community-based Latina HIV prevention program promoting healthy sexuality and gender equality, housed at Action for Boston Community Development, Health Programs at http://www.bostonabcd.org/programs/health-programs.htm#ent.
Gender, Culture, and Health Project: at Mauricio Gaston Institute, University of Massachusetts, Boston: (617) 287-5790, Ester Shapiro, Director; http://www.gaston.umb.edu.
National Latina Institute for Reproductive Health: a U.S. Latina reproductive health and rights organization; http://www.latinainstitute.org/mission.html.

Latin American Feminist and Women's Health Activism

Red de Salud de America Latina y el Caribe (Latin American and Caribbean
  Women's Health Network): activist network organizes regional campaigns,
  connects groups, publishes a magazine and online interactive fact sheet
  monitoring status of women at http://www.reddedsalud.web.cl.
ISIS Internacional: feminist documentation center and Internet site for networks
  on violence against women and on feminist media and communications;
  http://www.isis.cl.
Pan American Health Organization (PAHO): Latin American and Caribbean
  World Health's Organization regional network, webpage has information on
  the region; see especially their gender, health, and development resources at
  http://www.paho.org; see also their equity and health listserv, EQUIDAD@
  LISTSERV.PAHO.ORG.
Red de Educación Popular Entre Mujeres (Network for Women's Popular Education) (REPEM): publications emphasize women's health and economic empowerment; http://www.repem.ur.

Global Women of Color Feminist Organizations

Development of Women for a New Era (DAWN): a network of women scholars
  and activists from the economic South who engage in feminist research and
  analysis of the global environment and are committed to working for economic justice, gender justice, and democracy. DAWN works globally and
  regionally in Africa, Asia, the Caribbean, Latin America, and the Pacific on
  the themes of the political economy of globalization; political restructuring
  and social transformation; sustainable livelihoods; and sexual and reproductive health and rights, in partnership with other global NGOs and networks.
  Their webpage posts extensive information on activist projects, monitoring
  of global accords, and publications at http://www.dawn.org.fj/.
International Women's Health Coalition (IWHC): provides HERA (Health, Action, Empowerment, Rights and Accountability) action sheets on Cairo and
  Bejing agreements and monitoring, gender equity and empowerment, women
  and adolescents' sexual and reproductive rights and health, men's role and
  responsibility for sexual and reproductive rights and health, and abortion.
  Action sheets available at http://www.iwhc. org/hera/index.htm.

References

Acosta-Belen, Edna, and Christine Bose. 2000. "U.S. Latina and Latin American
  Feminisms: Hemispheric Encounters." Signs 25(4): 1113–19.
Alvarez, Sonia. 2000. "Translating the Global: Effects of Transnational Organizing on Local Feminist Discourses and Practices in Latin America." Meridians 1(1): 29–67.

———. 1998. "Latin American Feminisms 'Go Global': Trends of the 1990s and Challenges for the New Millenium." In *Re-Visioning Latin American Social Movements*, ed. Sonia Alvarez, Evelina Dagnino, and Arturo Escobar. Boulder, CO: Westview Press.

Alvarez, Sonia, Elizabeth Friedman, Maylei Blackwell, and Maryssa Navarro. 2003. "Encountering Latin American and Caribbean Feminisms." *Signs* 28(2): 537–79.

Basu, Amrita. 2000. "Globalization of the Local/Localization of the Global: Mapping Transnational Women's Movements." *Meridians* 1(Autumn): 68–84.

———. 1995. *The Challenge of Local Feminisms: Women's Movements in Global Perspective.* Boulder, CO: Westview Press.

Bonilla, Frank, Edwin Melendez, Rebeca Morales, and Maria de los Angeles Torres. 1998. *Borderless Borders: U.S. Latinos, Latin Americans, and the Paradox of Interdependence.* Philadelphia: Temple University Press.

Boston Women's Health Book Collective. 2000. *Nuestros Cuerpos, Nuestras Vidas.* New York: Siete Cuentos Editorial.

———. 1998. *Our Bodies, Ourselves.* New York: Simon & Schuster.

Chant, Sylvia, and Nikki Craske. 2003. *Gender in Latin America.* New Brunswick, NJ: Rutgers University Press.

Conway, Dennis, Adrian Bailey, and Mark Ellis. 2001. "Gendered and Racialized Circulation-migration: Implications for the Poverty and Work Experience of New York's Puerto Rican Women." In *Migration, Transnationalization, and Race in a Changing New York*, ed. Hector Cordero-Guzman, Robert Smith, and Ramon Grosfoguel. Philadelphia: Temple University Press.

Darder, Antonia. 2002. *Pedagogy of Love.* Boulder, CO: Westview Press.

Davis, Kathy. 2003. "Feminist Body/Politics as World Traveler: Translating Our Bodies, Ourselves." *European Journal of Women's Studies* 9(3): 223–47.

Freire, Ana Marie, and Donaldo Macedo, eds. 2000. *The Paulo Friere Reader.* New York: Continum Press.

Freire, Paolo. 2000. *The Paulo Freire Reader*, ed. Ana Maria Freire and Donaldo Macedo. New York: Continuum Press.

———. 1994. *Pedagogy of Hope.* New York: Continuum Press.

Gomez, Elsa. 1993. "Gender, Women and Health in the Americas." Pan American Health Organization. Scientific Publication #541, Washington, DC.

Hardy-Fanta, Carol. 2002. *Latino Politics in Massachusetts.* New York: Routledge Press.

Hurtado, Aida. 1996. *The Color of Privilege: Three Blasphemies on Race and Feminism.* Ann Arbor: University of Michigan Press.

Kabeer, Naila. 1999. "Resources, Agency, Achievements: Reflections on the Measurement of Women's Empowerment." *Development and Change* 30(3): 435.

Kaplan, Caren, Norma Alarcon, and Minoo Moallem. 1999. *Between Woman and Nation: Nationalisms, Transnational Feminisms, and the State.* Durham, NC: Duke University Press.

Kaplan, Caren, and Inderpal Grewal. 2002. "Transnational Practices and Interdisciplinary Feminst Scholarship: Refiguring Women's and Gender Studies." In *Women's Studies on its Own*, ed. Robyn Wiegman. Chapel Hill, NC: Duke University Press.

Kar, Snehendu, Catherine Pascual, and Kirstin Chickering. 1999. "Empowerment of Women for Health Promotion: A Meta-Analysis." *Social Science and Medicine* 49: 1431–60.

Kar, Snehendu, Catherine Pascual, Kirstin Chickering, and Tracy Hazelton. 2002. "Empowerment of Women for Health Development: A Global Perspective." *Journal of Health and Population in Developing Countries* 4(1), http://www.jhpdc.unc.edu/Journal41/empower.pdf.

Keck, Margaret, and Katherine Sikkink. 1998. *Activists Beyond Borders: Advocacy Networks in International Politics*. Ithaca: Cornell University Press.

Kickbusch, Iona. 2003. "The Contribution of the World Health Organization to a New Public Health and Health Promotion." *American Journal of Public Health* 93(3): 383.

Latina Feminist Group. 2002. *Telling to Live*. Durham, NC: Duke University Press.

Main, Shelly. 1997. "Our Feminist Institutions, Ourselves." *Sojourner* 23 (December): 10–12.

Malhotra, Anju. 2002. "Conceptualizing and Measuring Women's Empowerment as a Variable in International Development." Paper presented at workshop on "Measuring Empowerment: Cross-Disciplinary Perspectives," World Bank, Washington, DC.

Mendoza, Breny. 2002. "Transnational Feminisms in Question." *Feminist Theory* 3(3): 295–314.

Minkler, Meredith, and Nina Wallerstein, eds. 2004. *Community Based Participatory Research for Health*. San Francisco, CA: Jossey Bass.

Mohanty, Chandra. 2003. *Feminism Without Borders: Decolonizing Theory, Practicing Solidarity*. Chapel Hill, NC: Duke University Press.

Moya, Paula. 2002. *Learning from Experience: Minority Identities, Multi-Cultural Struggles*. San Francisco: University of California Press.

Naples, Nancy, and Manisha Desai. 2002. *Women's Activism and Globalization: Linking Local Struggles and Transnational Politics*. New York: Routledge.

Nieto, Sonia. 2003. *Affirming Diversity: The Sociopolitical Context of Multicultural Education*. Hanover, NH: Heineman.

Norsigian, Judy, Vilunya Diskin, Paula Doress-Worteres, Jane Pincus, Wendy Sanford, and Norma Swenson. 1999. "The Boston Women's Health Book Collective and Our Bodies, Ourselves: A Brief History and Reflection." *Journal of the American Medical Women's Association* 54(1): 35–40.

Ortiz, Fernando. 1940/1995. *Cuban Counterpoint: Tobacco and Sugar*. Durham, NC: Duke University Press.

Palomino, Nancy. 2002. "Citizenship and Women's Health." *Women's Health Journal*. http://www.fas.harvard.edu/womenstudy/events/palomino_citzandhealth.doc.doc.

Petchesky, Rosalind. 2003. *Global Prescriptions: Gendering Health and Human Rights*. London: Zed Books.

Petchesky, Rosalind, and Karen Judd. 1998. *Negotiating Reproductive Rights: Women's Perspectives Across Countries and Cultures*. London: Zed Books.

Ruzek, Sheryl, and Julie Becker. 1999. "The Women's Health Movement in the United States: From Grassroots Activism to Professional Agendas." *Journal of the American Women's Medical Association* 54(1): 4–8.

Sanchez, Patricia. 2001. "Adopting a Transnational Theory and Discourse: Making Space for a Transnational Chicana." *Discourse: Studies in the Cultural Politics of Education 22*(3): 375–81.

Sandoval, Chela. 2002. "Foreword: AfterBridge: Technologies of Crossing." In *This Bridge We Call Home: Radical Visions for Transformation*, ed. Gloria Anzaldua and Annemarie Keating, 21–26. New York: Routledge.

———. 2000. *Methodologies of the Oppressed*. Minneapolis: University of Minnesota Press.

Shapiro, Ester. 2005. "The Personal is Methodological: From Our Bodies Ourselves to Nuestros Cuerpos Nuestros Vidas."

———. 2002. "Family Bereavement after Collective Trauma: Private Suffering, Public Meanings and Cultural Contexts." *Journal of Systemic Therapy 21*(3): 81–92.

———. 2000. "Crossing Cultural Borders with Our Bodies, Ourselves: Linking Women's Health Education and Political Participation in Nuestros Cuerpos, Nuestras Vidas." In *Strategies for Change: Women's Organizations and the Building of Civil Society in the 21st Century: International Perspectives.* http://www.philanthropy.org/GN/KEN/gntext/fullview_economicrights_crossing_divides_shapiro.htm.

———. 2001. "Santeria as a Healing Practice: My Cuban Jewish Journey with Oshun." In *Healing Cultures: Art and Religion as Curative Practices in the Caribbean*, ed. Margarite Fernandez-Olmos. New York: Palgrave Press.

———. 1996a. "Exile and Professional Identity: On Going Back to Cuba." *Cultural Diversity and Mental Health 2*(1): 21–33.

———. 1996b. "Family Development in Cultural Context: Implications for Prevention and Early Intervention with Latino families." *New England Journal of Public Policy 11*(2): 113–28.

———. 1994, 2005. *Grief as a Family Process: A Developmental Approach to Clinical Practice*. 2nd ed. New York: Guilford Press.

———. 1994b. "Finding What Had Been Lost in Plain View." In *Bridges to Cuba, Michigan Quarterly Review*, ed. Ruth Behar and Jose Leon, 579–89

Shapiro, Ester, and Jennifer Leigh. 2005. "Toward Culturally Competent Feminist Leadership: Assessing Outcomes in Diverse Contexts." In *Cultural Diversity and Feminist Leadership*, ed. Jean Lau Chin. Washington, DC: American Psychological Association.

Shepard, Bonnie. 2003. *NGO Advocacy Networks in Latin America: Lessons From Experience in Promoting Women's and Reproductive Rights*. University of Miami: North/South Center Press, http://www.miami.edu/nsc/publications/pub-ap-pdf/61AP.pdf.

———. 2002. " 'Let's Be Citizens, Not Patients!' Women's Groups in Peru Assert Their Right to High Quality Reproductive Healthcare." In *Responding to Cairo: Case Studies of Changed Practice in Reproductive Health and Family Planning*, ed. Nicole Haberland and Diana Meacham. New York: Population Council.

Shohat, Ella. 2002. "Area Studies, Gender Studies, and the Cartographies of Knowledge." *Social Text 20*(3): 67–78.

Stephen, Lynn. 1997. *Women and Social Movements in Latin America: Power from Below*. Austin: University of Texas Press.

Thayer, Millie. 2001. "Transnational Feminism: Reading Joan Scott in the Brazilian Sertao." *Ethnography* 2(2): 243–71.

———. 2000. "Traveling Feminisms: From Embodied Women to Gendered Citizenship." In *Global Ethnography: Forces, Connections and Imaginations in a Postmodern World*, ed. Michael Burawoy, Joseph Blum, Sheba George, Zsuzsa Gille, Teresa Gowan, Lynne Haney, Maren Klawiter, Steve Lopez, Sean Riain, and Millie Taylor. Berkeley: University of California Press.

Torres, Maria de los Angeles. 1998. "Transnational Political and Cultural Identities: Crossing Theoretical Borders." In *Borderless Borders: U.S. Latinos, Latin Americans, and the Paradox of Interdependence*, ed. Frank Bonilla, Edwin Melendez, Rebecca Morales, and Maria de los Angeles Torres, 169–82. Philadelphia: Temple University Press.

Torres, Maria Idali, and George Cernada. 2003. *Sexual and Reproductive Health Promotion in Latino Populations: Parteras, Promotoras y Poetas Case Studies Across the Americas*. Amityville, NY: Baywood Publishing Co.

Tropicana, Carmelita. 2000. *I, Carmelita Tropicana*. Boston: Beacon Press.

Velez-Ibanez, Carlos, and Anna Sampaio, eds. 2002. *Transnational Latina/o Communities: Politics, Processes and Cultures*. Lanham, MD: Rowman and Littlefield.

Warren, Alice E. Colon. 2003. "Puerto Rico Feminism and Feminist Studies." *Gender and Society* 17(5): 664–90.

Women's Health Project. 1996. *The South African Women's Health Book*. London: Oxford University Press.

Yuval-Davis, Nira. 1999. "The 'Multi-Layered Citizen': Citizenship in the Age of 'Glocalization.'" *International Feminist Journal of Politics* 1(1): 119–36.

Zavella, Patricia. 2002. "Engendering Transnationalism in Food Processing: Peripheral Vision on Both Sides of the U.S.-Mexican Border." In *Transnational Latina/o Communities: Politics, Processes and Cultures*, ed. Carlos Velez-Ibanez and Anna Sampaio. Lanham, MD: Rowman and Littlefield.

CHAPTER FIVE

Including Every Woman: The All-Embracing "We" of *Our Bodies, Ourselves*

ZOBEIDA E. BONILLA

As tone and voice editor of the 8th edition of *Our Bodies, Ourselves* (*OBOS*), my task was to read the draft chapters for inclusive language and content, bearing in mind issues such as cultural and ethnic diversity, socioeconomic class, demographic cohorts, religion and belief systems, health traditions, gender and sexual orientation, and disability. Keeping in perspective that it is a gigantic effort to present the gamut of health needs and concerns of All women in a single book, I commenced my encounter with the "all-embracing we"—the idea of a "we" that is inclusive—in the personal stories, viewpoints, and health information presented throughout the book. From "Environmental and Occupational Health" to "Abortion," from "Childbirth" to "Midlife and Menopause," my task was to ensure that a variety of voices were represented and that the chapters' language was sensitive to the multiplicity of health issues of women from disparate backgrounds.

Before I could read the draft chapters in the upcoming 8th edition of *OBOS* for this purpose, it seemed important to learn how the all-embracing "we" had changed over time to determine what would be new and distinct in this edition. The 8th edition of *OBOS* is the second time that this influential book on women's health includes a tone and voice editor on its team (which included about 500 writers, readers, and editors for this edition). A tone and voice editor was part of the team for the first time during the production of the 1998 edition of *OBOS* (Whelan and Sanford 2003a). The idea of having a tone and voice editor emerged from "the need to bring in diverse viewpoints and voices" and the desire for the "revision/update to include and be shaped by the voices of a wider range of communities" (Whelan and Sanford 2003b, 5).

This essay is divided into two main sections. The first section provides a brief review of changes in the "we" from the 1970s to the late 1990s and *OBOS*'s struggle for inclusiveness. The second section describes the issues I faced in dealing with representation of different women through the use of pronouns, the construction of the other, the incorporation of personal experiences, and the presentation of medical information.

Originally published in the spring 2005 issue (vol. 17, no. 1).

Including Every Woman: The Centrality of the "We" and the Struggle for Inclusiveness

The use of the word *we* in *OBOS* has been a fundamental feature of the book, which has given *OBOS* an accessible and caring tone and a more inviting and embracing voice (Whelan and Sanford 2003b). In the early 1970s the title of the book underwent an initial transformation from *Women and Their Bodies* to *Women and Our Bodies*, then changed to *Our Bodies, Ourselves* (Kahn 1995). This change in the title suggests a shift toward a more inclusive "we," with women placed at the center of knowledge about their own health and bodies. These initial changes in the title of the book were directly related to the original authors' reflection and discussions about their individual encounters with the medical system, their personal knowledge about their bodies, and their frustrations with health care settings where they were treated in a "condescending, paternalistic, judgmental, and uninformative" way (Norsigian et al. 1999, 35; Norsigian 1998).

The editions of *OBOS* in the early 1970s remained focused for the most part on a "we" that was composed of young, educated, middle-class, white women: "We are white, our ages range from 24 to 40, most of us are from middle-class backgrounds and have had at least some college education, and some of us have professional degrees. We are white middle-class women, and as such can describe only what life has been for us" (BWHBC 1973, cited in Morgan 2002, 17). Although the original "we" did not directly include women of color, women with disabilities, or older women, for example, throughout the various editions of *OBOS* the Boston Women's Health Book Collective (hereafter referred to as the Collective) has struggled to reach a more embracing "we":

> [L]ike many groups initially formed by white women, we have struggled against society's, and our own, internalized presumption that middle-class white women are representative of all women and thus have the right to define women's health issues and set priorities. This assumption does a great injustice by ignoring and silencing the voices of women of color, depriving us all of hard-won wisdom and crucial, lifesaving information. (Pincus 1998)

By the late 1970s and early 1980s, *OBOS* had expanded its voices and the health issues discussed in its pages, thus reflecting the broadened awareness of the organization about the way in which women of diverse backgrounds experience health and illness (Kahn 1995; Morgan 2002).

The themes addressed in the early editions of *OBOS*—reproductive health, relationships, abortion rights, sexuality, pregnancy, and childbirth—reflect the concerns of a young Collective (Houck 2003) and defined the "we" represented in these editions. The subject of menopause, for example, did not appear until the end of the 1970s, and occupational health did not receive attention until the 1984 edition of the book (Kahn 1995). The efforts to be more inclusive were accentuated in *OBOS* 1998, which for the first time put photos of diverse women on its cover. In this edition of *OBOS* more women of color were engaged in producing the book and critically reviewing the chapters (Pincus 1998). As the following quote from the body image chapter in *OBOS* 1998 illustrates, the "we" includes women from various populations:

> We are wounded when a physical characteristic or set of characteristics is loaded with negative expectations. If we have black skin and African features, or olive skin and Asian features, or dark curly hair and a prominent nose as do many Jews and Arabs, or if we have a visible disability, or if we are perceived as "overweight," our experiences from an early age may be marked by other people's negative reaction to our physical selves. We may have come to dislike, mistrust, or even hate our bodies as a result, feeling that they, rather than the society we live in, have betrayed us. (Iazetto, King, and Yanco 1998, 34)

In 2000 *Nuestros Cuerpos, Nuestras Vidas (NCNV)*, literally translated as *Our Bodies, Our Lives*, was published, becoming the first cultural adaptation of *OBOS* produced by the Collective.[1] Although *OBOS* has been translated into sixteen other languages as a result of projects initiated by women's health groups from other countries using *OBOS* as a model, the publication of *NCNV* marked a very important step in the journey toward inclusiveness. The Collective initiated this effort; invested time, energy, and resources; and assembled an outstanding team of Latinas who worked from within the organization with the goal of making *OBOS* more culturally relevant and accessible to a growing segment of our society. The "we" continued to grow as *OBOS* continued to embrace a wider audience and expanded collaborations with women's health groups to reflect the issues of a more diverse community (Norsigian 1998).

OBOS has also expanded its voice by addressing a larger set of health issues relevant to a broader female audience, extending its contents to include, for example, health concerns that are specific to female workers; addressing health risks associated with geography, the environment, racism, and poverty; and expanding the discussion of the health needs of women who were often marginally mentioned in earlier editions such as immigrant women (BWHBC 1984; BWHBC 1992; BWHBC 1998). Furthermore, *OBOS* has broadened the voices in the text by addressing and valuing the impact of diverse health traditions and the role of spirituality in our experiences of health and disease (Kahn 1995).

The transformation in the title of the chapter on lesbianism throughout the various editions of *OBOS* offers an example of the Collective's aim for the all-embracing "we." Initially, the chapter was entitled "Homosexuality," but in 1973 it was changed to "In Amerika They Call Us Dykes." According to Robbie P. Kahn, the use of the word *dykes* in the chapter's title is a "defiant stance," "an attempt to transcend the slang," and a way to challenge the current sociopolitical structures (1995, 329). This radical change is also an important moment in the growth of the all-embracing "we," when women who faced discrimination because of their gender identity or sexual orientation were recognized and included in their own right and with their own voices and self-definitions. In the 1984 edition the chapter is called "Loving Women: Lesbian Life and Relationships," while in 1998 the chapter is simply entitled "Relationships with Women." In the 1984, 1992, and 1998 editions the chapter is part of a larger section that deals with, among other issues, relationships with men and mutuality among men and women. In the 2005 edition, the section "Relationships and Sexuality" opens the discussion with the chapter "Gender Identity and Sexual Orientation," which is followed by the chapters "Relationships with Men," "Relationships with Women," and "Sexuality."

Throughout the years the changing title has created a larger space where multiple identities can be found and are welcomed. The "we" of this chapter has become more receptive, allowing for more women to feel that the chapter speaks to them. A space was created where both words and the embodiment of the words became more comfortable and acceptable as a direct result of larger societal changes and the contribution of the women's health movement (Kahn 1995). In the 2005 edition the "we" in the unit further recognizes the multiplicity of identities and sexual orientations. It continues to challenge the traditional sex roles and includes a provocative cutting-edge discussion on the fluidity of gender and sexual orientation, as well as on important health concerns.[2]

Not only has a larger space been created for a careful discussion about sexual orientation and gender, but also a larger space has been created where the health issues and needs of more women are recognized, included, and examined. With each edition of *OBOS* we see more voices and new perspectives, as well as a more challenging "we" created in the midst of the increased tensions that come as part of the process of welcoming diversity, defining which health issues of women from multiple backgrounds to include, and embracing inclusiveness (Pincus 1998, 21–3).

Tone and Voice in *OBOS* 2005

The continuous expansion of *OBOS*'s voices and the more sensitive and respectful tone in *OBOS* has been, in part, influenced by the growth in the diversity of this nation, the relevance of *OBOS* to women's health initiatives in the national and international arenas (see Sow and Bop 2004), and the way in which medical and scientific knowledge is reconstructing old and creating new frontiers of health and pathologies. In 1998, when a tone and voice editor was first a team member, the editorial guidelines alerted writers and editors to instances when the word *we* could be used inappropriately or would make claims beyond what would be universally shared by most women (Whelan and Sanford 2003a). As tone and voice editor of *OBOS* 2005, my main task was to ensure that the voices of as many women as possible were included in the text and that their representations were respectful and as accurate as possible. Seeking to expand the voices of a younger audience and to address the needs of immigrant women in particular, it was my task to see that the experiences of these two groups were included and/or expanded from the previous editions.

The first step in my overall task was to develop a set of tone and voice guidelines to alert the editors of possibly sensitive subjects and to bring consistency to the use of terms and descriptors.[3] These guidelines included seven categories in which particular attention to language and representation of diverse groups of women could be needed. The seven categories were: (1) ethnicity/race; (2) disability issues; (3) ageism; (4) sexual orientation and gender identity; (5) medicalization; (6) violence against women; and (7) religious and cultural background. For example, preference to national origins and names of groups was given when addressing cultural, ethnic, or racial backgrounds. In addressing women with disabilities, the focus was on the woman's individuality, avoiding terms and expressions that defined the person as "disabled" in addition to avoiding contrasting terms such as *normal*. Attempts were made to be as inclusive as possible when addressing the needs of groups such as immigrant women, younger women, and lesbians by making the chapters throughout the book more relevant and accessible to a larger audience instead of just "mentioning" the needs of special groups. Throughout the text it was important to ensure that women's choices regarding health care and therapies were respected. An effort was made to avoid terms and descriptions that judge women's choices, yet to critique the medicalization of women's bodies and present the information needed to make informed decisions. The role of spirituality and cultural background in keeping women healthy was acknowledged as well. It was also important to present the assets of cultural and religious diversity, as well as the role of different healing and medical traditions in the health and well-being of women.

In addition to keeping these categories in perspective as I read the chapters, I specifically evaluated the presence or absence of issues and narratives addressing the needs of younger women and immigrant women. One of *OBOS*'s distinguishing features is the use of narratives and personal stories along with medical information to present the health concerns of women. The narratives needed to be as representative as possible of women of diverse backgrounds and generations, while the information needed to speak to as many women as possible. The draft of the chapter "Environmental and Occupational Health," for example, did not address young women workers directly, a group of employees who may be at higher risk than older, more experienced workers for occupational hazards, underpayment, and exploitation. In this case the "we" needed to be expanded to include directly the voices of those young women workers.

Wrestling with pronouns, terminology, and descriptors in the construction of risk, health, and illness was another challenge that I encountered. It was important that the medical information and the narratives addressed risks and illness without inappropriately creating a face of disease that was young, ethnic, or stressing some other stereotype. Yet, it remained imperative that the facts were stated accurately and that women were informed of risks, options, and choices. For example, the use of the pronouns *we, us, you,* and *they* in the "Sexually Transmitted Infections" (STIs) chapter initially situated younger women and women of color as "the other" in the chapter, something that happened in many instances throughout the first drafts of the book. In an early version of the new chapter on STIs, the terms *we* and *us* were used when talking about the risks of STIs among lesbian and older women. However, when explaining issues and risks related to younger women and women of color these groups were addressed as *you* or *they*, creating a selective use of *we* that needed to be corrected. Another example from the same chapter was related to the potential omission of important factors influencing access to health services and treatment options for groups such as women with limited English proficiency and immigrant women. In these cases, I expressed my concerns about potentially not fully including the "we" that immigrant women constitute.

Some terms, such as the descriptor *women of color*, brought up concerns. Even though we decided to use it in some cases, we recognized the ways that particular term can be problematic. In my role as tone and voice editor I struggled with issues such as appropriate inclusion, accurate representations, and the multiple meanings of the term. The use of *women of color* as a descriptive category to identify health issues of women from multiple backgrounds can be challenging because of the diversity of the many groups that are included under the category. This idea is particularly important as it relates to health issues and risk factors since many women who might not identify themselves as "women of color" are classified as such by outside observers and often included in reports that inform texts like *OBOS.* By our national origin, cultural and linguistic background, or race—and not always by the color of our skin—

Latinas, Asians, African Americans, Native Americans, Africans, and other women have been placed in a category of risk or in a statistic that may situate us in the *women of color* descriptor. There is a possibility of the term not reaching and/or missing women who might not see themselves described by the subjective interpretation of skin color or represented in the history of the term. In these cases, and when permitted, the clearest and most specific name of the group, often based on self-identification, national and cultural origins, and racial and ethnic affiliations, was preferred.

Listening to the tone of the text was about sensibility and respect for a woman's personal encounters with her own body and the medical traditions and health therapies that she decided to follow. The continuous expansion of *OBOS*'s voices requires a conscious effort to look between the lines and behind the words at the way in which the nuanced tone and voice of the printed text depicts the other, acknowledging in the process internalized assumptions and stereotypes. In some instances the tone of the draft chapter became judgmental of the therapies and health choices that women may have followed as informed consumers of health care. In these cases it was my role to ask how the critique of overmedication would make women who have used conventional medicine feel: "bad," "guilty," "concerned"? Would extending the voices, the flexibility, and the sensibilities of the tone in the text be watering down the radical criticism of the medicalization of women's bodies? I would argue that it can act to extend the frontiers of criticism and acknowledge the many individual women, advocates, and families who have learned to fight the medicalization of women's bodies from inside the medical establishment; have fought for access to needed health services; and have made health professionals and researchers rethink and improve existing medical protocols and interventions.

Conclusion: *OBOS* Embracing the Challenges of Diversity

Throughout eight editions, *OBOS* has embraced the challenge of diversity, the increasing complexity of medical knowledge and technological advances, and the reconstruction and deconstruction of social and medical bodies that have demanded the expansion of borders, categories, understandings, and sensibilities in the text. However, it has not been without pains that *OBOS* has become a more inclusive text. During the process of learning about the all-embracing "we" of *OBOS* over time—a "we" situated in the larger context of the history of the women's health movement (Rodriguez-Trias 1999; Ruzek and Becker 1999)—and by editing the text for tone and voice, it became clear to me that the all-embracing "we" has advanced tremendously over the years. The Collective has invited the collaborations, perspectives, and contributions of diverse women, thus making OBOS more relevant, responsive, and attentive to the health needs of a larger audience, and helping advance the women's health agenda in a more inclusive way.

Notes

Thanks to Heather Stephenson, managing editor of the 8th edition of *Our Bodies, Ourselves*, for suggesting this title.

1. The Collective's efforts to share information in *OBOS* with women in Latin America and other Latinas in the United States date back to 1976, when a literal translation of *OBOS* into Spanish was first produced (BWHBC 2000).

2. See reports by Lindsey and McPherson in this anthology for further discussion of this topic.

3. These guidelines were developed from input received from *OBOS*'s postreaders, Heather Stephenson, Judy Norsigian, Kiki Zeldes, and Sally Whelan; web-based research; and suggestions gathered at the revisers' meeting of February 12, 2004.

References

Boston Women's Health Book Collective (BWHBC). 2005. *Our Bodies, Ourselves: A New Edition for a New Era.* New York: Simon & Schuster.
———. 2000. "Introducción." *Nuestros Cuerpos, Nuestras Vidas: La Guía Definitiva para la Salud de la Mujer Latina.* New York: Siete Cuentos Editorial.
———. 1998. *Our Bodies, Ourselves for the New Century: A Book by and for Women.* New York: Simon & Schuster.
———. 1992. *The New Our Bodies, Ourselves: A Book by and for Women,* Updated and Expanded for the 1990s. New York: Simon & Schuster.
———. 1984. *Our Bodies, Ourselves: A Book by and for Women.* New York: Simon & Schuster.
———. 1973. *Our Bodies, Ourselves: A Book by and for Women.* New York: Simon & Schuster.
Houck, Judith A. 2003. "What Do These Women Want?:" Feminist Responses to Feminine Forever, 1963–1980." *Bulletin of the History of Medicine* 77(1): 103–32.
Iazetto, Demetria, Linda King, and Jennifer Yanco. 1998. "Chapter One: Body Image." In *Our Bodies, Ourselves for the New Century: A Book by and for Women,* 33–43. New York: Simon & Schuster.
Kahn, Robbie Pfeufer. 1995. "The Maternal Body Bound." In *Bearing Meaning: The Language of Birth,* 291–357. Chicago: University of Illinois Press.

Morgan, Sandra. 2002. *Into Our Own Hands: The Women's Health Movement in the United States, 1969–1990.* New Brunswick: Rutgers University Press.

Norsigian, Judy. 1998. Response pancl, "The History and Future of Women's Health," Seminar Highlights. Retrieved September 23, 2004, from: http://www.4woman.gov/owh/pub/history/responseB.htm.

Norsigian, Judy, Vilunya Diskin, Paula Doress-Worters, Wendy Sanford, and Norma Swenson. 1999. "The Boston Women's' Health Book Collective and Our Bodies, Ourselves: A Brief History and Reflection." *Journal of the American Medical Women's Association* 54(1): 35–9.

Pincus, Jane. 1998. "Introduction." In *Our Bodies, Ourselves for the New Century: A Book by and for Women,* 21–23. New York: Simon & Schuster.

Rodríguez-Trias, Helen. 1999. "If Women's Health Movements Is the Topic, Have We Arrived?" *Journal of the American Medical Women's Association* 54(1): 2–3.

Ruzek, Sheryl Burt, and Julie Becker. 1999. "The Women's Health Movement in the United States: From Grass-Roots Activism to Professional Agendas." *Journal of the American Medical Women's Association* 54(1): 4–8.

Sow, Fatou, and Codou Bop, eds. 2004. *Notre Corps, Notre Sante: La Sante et la Sexualite des Femmes en Afrique Subsaharienne.* Paris: L'Harmattan.

Whelan, Sally, and Wendy Sanford. 2003a. *OBOS Update Manual.* Boston Women's Health Book Collective, Boston, MA.

———. 2003b. *OBOS Update Manual: Appendices.* Boston Women's Health Book Collective, Boston, MA.

PART TWO   **Lesbians**

CHAPTER SIX

Reexamining Gender and Sexual Orientation:
Revisioning the Representation of Queer
and Trans People in the 2005 Edition of
Our Bodies, Ourselves

ELIZABETH SARAH LINDSEY

Big Platform Shoes to Fill

When Heather Stephenson asked me to revamp what had been a four-page introduction on gender and sexual orientation into a full-length chapter in the 2005 edition of *Our Bodies, Ourselves* (*OBOS*), I was flattered, elated, and absolutely terrified. *OBOS* is, as Heather lovingly refers to it, the bible on women's health of the late-twentieth century, and I am 24 years old, just two years out of college. I am also an anti-authoritarian African American high femme dyke from a working poor family. I do not fit what I and many others in my peer group see as the target audience for *OBOS*—white middle-class women who grew up reading this book and their teenage daughters. Yet when Heather asked me to write this chapter, I tearfully accepted because I realized that *OBOS* was committed to expanding the breadth and depth of its audience by becoming more inclusive of young women, women of color, and trans and queer people.

Challenging and Honoring the Past

Before I began to work on my chapter, I decided to research the representation of queer and trans people in earlier editions of *OBOS*. In one of the first editions of the book published more than 30 years ago, the chapter on lesbians was titled "In Amerika They Call Us Dykes" (BWHBC 1973). There were a few major themes that ran through this section. First, the writers of the chapter self-disclosed that they were all middle-class white women. They wrote the chapter as a collective, and some were out of the closet while others were deeply burrowed within. Another interesting theme, one that I don't hear echoed among the young political queers that I know, was that deciding to embrace one's lesbianism was a decidedly political and feminist choice. Many of the writers in the chapter suggested that becoming queer was the next logical step in their politici-

Originally published in the spring 2005 issue (vol. 17, no.1).

zation as feminists. Consequently, choosing to be a lesbian (or at least live and/or come out as one) was also equated with a conscious rejection of men and "male" values, such as oppression and patriarchal domination within interpersonal relationships. Also, anyone who was not gendered as a woman in this particular lesbian context—butches, transgendered people, and even femmes—was completely invisible from the discussion. In fact, gender expression and identity were hardly discussed in the chapter.

As I read through the chapter, my first impulse was to discount it as politically and socially backward, the words of lesbians whose lives could not possibly have any connection to my own struggles as a femme, a woman of color, a dyke who dates and loves butches and tranny boys and trans men, a woman who grew up working poor. However, as I began to write my chapter, my respect and appreciation for the authors of this chapter grew. These women lived in a world in which "coming out" was not something proudly flaunted on primetime television. To be themselves, they gave up their families, their careers, and their friends. They recognized that they came from privileged positions in society and did not hesitate to admit to their shortcomings. Moreover, women across the country tell me that this chapter saved their lives. While I do lead a different life in a different time, I realized that I share with these dyke pioneers the same desire to be heard.

New Voices and New Themes for a New Generation

Though my chapter is fairly short (about thirteen pages in the book), it includes introductions and definitions of topics such as gender identity, sexual orientation, bisexuality, coming out, queer and trans communities, and homophobia and transphobia. My hope, and the hope of the *OBOS* editors, is that people from a wide range of backgrounds and identities can pick up this chapter and walk away with a basic understanding of the difference between gender and sexual orientation, the idea that gender is not always determined by sex, and at least an overview of some of the issues faced by lgbtqi (lesbian, gay, bisexual, transgender, queer, and intersexed) individuals.

The first basic question that I asked myself as I sat down to write my chapter was "What does it mean to be a woman?" *OBOS* bills itself as "by women for women," but who does that really include? People born biologically female? People born biologically female who still identify as women? People who identify as women regardless of their sex at birth? It was never a question for me that in my chapter "woman" includes anyone and everyone who has at one time or does currently identify or live as a woman. We all need information on health, sex, feminism, and relationships, even if our lives and struggles look completely different. More important, in this first edition of *OBOS* to which a new generation might be exposed, it is essential to include and expand the section on trans people.

Word choice and language posed some of the most trying issues in writing this chapter. How to describe, in accessible language, such complicated and personal issues as one's gender identity or the choice to medically transition or how a searing homophobic or transphobic remark can damage our psyches? How to define words like *transgender* or *transsexual* or *queer*—loaded words that some of us claim, others of us do not, and some do not even recognize or understand. I am not trans-identified. As a femme, I pass for straight on a daily basis, and I do not experience queer and trans bashing when I walk down the street by myself. Writing from this relatively privileged position, I felt that it was of the utmost importance that my language was inclusive and respectful. The editors and I decided to use the broadest language we could find, emphasizing often that we all have the right to choose whether or not we want to use labels and which labels we want to use. However, as we struggled to use inclusive language, contradictions and subtleties arose that we could not always adequately address. For example, I discuss at length the idea that there are many genders and that our sex does not determine our gender. And then, a page or two later, I discuss bisexuality, a term that reasserts the two-gender paradigm. Another example—I use the word queer repeatedly in my chapter with nary a mention of the history and class and race background of the term. There was not time and space to describe the complexity of my choice and why I chose to use that word, despite its history. In the future I hope that space and time allow for a more nuanced examination of the complexities of gender and sexuality within this book.

Coming out was another topic that I grappled with while writing this chapter. In the mainstream media, both gay and straight, coming out is portrayed in an extremely idealized and simplistic way. The gay person, always white and middle class, decides that he or she is gay, tells families and friends, might experience a little homophobia but none too pernicious, and ends up marching proudly down the main thoroughfare of a progressive major metropolitan area during the exuberant gay pride parade with a rainbow flag in one hand and a life partner in the other. Though this representation may seem fairly innocuous and hopeful to some, it is far from reality for many. Queer and trans people of color oftentimes have to make the agonizing choice between coming out in a mainstream way and losing touch and support from our communities of color or facing racism within white gay spaces. For the working class and working poor, coming out in our communities and at our workplaces can mean losing the only means that we have to support our families. In my chapter, I emphasized that coming out looks very different in different spaces. For some, it might mean telling our closest friends, or having a queer life in one sphere and a straight life with relatives. It might mean dressing up in racy lingerie while at home and wearing loose jeans and a hoodie on the street. While the world might be easier for queers if we could all live like "Will & Grace," the diversity of our struggles and our communities means that we look and act queer and trans in countless ways.

An Outpouring of Support

The most exhilarating and touching part of the process of writing my chapter was the astounding e-mail response that I received in a call for submissions of anecdotes for my chapter. Each chapter in *OBOS* combines information about various topics with anonymous quotes from women sharing their experiences with the topic. I decided that I wanted new quotes from people reflecting the issues that we face today. For this reason, I composed a short e-mail asking for queer and trans people to tell me their stories about coming out as queer or trans, their experiences living as queer and trans people, as queer and trans people of color, of differing abilities, class backgrounds, and politics. I sent this e-mail to a network of about 30 or 40 of my queer and straight friends, who then passed it on to their networks. To this day, close to a year later, I am still receiving submissions. I have received more than 200 responses from the United States, the United Kingdom, Australia, the Netherlands, Canada, and Belgium. People were hungry to have a voice in this famous book. Many remained skeptical that *OBOS* would accurately and sensitively convey their issues, but they submitted their stories nonetheless.

As a queer person of color, reading the barrage of e-mails daily from queer and trans people around the world was an extremely emotional and personal experience. The stories of social isolation that many people shared were heartbreaking and sobering. I live in Philadelphia and came out at a progressive, elite liberal arts college, and I am lucky enough to have a family that supports me. Queer people not having anyone else to talk to, not having access to community centers or gayborhoods or even bars, trans people living deeply closeted for years and years in fear for their lives—this is our experience in America and beyond. I was struck by how easily I could forget that my situation is a rare and privileged one.

In addition to social isolation, there were a few other recurring themes in the responses to my call. Many trans people wrote about their negative experiences with the women's health movement and health care providers, a topic that *OBOS* is addressing for the first time in this new edition. Coming out as lesbian, gay, bisexual, or transgender was another prevalent theme. Stories ranged from the tranny boy who comes out to his accepting mother as they make spaghetti sauce together to the lesbian whose father suspects she's gay and reminds her that he "does not want a fucking faggot for a daughter."

One topic mentioned numerous times that I found unsurprising and, at the same time, enraging was the prevalence of transphobia in lesbian communities. More specifically, a number of trans women wrote to me about their attempts to take part in lesbian and women's communities only to experience blatant discrimination within these spaces. Their stories often followed the same trajectory: after struggling for years, these women decide to come out as trans and soon after begin to seek out community. Assuming that a gay community would accept them because of shared struggles, the women attempted over and over again to enter into women's coffeehouses, festivals, support groups, bars, and clubs only to be repeatedly rebuffed and humiliated. The frequency of these stories conveys, to me, the magnitude of the need for increased education on trans issues within many lesbian communities.

Looking toward the Future

In 2005 edition of *OBOS*, queer and trans issues are incorporated more fully throughout the text, from discussions on lesbian parenting in the parenting chapters to the inclusion of trans issues in sections about mammograms, and exams of the breasts and uterus. Of course, I would have loved to have seen more trans and queer people taking part in the creation of the book on every level. Throughout *OBOS*, each writer uses the *we* and *us* pronouns. This is a political choice from the early editions of the book. The editors encourage the chapter writers to use these inclusive pronouns to give readers a sense that the book really is by them and for them. However, I think that this practice needs to be more closely examined. As I wrote my chapter, I felt extremely uncomfortable writing as if I belonged to groups such as trans and genderqueer communities or people with disabilities, who face struggles that I have never lived and that I can never truly understand. It is problematic to have someone speak "for" another person, let alone "as" another person. Before the next edition of the book goes into production, I hope that the writers and editors reexamine this language policy and the politics of personal privilege and the power of voice that influence it.

I have learned and I have grown so much through writing this chapter. I have felt empowered by Heather Stephenson and my fellow coauthors at

OBOS to make change through my words. This book is imbued with encouraging voices reminding us all that we have a right to live our lives and in our bodies in the ways that are healthiest and most empowering to us, as queers, as trans people, as people of color, and as women.

Reference

Boston Women's Health Book Collective (BWHBC). 1973. *Our Bodies Ourselves: A Book by and for Women.* New York: Simon & Schuster.

CHAPTER SEVEN

Ignored, Overlooked, or Subsumed: Research on Lesbian Health and Health Care

SUE V. ROSSER

In health care research, diagnosis, and treatment lesbians have usually been ignored. The norm for research, diagnosis, and treatment of health and disease in the United States is the white heterosexual middle-class male. Health care for heterosexual women and homosexual men has been researched less since both deviate from the norm. Doubly distanced from the heterosexual male norm, lesbian health care and disease issues have failed to receive funding and study (Robertson).

When lesbians are recognized, they are often subsumed as a subset of women or homosexuals where heterosexual females (Bernhard and Dan; Stevens and Hall, "Stigma") or homosexual males (Trippet and Bain) become the respective norms against which lesbians are measured. The implicit assumption underlying the failure to recognize health care issues for lesbians is either that lesbians do not exist, that lesbians have precisely the same health care issues as heterosexual females, or, in rare cases, that lesbians share the same health care issues as male homosexuals (Trippet and Bain). This ignoring or subsumption of lesbian health care issues becomes exacerbated by homophobia on the part of health care professionals. Not only does homophobia discourage lesbians from seeking necessary health care, but it also prevents health care workers from tying appropriate diagnoses and treatments to risk behaviors.

The Status of Research on Women's Health

Women's health in the United States has been defined with the white middle-class heterosexual male as the norm for research, diagnosis, and treatment of diseases. This definition of the norm is revealed in the exclusion of women from drug testing, the definition of some diseases that affect both sexes as male diseases, the insufficient study of conditions specific to females, and the ignoring of women's experiences.

Since it is clear that many diseases have different frequencies (heart diseases, lupus), symptoms (gonorrhea), or complications (most sexually transmitted diseases) in the two sexes, scientists should routinely consider and test for the presence or absence of differences based on gender in any

Originally published in the summer 1993 issue (vol. 5, no. 2).

hypothesis being tested. For example, when exploring the metabolism of a particular drug, one should routinely run tests on both males and females. Four dramatic, widely publicized recent examples demonstrate that sex differences are *not* routinely considered as part of research questions asked. In a longitudinal study of the effects of cholesterol-lowering drugs, gender differences were not tested since the drugs were tested on 3,806 men and no women (Hamilton). The Multiple Risk Factor Intervention Trial (1990) examined mortality from coronary heart disease in 12,866 men only. The Health Professionals Follow-up Study (Grobbee et al.) looked at the association between coffee consumption and heart disease in 45,589 men. In a similar test of the effects of aspirin on cardiovascular disease, which is now used widely by the pharmaceutical industry to support "taking one aspirin each day to prevent heart attacks," 22,071 males and no females were included (Steering Committee).

Some diseases that affect both sexes are defined as male diseases. Heart disease is the best example of a disease that has been so designated because of the fact that heart disease occurs more frequently in men at younger ages than women. Therefore, most of the funding for heart disease has been appropriated for research on predisposing factors for the disease (such as cholesterol level, lack of exercise, stress, smoking, and weight) using white middle-aged middle-class males.

This "male disease" designation has resulted in very little research being directed toward high-risk groups of women. Heart disease is a leading cause of death in older women (Kirschstein), and women live an average of 8 years longer than men (Boston Women's Health Book Collective). It is also frequent in poor black women who have had several children (Manley et al.). Virtually no research has explored predisposing factors for these groups who fall outside the disease definition established from an androcentric perspective. Recent data indicate that the designation of AIDS as a disease of male homosexuals and drug users has led researchers and health care practitioners to fail to understand the etiology and diagnosis of AIDS in women (Norwood). Women constitute the group in which AIDS is currently increasing most rapidly and women appear to manifest AIDS with different symptoms from those of men. However, until January 1993 the Centers for Disease Control (CDC) Case Definition failed to include gynecological conditions and other symptoms related to AIDS in women.

Research on conditions specific to females receives low priority, funding, and prestige. Some examples are dysmenorrhea, incontinence in older women, and nutrition in postmenopausal women. The effects of exercise level and duration on the alleviation of menstrual discomfort and length and sustained exposure to visual display terminals (VDTs), which has resulted in the "cluster pregnancies" of women giving birth to deformed babies in certain industries, have also received low priority.

Suggestions of fruitful questions for research based on the personal experience of women have also been ignored. In the health care area, women have often reported (and accepted among themselves) experiences that could not be documented by scientific experiments or were not accepted as valid by the researchers of the day. For decades, dysmenorrhea was attributed by most health care researchers and practitioners to psychological or social factors despite the reports from an overwhelming number of women that these were monthly experiences in their lives. Only after prostaglandins were "discovered" was there widespread acceptance among the male medical establishment that this experience reported by women had a biological component (Kirschstein). Health care practitioners must treat the majority of the population, which is female, based on information gathered from clinical research in which drugs may not have been tested on females, in which the etiology of the disease in women has not been studied, and in which women's experience has been ignored.

Heterosexual Assumptions of Obstetrics and Gynecology

Ironically, obstetrics/gynecology, the medical specialty centered exclusively on women's health issues, also derives its norms from the heterosexual male. The major focus of obstetrics and gynecology is dealing with issues surrounding procreation and heterosexual activity. The centering of women's health in obstetrics/gynecology defines women's health care in terms of their relationships with men. Most women first consult an ob/gyn when they become or are thinking of becoming heterosexually active. The possibility of future problems with procreation, difficult periods, the absence of periods, or other problems surrounding menarche bring other women to consult a gynecologist before they become heterosexually active. For many women, the obstetrician/gynecologist becomes the primary care physician and reproduction becomes a major focus for health care.

Significant amounts of time and money are expended on clinical research on women's bodies in connection with aspects of reproduction. Up until the 1970s considerable attention was devoted to the development of contraceptive devices for females rather than for males (Cowan; Dreifus). Furthermore, substantial clinical research has resulted in increasing medicalization and control of pregnancy, labor, and childbirth. Feminists have critiqued the conversion of a normal, natural process controlled by women into a clinical, and often surgical, procedure controlled by men (Ehrenreich and English; Holmes et al.). More recently, the new reproductive technologies such as amniocentesis, in vitro fertilization, and artificial insemination have become a major focus as means are sought to overcome infertility. Feminists have warned of the extent to which these technologies place pressure on women to produce the "perfect" child while placing control in the hands of the male medical establishment (Arditti et al.; Corea and Ince; Corea et al.; Hubbard).

These examples suggest that considerable resources and attention are devoted to women's health issues when those issues are directly related to men's interest in controlling the production of children. Contraceptive research may permit men to have sexual pleasure without the production of children; research on infertility, pregnancy, and childbirth has allowed men to assert more control over the production of more "perfect" children and over an aspect of women's lives over which they previously held less power.

Defining women's health in terms of men's interests and norms has done more than promote the overmedicalization of normal processes such as pregnancy and childbirth. It has led to insufficient and underfunding of most aspects of women's health not directly related to procreation and heterosexual activity. For example, one of the factors contributing to the rising incidence of breast cancer is the fact that breast cancer is a women's health issue but does not fit the traditional "territory" of obstetrics/gynecology. Obstetrics/gynecology has usually focused on the part of women's reproductive system located below the waist. Although the breasts are related through lactation to procreation and often also involved in heterosexual activity, they are not part of the territory below the waist—the ovaries, oviduct, uterus, vagina, or urethra and their associated glands—traditionally seen as the focus of obstetrics/gynecology.

Similarly, other aspects of women's health only tangentially related to procreation and heterosexual activity have received little attention. For example, incontinence and nutrition in older women have received little funding or study. Dysmenorrhea and the effects of exercise on alleviating cramps are also insufficiently studied. Although menopause has received little attention and few research dollars, most menopausal research has centered on hormone replacement therapy (HRT). Now much research on HRT is carried out in conjunction with osteoporosis prevention and because of its positive effects for atherosclerosis prevention, but the initial interest in the use of HRT sprang partially from the desire to alleviate difficulties with vaginal dryness and painful heterosexual intercourse.

Given the difficulty of drawing attention to women's health issues not directly related to procreation and sexual activity for heterosexual women, it is not surprising that virtually no research has explored lesbian health issues. Thought of as homosexuals and thus defined in opposition to their heterosexual counterparts, lesbians naturally become excluded from obstetrics/gynecology, the medical specialty devoted to women's health.

Effects of the Failure to Study Lesbian Health Issues on Both Lesbians and Nonlesbians

Very little health care research has included separate studies of health care issues for lesbians. The Santa Cruz Women's Health Collective, the Radicalesbians Health Collective (O'Donnell et al.), some women's health groups, such as the National Women's Health Network, and some studies (Eliason, Donelan, and Randall; Robertson) have suggested differences in health and disease processes in lesbians and nonlesbians. For example, it is clear that lesbians have a much lower incidence of certain diseases such as cervical cancer. Heterosexual intercourse permits the transmission of herpes, trichomoniasis, chlamydia, and the human papilloma virus (HPV) thought to be major causes of cervical cancer. Beginning intercourse at an early age also increases the chances of cervical cancer (Boston Women's Health Book Collective). Cervical cancer is nonexistent in celibate women and rare in lesbians who have engaged in limited heterosexual intercourse or are not at risk from other factors such as diethylstilbesterol (DES) exposure and smoking.

In contrast, lesbians may be at higher risk for certain other diseases such as breast cancer and uterine cancer. Dr. Suzanne Haynes of the National Cancer Institutes estimates that one in three lesbians may develop breast cancer during their lifetimes because they are more likely than other women to fall into high-risk categories for the disease (Campbell). Women who have never had children are at an almost 80 percent greater risk for breast cancer than women who have had children; it may be inferred that lesbians are at increased risk for the disease because lesbians are less likely to have children than their heterosexual sisters. Women with a higher body fat content have about a 55 percent greater risk of developing breast cancer; since overweight conditions are more acceptable in the lesbian community, this may present an additional risk factor for breast cancer among lesbians. Because of the need for Pap smears in order to receive birth control pills and a higher incidence of veneral diseases, heterosexually active women seek gynecological exams approximately every eight months. In contrast, lesbian women seek gynecological exams about every twenty-one months. Since gynecological examinations include mammograms and breast examinations by physicians, lesbians are subject to these mechanisms for early detection of breast cancer at less frequent intervals than heterosexually active women (Campbell). These health factors, plus evidence that alcohol intake and smoking, factors that increase the risk of breast cancer and have been shown by some studies (Hall, "An Exploration"; Buenting) to be higher in lesbians than nonlesbians, led Haynes to theorize the one-in-three rate for breast cancer in lesbians (Campbell).

Despite these increased risks, no federal research dollars have targeted lesbian health issues as their focus of study. Even the newly founded Office of Research on Women's Health at the National Institutes of Health has not earmarked any of its $500 million Women's Health Initiative to exploring lesbian health research (Medical News and Perspectives).

Failure to identify and fund separate studies of lesbian health issues usually results in lesbians being lumped with heterosexual women in studies of women's health issues. Combining lesbians and heterosexual women may obscure not only the true incidence but also the cause of a disease. In addition to the higher rates of cervical cancer among heterosexual women, the likelihood of most sexually transmitted diseases, including gonorrhea, syphilis, herpes, and chlamydia, being transmitted from males to females during heterosexual activity is dramatically greater than the likelihood of transmission through lesbian contact. Although transmission of such sexually transmitted diseases between lesbians does occur, the incidence is minuscule compared to transmission between male homosexuals, males and females, and females and males during heterosexual activities.

When lesbians are lumped with heterosexual women in studies of the incidence and/or the causes of sexually transmitted diseases or other gynecological problems from which lesbians are exempt or at low risk because they do not engage in heterosexual intercourse, both lesbians and nonlesbians suffer. Defining such studies generally as research on "women's health issues" rather than "health issues for women engaging in heterosexual sex" leads the general population and some health care workers to think that lesbians are at risk for diseases that they are unlikely to contract, while obscuring the true risk behavior for heterosexual women.

The Status of Research on Homosexual Health

When women are defined as homosexual, the norm for lesbian health care issues continues to be the male. Lesbians are assumed to be a subset of or very similar to male homosexuals (Anderson; Corbett et al.; Hudson and Ricketts). Since male homosexuals are typically distinguished by their deviation from the male heterosexual norm, lesbians again find themselves doubly distanced from the norm. Lesbians are neither heterosexual nor male. Recognition of lesbians, while defining them as homosexuals, nonetheless typically results in lesbian health issues continuing to be overlooked or ignored. For example, most current funding for homosexual health care issues is directed toward the study of AIDS. Although most lesbians politically support the issue of funding AIDS research for society in general, for their male homosexual brothers in whom the epidemic is rampant (Shilts), and for their heterosexual sisters, who represent the group where AIDS is currently increasing most rapidly in the United States (Anastos and Marte), they receive few direct benefits of this research. Lesbians represent the group engaging in behaviors that put them at lowest risk for contracting AIDS.

A related confusion arises when lesbians are not listed as a separate statistical category for frequency of diseases. The Centers for Disease Control does not list lesbians as a separate category in its groups for AIDS infection; homosexual men, bisexual men, and adult men are listed separately (Curran et al.). Men are listed not only by sexual orientation but are further subdivided by intravenous drug use and race.

The statistics on all women collected by the CDC for HIV infection are not as complete as those collected for men. For example, no distinct category for women at double risk from infection as IV drug users and partners of infected men exists as it does for men. This may be responsible for the results suggesting that a significantly higher percentage of women (9 percent) than men do not understand the source of their AIDS infection (Anastos and Marte). This sloppy statistical reporting may lead to false complacency for women who engage in heterosexual relations with men in which women may not be aware of their partner's risk-taking behavior.

The failure to separate out lesbians as a distinct group for statistics on AIDS leads the public to false understandings of the risk behaviors causing AIDS. It may partially explain the misunderstanding by the public and even by 20 percent of nurse educators (Randall) that lesbians transmit AIDS. Lumping lesbians, celibate women, and heterosexually active women together obscures the increased risk of AIDS to women engaged in heterosexual activity, since lesbians and celibate women have virtually no risk for AIDS from sexual activity. In a few cases female-to-female transmission has been suggested through an IV-drug HIV-infected woman transmitting the virus through traumatic sex practices where the skin is broken (Monzon and Capellen). Lesbians may also be vulnerable to HIV infection via artificial insemination from an infected donor as well as from blood transfusions.

This inappropriate lumping may be partially responsible for the fact that women engaged in heterosexual sex represent the group in which AIDS is increasing most rapidly now. It also reinforces the initial mistake made in AIDS research in this country when AIDS was identified by group rather than risk behaviors. The initial designation of AIDS as a gay male disease, followed by the inclusion of IV drug users and Haitian immigrants, led to a plethora of problems resulting in lack of funding and study of AIDS and its transmission (Shilts) and diagnosis in many populations. This led the general public to believe that being a homosexual, rather than engaging in risk behaviors, causes AIDS.

Other health issues significant for the homosexual population may result in lesbians receiving diagnosis and treatment that is less appropriate for them because the male has been chosen as the norm. Alcoholism, a problem for lesbians as well as male homosexuals, is thought to be underdiagnosed and undertreated in the lesbian community. Some studies (Fifield et al.; McKirnan and Peterson, "Alcohol and Drug Use"; Saghir and Robins) suggest that the drinking patterns of lesbians are more consistent with national norms for male drinkers than female drinkers (Fifield et al., McKirnan and Peterson, "Alcohol and Drug Use," Psychosocial and Social Factors"; McNally; Hall, "An Exploration"). Much of the study of alcoholism in homosexual populations has used the gay bar as a source for estimating and diagnosing the incidence of alcoholism (Hall, *Lesbians and Alcohol*). Limited research (Luly; Weathers) suggests that many lesbians, particularly in some geographic areas, such as the South, and from the upper and middle socioeconomic classes, may not frequent lesbian bars. This does not mean that they are not drinking elsewhere and may not be suffering from alcoholism. Similarly the twelve-step treatment, the model considered to be most successful for treating alcoholics, was developed by two men using themselves (white middle- to upper-class heterosexuals) as the norm. Feminists have critiqued the confrontation aspects of the model as less appropriate for many women who seek to avoid conflict (Tallen; Muller; Hall, "An Exploration"). The self-revelation aspects of the model and involvement of the spouse in Al-Anon or codependent groups are less appropriate for lesbians who are likely neither to have a spouse nor to reveal much about their personal life in a lesbophobic society (Deevey and Wall). In some cases, Alcoholics Anonymous (AA) is not sensitive to painful prior events such as rape, incest, battering, or other traumas for which alcohol or drug use becomes a symptom (Hall, "An Exploration").

The use of the white heterosexual male as the norm for health care issues has resulted in a lack of information about health and disease processes of lesbians. The main people damaged by this lack of information are lesbians. Being ignored has led to ignorance of themselves with regard to some crucial health care issues. Ironically, lesbians being ignored or subsumed under "women's" or "homosexuals'" health issues also hurts nonlesbians, especially heterosexual women who then fail to understand the significance of risk behaviors or lifestyle choices for health and disease processes.

Health Care Issues Defined by Lesbians

Inappropriate inclusion of lesbians in studies and statistics of women's health problems such as cervical cancer and homosexual health problems such as AIDS has consequences beyond obscuring the true risk behavior causing these diseases. Failure to separate lesbian health issues means that health issues as defined from lesbian experience have not been explored. The absence of this focus implies that research on health issues important to lesbian women, and that may be increasingly important for elderly, widowed, or celibate heterosexual women for whom it is no longer appropriate to define health around procreation and heterosexual activity, has not been undertaken.

For example, studies of ways to diagnose endometriosis in women not engaging in heterosexual intercourse or trying to become pregnant may reveal information previously unexplored about the symptoms of endometriosis. An examination of the effects of bodybuilding, karate, and self-defense in helping women to ward off attacks and battering may be as important for women's health as contraception. As more funds are allocated to the up until now insufficiently studied aspects of menopause, attention to the models of communities of women living together as they age may be more important than studies of the empty-nest syndrome in a society where many women have few children and the aging population is primarily female.

Lesbians as a Model

Overlooking lesbians in research design ignores the possibility that the lesbian may be the best model for exploring some aspects of women's health. In their attempts to find self-definition and reject many of the definitions and needs projected onto them by the surrounding culture, lesbians have become aware that most institutions use the white middle-class heterosexual male as the norm. Lesbians have struggled to define themselves in a patriarchal culture by asking what their experience has been and what their needs are. This struggle provides them with a beginning for a female-centered model of health care. Lesbians and the lesbian community seek alternatives to male-focused systems. A model for health care research in which the health and disease processes of women's bodies are examined without a focus on contraception, sexually transmitted diseases, pregnancy, childbirth, and accommodation of sexual functions to fit men's needs opens the door for a model for women's health and disease free from the gynecological complications normally imposed by heterosexual activity. This model would provide baseline data for normal health events such as menarche, menopause, and aging, as well as disease processes, in the absence of reproductive complications. Applicable particularly to lesbians, it would also apply well to the large numbers of celibate and heterosexual women without children.

Ignoring lesbians in general in research designs and discussions of health issues overlooks and obscures particular diversities among lesbians. With the exception of their sexual orientation, lesbians demonstrate as much variety with regard to race, class, occupation, and age as their heterosexual sisters. Indeed, many lesbians also share a history of heterosexual experiences. Many married, either before they recognized their sexual orientation or as an attempt to conform to the pressures for compulsory heterosexuality in this society. Many lesbians are biological parents, their children having been conceived while in a heterosexual relationship or through artificial insemination. Studies using lesbians must pay attention to these diverse factors and their implications for health in order to avoid the similar confounding among variables that occurs when lesbians are lumped with heterosexual women or male homosexuals.

Diversity among Lesbians

Attention to lesbians as a group and the diversity among lesbians (West; Gomez and Smith) should lead to cleaner research designs with less conflation of variables. For example, a study of lesbians who have never had heterosexual sex compared with those who have for varying lengths of time might definitively establish the duration of heterosexual activity correlated with cervical cancer.

Rethinking the differences among lesbians also reveals situations when sexual orientation should not be used to distinguish among women. For example, to study the role of childbearing in preventing breast cancer, childless lesbians should be grouped with childless heterosexual, bisexual, or celibate women for comparison with women from those groups who have borne children. Similarly, studies of cervical cancer should combine heterosexual and lesbian women who have never had intercourse for comparison with women who have had intercourse regardless of their present sexual orientation. This attention to diversity shifts the focus from inappropriate groups to risk behaviors.

A different aspect of diversity recognition includes understanding that some lesbians may have more difficulty than others in dealing with their sexual orientation in a homophobic society. This may have direct effects on health care research, particularly research based on clinical or case data (Swanson et al.). Extant literature on lesbian health, particularly mental health, is likely to include an overrepresentation of lesbians who have problems (Morin; Stevens). Their representation in the literature as lesbians in many cases reflects some disclosure (through self or referral) that lesbianism is perceived as part of or related to their health problem.

Overexamination and research centered on the lesbian population seeking or referred for counseling and therapy have possibly led to misperceptions about the prevalence and severity of problems that sexual orientation causes for lesbians (Freedman; Smith et al., "Healthcare Attitudes"; Stevens and Hall, "Stigma"). Since lesbians having fewer problems tend not to seek help, they are underrepresented in the literature or unknowingly lumped with heterosexual women. Presumably the pattern of overrepresentation of lesbians with problems and underrepresentation of lesbians without problems documented in psychology has been repeated for other aspects of health. This pattern provides health care practitioners and the general population with a false picture of the prevalence of diseases and difficulties in the lesbian population.

Stress in Lesbians

The overrepresentation/underrepresentation dilemma may also obscure the role that social and psychological factors play in physical disease processes. The role that stress plays in a number of diseases, such as cardiovascular disease, ulcers, skin allergies, lupus, and even cancer, has been well documented (Selye; Haynes and Feinleib). Although most lesbians view their sexual orientation as a positive force in their lives, many would admit that being a lesbian in a homophobic society is quite stressful (Underhill and Ostermann), particularly for lesbians of color who fight racism and sexism (Lorde; Smith). The role that this stressor, in comparison to other stressors, plays in diseases more prevalent in the lesbian population needs to be studied. In order to evaluate this role, a lesbian population needs to be clearly identified and interdisciplinary methods from the social sciences and natural sciences need to be utilized to elucidate the relationship between stress and disease in lesbian lives.

Jean Hamilton has called for interactive models that draw on both the social and natural sciences to explain complex problems:

> Particularly for understanding human, gender-related health, we need more interactive and contextual models that address the actual complexity of the phenomenon that is the subject of explanation. One example is the need for more phenomenological definitions of symptoms, along with increased recognition that psychology, behavioral studies, and sociology are among the "basic sciences" for health research. Research on heart disease is one example of a field where it is recognized that both psychological stress and behaviors such as eating and cigarette smoking influence the onset and natural course of a disease process. (IV-62)

Such interdisciplinary methods might be useful for studying the role of stress in various diseases in the lesbian population.

Interactions between Lesbians and Health Care Professionals

Ignoring lesbian health issues in research has led to inappropriate diagnoses and treatments for lesbians. For many health care practitioners, the absence of lesbians as a group from studies and discussions of lesbian health care literature has been translated into the assumption that no lesbians seek health care service or that heterosexual activity should be assumed for all patients. In fact a significant issue that hinders many lesbians from seeking health care is homophobia or insensitivity on the part of health care practitioners.

Historically within the twentieth century, lesbians have been characterized by the medical profession as sick, dangerous, aggressive, tragically unhappy, deceitful, contagious, and self-destructive (Bergler; Caprio; Romm; Socarides; Wilbur; Wolff). Defined as a disease at the turn of the century, lesbianism was characterized by health care professionals until the early 1980s through an emphasis on etiology, diagnosis, and cure (Morin; Schwanberg, "Changes in Labeling," "Attitudes towards Homosexuality"; Watters).

Not surprisingly, many health care professionals hold extremely homophobic attitudes, which they reflect in their interactions, diagnoses, and treatments of lesbian patients. In a recent review of research related to lesbians' experiences with health care during the past twenty years, Patricia Stevens discovered nine studies about health care providers' attitudes toward lesbian clients. All nine studies (Douglas et al.; Eliason and Randall; Garfinkle and Morin; Levy; Liljestrand et al.; Mathews et al.; Randall; White; Young) uncovered significant homophobic attitudes on the part of health care professionals. Particularly revealing are relatively recent studies. A 1986 convenience sample of 1,000 MDs in San Diego found that 23 percent were severely homophobic (Mathews et al.); surgeons, gynecologists, and family practice MDs were most homophobic. This same study demonstrates the direct effects of these attitudes on their treatment of gay and lesbian clients: 40 percent were uncomfortable with treating gays and lesbians; 30 percent opposed admitting gays and lesbians to medical schools; 40 percent would not refer clients to gay or lesbian colleagues. A 1988 study of nurses uncovered that 64 percent of RNs hold negative attitudes such as pity, disgust, unease, embarrassment, fear, and sorrow toward gays and lesbians (Young); 50 percent of RNs with these feelings stated that they had no desire to change (Young). Studies of nursing educators (Randall) and nursing students (Eliason and Randall) reveal similar homophobic attitudes, which are correlated with medical misinformation such as the belief of 20 percent of nursing educators (Randall) and 28 percent of students (Eliason and Randall) that lesbians transmit AIDS.

Lesbians directly experience the homophobic attitudes of health care professionals. These experiences range from an assumption of heterosexuality on the part of the health care provider (Dardick and Grady; Johnson and Palermo; Reagan; Stevens and Hall, "Stigma") through a negative reaction (72 percent of respondents) when patients disclosed their sexual preference (Stevens and Hall, "Stigma") to attempts to cure their lesbian-ism (Glascock, *Access, Lesbians*).

Most lesbians believe their health care would be of higher quality if they could safely disclose their lesbian identity (Cochran and Mays; Hume; Smith et al.; Stevens and Hall "Abusive Health Care," "Stigma"). However, the majority of lesbians (Cochran and Mays; Glascock, *Access, Lesbians*; Hume; Olesker and Walsh) did not disclose because of fears and experiences of mistreatment, intimidation, humiliations, and lack of safety in health care interactions (Stevens).

The inability to disclose their sexual identity coupled with the nega-tive reactions they must undergo when they do, leads many lesbians to delay seeking health care (Bradford and Ryan; Deevey; Stevens and Hall, "Stigma"; Zeidenstein). Distrusting mainstream health care (Deevey), many lesbians are likely to seek help for a health problem from lesbian friends rather than health care professionals (Saunders et al.) or seek re-ferral from a friend to a supportive health care professional. In addition to the failure of mainstream health care to meet the needs of lesbian women, a 1992 study revealed other reasons lesbians do not seek health care from traditional sources: "(a) low-cost, natural, or alternative care is not provided; (b) holistic care is not provided; (c) little preventive care and education are provided; (d) communication and respect are lacking; and (e) few women-managed clinics are available" (Trippet and Bain, 148).

Assuming a heterosexual orientation, many obstetricians/gynecolo-gists routinely begin examinations of women aged 16–55 by asking ques-tions about the kind of contraception the woman uses (Glascock; Stevens and Hall) and whether it is working successfully. They require all of their patients to have yearly Pap smears, without first ascertaining whether or not the woman is at risk for cervical cancer. A yearly Pap smear may waste time and money for a woman who has never engaged in heterosex-ual intercourse or other behaviors that put her at risk for cervical cancer.

Because of the assumption of most health care practitioners of the het-erosexual norm, many lesbians and celibate women refuse routine exami-nations or delay seeking treatment for serious symptoms (Bradford and Ryan; Deevey; Stevens and Hall, "Stigma"; Zeidenstein) because they find the questions about contraception and heterosexual activity to be distaste-ful. Diseases such as endometriosis are unlikely to be diagnosed in lesbi-ans if the practitioner uses pain during intercourse as the major criterion for diagnosis. Some lesbians fear that revealing their sexual orientation to a health care practitioner may lead to loss of jobs or children if this infor-mation is recorded in medical records that may become available to em-ployers or social service workers (Glascock, *Access, Lesbians*; Hume; Ste-vens and Hall, "Abusive Health Care," "Stigma").

Less Homophobic Approaches for Practitioners

Health care practitioners may avoid some of this discomfort and fear (as well as educating all of their patients to varieties of sexual orientation) by presenting different health risks for different groups. A practitioner might begin an initial, general examination by indicating that, depending on the patient's sexual activities, she may be at risk for different health problems. For example, if she is currently engaging in heterosexual intercourse and does not wish to become pregnant, she should use some contraceptive device. Prevention of sexually transmitted diseases, including AIDS is likely to be an issue for her, depending on the nature of her relationship with her partner(s). She should definitely have a yearly Pap smear. If she has never engaged in heterosexual intercourse and is not planning to do so in the near future, contraception and yearly Pap smears are not necessary for her unless she has other risk factors such as being a diethylstilbestrol (DES) daughter. It is also less likely that she will need protection against sexually transmitted diseases (STDs). If she has engaged in heterosexual intercourse in the past, but is not now doing so and does not plan to in the near future, then contraception and STD prevention may not be an issue for her, but she should have a Pap smear now and at three-year intervals.

Similar approaches might be taken for discovering whether or not the woman has had children and the risks this poses for breast cancer, uterine cancer, and endometriosis. This approach does not assume a heterosexual or a lesbian norm. It educates the patient about risk behaviors that may lead to increased incidence of certain diseases, thus providing her with more accurate information. It also educates the public about diversity with regard to sexual orientation in the population. In order for a practitioner to use this approach, she or he must be educated to recognize that lesbians do exist and to be knowledgeable about their health issues.

Public health campaigns to educate women about health promotion and disease prevention need to be oriented toward risk behaviors with the recognition that women have diverse sexual orientations. Public service announcements that encourage every woman to have a Pap smear every year do not focus on risk behaviors. They assume that all women engage in heterosexual activity and inadequately convey to the public the risk behavior responsible for cervical cancer. These announcements repeat for public information the initial mistakes in research design that define women in relationship to sexual activity with men.

Even when health care practitioners are aware that lesbians exist, they may not recognize diversity among lesbians. Assuming the accuracy of stereotypes, partially derived from medical literature (Morin), according to which lesbians dress in more masculine clothing, occupy certain occupations, or exhibit "butch" mannerisms may lead health care practitioners to think that they can spot a lesbian and modify their questions and examination for the health care issues for which she is at risk. Since lesbians exhibit considerable variation with regard to race, occupation, mode of dress, appearance, and history of previous sexual activity and pregnancy, ignoring the diversity among lesbians also leads to inappropriate treatment and diagnosis. Asking questions to reveal risk factors rather than assuming a norm for heterosexuality or lesbianism is the only way to ensure accurate diagnosis and appropriate treatment.

When a woman does reveal her sexual orientation to the health care practitioner, she must be cautious not to assume that this automatically means that the woman engages in a particular risk behavior. Risk behaviors, such as anal intercourse, not homosexuality itself, put male homosexuals at risk for HIV. Similarly, not engaging in heterosexual or anal intercourse, not simply current sexual orientation, puts lesbians at less risk for cervical cancer than women who engage in those activities.

A major reason that AIDS has reached epidemic proportions in the United States was the initial mistake made in identifying groups at risk for the disease rather than specific risk behaviors. The campaign against AIDS has been even less successful in the Hispanic community. Although multiple reasons exist for the failure, a substantial reason is that the prevention campaign described sexual practices used by male homosexuals or bisexuals as risky. Many Hispanic men who engage in anal sex with other men do not identify that behavior as a "sexual practice used by male homosexuals or bisexuals." Since these men also engage in heterosexual intercourse with their wives and/or girlfriends, they do not identify themselves as male homosexuals or bisexuals. As health care practitioners recognize lesbianism and help to define and educate themselves and the public about lesbian health care issues, they must be aware of problems of labeling by group rather than describing behaviors.

Conclusion

Describing specific risk behaviors rather than ascribing them to lesbians because of their sexual orientation will open the way for a better understanding of lesbian health care issues without reinforcing the status quo of ignorance and oppression from homophobia. The current condition of ignoring lesbians and their health care needs must not continue. It is tragic for lesbians who remain ignorant about their own health care issues; health care practitioners and the nonlesbian population also suffer. When lesbians are ignored in research design it may lead to their inappropriate inclusion or exclusion from studies of health issues; this obscures the true incidence and cause of some diseases for both lesbian and nonlesbian women. Inappropriate inclusion or exclusion from populations sampled may be translated into inaccurate diagnosis and treatment. Precious resources may be unnecessarily wasted in overprescribing tests such as Pap smears and tests for STDs.

As women's health initiatives are being brought to the fore and as more money is targeted for study of women's health issues, lesbians must be recognized as a group of women who have significant and insufficiently studied health needs. Lesbians have fought for funding and study of women's health in general. Homosexuals have demonstrated limited success in receiving funding for the study of diseases such as AIDS that have a significant impact on the health of male homosexuals. Many lesbians have joined their homosexual brothers in fighting homophobia about AIDS, caring for AIDS patients, and bringing political pressure for AIDS research dollars. Male homosexuals must also join lesbians in recognizing that health issues for lesbians represent another facet of homosexual health that deserves attention.

Previously defined by the male, heterosexual norm, both women and male homosexuals have struggled for their own health agendas and should be understanding of the need for lesbians to define their own health needs. Lesbian health needs cannot be defined exclusively by either women's health needs or homosexual health needs. Overlapping both groups in many respects, but separate from each in some respects, lesbians are women with a homosexual orientation. Lesbian health issues deserve study and definition based on lesbian experience.

References

Anastos, Kathyrn, and Carola Marte. "Women—Missing Persons in the AIDS Epidemic." *Health PAC Bulletin 19* (1989): 6–13.

Anderson, Carla L. "The Effect of a Workshop on Attitudes of Female Nursing Students Toward Male Homosexuality." *Journal of Homosexuality 7* (1981): 57–69.

Arditti, Rita, Renate D. Klein, and Shelley Minden. *Test Tube Women: What Future for Motherhood?* London: Pandora Press, 1984.

Bergler, E. *Homosexuality: Disease or a Way of Life?* New York: Hill and Wang, 1957.

Bernhard, Linda, and Alice Dan. "Redefining Sexuality from Women's Own Experiences." *Nursing Clinics of North America 21* (1986): 123–36.

Boston Women's Health Book Collective. *The New Our Bodies, Ourselves: Updated and Expanded for the 90's.* New York: Simon & Schuster, 1992.

Bradford, J., and C. Ryan. *The National Lesbian Health Care Survey.* Washington, DC: National Lesbian and Gay Health Foundation, 1988.

Buenting, Julie A. "Health Life-Styles of Lesbian and Heterosexual Women." *Health Care for Women International 13* (1992): 165–73.

Campbell, Kristina. "1 in 3 Lesbians May Get Breast Cancer, Expert Theorizes." *Washington Blade* 2 October, 1992: 1, 23.

Caprio, F.S. *Female Homosexuality: A Psychodynamic Study of Lesbians*. New York: Citadel, 1954.

Cochran, S.D., and V.M. Mays. "Disclosure of Sexual Preference to Physicians by Black Lesbian and Bisexual Women." *Western Journal of Medicine 149* (1988): 616–19.

Corbett, Sherry L., Richard R. Troiden, and Richard A. Dodder. "Tolerance as a Correlate of Experience with Stigma: The Case of the Homosexual." *Journal of Homosexuality 3* (1977): 3–13.

Corea, Gena, Jalna Hanmer, Betty Hoskins, Janice Raymond, Renate Duelli Klein, Helen B. Holmes, Madhu Keshwar, Robyn Rowland, and Roberta Steinbacker, eds. *Man-made Women: How New Reproductive Technologies Affect Women*. Bloomington: Indiana University Press, 1987.

Corea, Gena, and Susan Ince. "Report of a Survey of IVF Clinics in the USA." In *Made to Order: The Myth of Reproductive and Genetic Progess*, ed. Patricia Spallone and Deborah L. Steinberg. Oxford: Pergamon Press, 1987. 133–45.

Cowan, Belinda. "Ethical Problems in Government-Funded Contraceptive Research." In *Birth Control and Controlling Birth: Women-Centered Perspectives*, ed. Helen Holmes, Betty Hoskins, and Michael Gross. Clifton, NJ: Humana Press, 1980. 37–46.

Curran, James W., Harold W. Jaffe, Ann M. Hardy, W. Meade Morgan, Richard M. Selik, and Timothy Dondero. "Epidemiology of HIV Infection and AIDS in the United States." *Science 239* (1988): 610–16.

Dardick, L., and K.E. Grady. "Openness between Gay Persons and Health Professionals." *Annals of Internal Medicine 93* (1980): 115–19.

Deevey, Sharon. "Older Lesbian Women: An Invisible Minority." *Journal of Gerontological Nursing 16*(5) (1990): 35–39.

Deevey, Sharon, and Lana Wall. "How Do Lesbian Women Develop Serenity?" *Health Care for Women International 13*(2) (1992): 199–208.

Douglas, C.J., C.M. Kalman and T.P. Kalman. "Homophobia among Physicians and Nurses: An Empirical Study." *Hospital and Community Psychiatry 36* (1985): 1309–11.

Dreifus, Claudia. *Seizing Our Bodies*. New York: Vintage Books, 1978.

Ehrenreich, Barbara, and Deirdre English. *For Her Own Good*. New York: Anchor Press, 1978.

Eliason, Michelle, Carol Donelan, and Carla Randall. "Lesbian Stereotypes." *Health Care for Women International 13*(2) (1992): 131–44.

Eliason, Michelle J., and Carla E. Randall. "Lesbian Phobia in Nursing Students." *Western Journal of Nursing Research 13* (1991): 363–74.

Fifield, L.H., D.J. Latham, and C. Phillips. *Alcoholism in the Gay Community: The Price of Alienation, Isolation and Oppression*. Los Angeles: A Product of the Gay Community Services Center, 1977.

Freedman, M. "Homosexuals May Be Healthier Than Straights." *Psychology Today* March 1975.

Garfinkle, E.M., and S.F. Morin. "Psychologists' Attitudes toward Homosexual Psychotherapy Clients." *Journal of Social Issues 34* (1978): 101–12.

Glascock, E.L. "Access to the Traditional Health Care System by Nontraditional Women: Perceptions of a Cultural Interaction." Paper presented at the annual meeting of the American Public Health Association, Los Angeles, November 1981.

———. "Lesbians Growing Older: Self-Identification, Coming Out, and Health Concerns." Paper presented at the annual meeting of the American Public Health Association, Dallas, November 1983.

Gomez, Jewelle, and Barbara Smith. "Taking the Home Out of Homophobia: Black Lesbian Health." In *The Black Women's Health Book: Speaking for Ourselves*, ed. Evelyn C. Hite. Seattle, WA: Seal Press, 1990. 198–213.

Grobbee, D.E., E.B. Rimm, E. Giovannucci, G. Coldits, M. Stamfer, and H.W. Wille. "Coffee, Caffeine, and Cardiovascular Disease in Men." *New England Journal of Medicine 321* (1990): 1026–32.

Hall, Joanne M. "An Exploration of Lesbians' Images of Recovery from Alcohol Problems." *Health Care for Women International 13*(2) (1992): 181–98.

———. "Lesbians add Alcohol: Patterns and Paradoxes in Medical Notions and Lesbian Beliefs." *Journal of Psychoactive Drugs. 25*(2) (1993): 109–19.

Hamilton, Jean. "Avoiding Methodological Biases in Gender-Related Research." In *Women's Health Report of the Public Health Service Task Force on Woman's Health Issues*. Washington, DC: U.S. Department of Health and Human Services Public Service, 1985.

Haynes, S.G., and M. Feinleib. "Women, Work and Coronary Heart Disease: Prospective Findings from the Framingham Heart Study." *American Journal of Public Health 70*(2)(1980): 133–41.

Holmes, Helen, Betty Hoskins, and Michael Gross, eds. *Birth Control and Controlling Birth: Women-Centered Perspectives*. Clifton, NJ: Humana Press, 1980.

Hubbard, Ruth. *Politics of Women's Biology*. New Brunswick, NJ: Rutgers University Press, 1990.

Hudson, Walter W., and Wendell Ricketts. "A Strategy for the Measurement of Homophobia." *Journal of Homosexuality 5* (1980): 357–72.

Hume, B.J. "Perspectives on Women's Health: Disclosure Decisions, Needs, and Experiences of Lesbians." M.A. thesis, Yale University, 1983.

Johnson, S., and J. Palermo. "Gynecological Care for the Lesbian." *Clinical Obstetrics and Gynecology 27* (1984): 724–30.

Kirschstein, Ruth L. *Women's Health: Report of the Public Health Service Task Force on Women's Health Issues*. Vol. 2. Washington, DC: U.S. Department of Health and Human Services Public Health Service, 1985.

Levy, T. "The Lesbian: As Perceived by Mental Health Workers." Ph.D. diss. California School of Professional Psychology, 1978.

Liljestrand, Petra, Ernest Gerling, and Patricia Saliba. "The Effects of Social Sex-Role Stereotypes and Sexual Orientation on Psychotherapeutic Outcomes." *Journal of Homosexuality 3*(4) (1978): 361–72.

Lorde, Audre. *Sister Outsider*. Trumansberg, NY: Crossing Press, 1984.

Lluy, Margaret. "Alcohol Use Among Lesbians." Ph.D. diss. University of South Carolina, 1991.

Manley, Audrey, Jane Lin-Fu, Magdalena Miranda, Allan Noonan, and Tanya Parker. "Special Health Concerns of Ethnic Minority Women in Women's Health." *Report of the Public Health Service Task Force on Women's Health Issues*. Washington, DC: U.S. Department of Health and Human Services, 1985. II-37-II-47.

Mathews, W.C., M.W. Booth, J.D. Turner, and L. Kessler. "Physicians' Attitudes Toward Homosexuality: Survey of California County Medical Society." *Western Journal of Medicine* (1986): *144*: 106–10.

McKirnan, D.J., and P.L. Peterson. "Alcohol and Drug Use Among Homosexual Men and Women: Epidemiology and Population Characteristics." *Addictive Behaviors 14* (1989): 545–53.

———. "Psychosocial and Social Factors in Alcohol and Drug Abuse: An Analysis of a Homosexual Community." *Addictive Behaviors 14* (1989): 555–63.

McNally, E.B. "Lesbian Recovering Alcoholics in Alcoholics Anonymous: A Qualitative Study of Identity Transformation." Ph.D. diss. New York University, 1989.

Medical News and Perspectives. "Women's Health Initiative Leads Way as Research Begins to Fill Gender Gaps." *Journal of the American Medical Association 267* (1992): 169–70.

Monzon, O.T., and J.M.B. Capellan. "Female-to-Female Transmission of HIV." *Lancet 1987 2* (1987): 40.

Morin, S.F. "Heterosexual Bias in Psychological Research on Lesbianism and Male Homosexuality." *American Psychologist 32* (1977): 629–37.

Muller, Charlotte F. *Health Care and Gender.* New York: Russell Sage Foundation, 1990.

Multiple Risk Factor Intervention Trial Research Group. "Mortality Rates after 10.5 Years for Participants in the Multiple Risk Factor Intervention Trial: Findings Related to a Prior Hypothesis of the Trial." *Journal of the American Medical Association 236* (1990): 1795–1801.

Norwood, Chris. "Alarming Rise in Deaths." *Ms.* July 1988: 65–67.

O'Donnell, Mary, Val Loeffler, Katev Pollack, and Ziesal Saunders. *Lesbian Health Matters: A Resource Book about Lesbian Health.* Santa Cruz, CA: Santa Cruz Women's Health Collective, 1977.

Olesker, E., and L.V. Walsh. "Childbearing among Lesbians: Are We Meeting Their Needs?" *Journal of Nurse-Midwifery 29*(5) (1984): 322–29.

Radicalesbians Health Collective. "Lesbians and the Health Care System." In *Out of the Closets: Voices of Gay Liberation*, ed. K. Joy and A. Young. New York: Harcourt, Brace Jovanovich, 1977.

Randall, Carla E. "Lesbian Phobia among BSN Educators: A Survey." *Journal of Nursing Education 28* (1989): 302–6.

Reagan, P. "The Interaction of Health Professionals and Their Lesbian Clients." *Patient Counselling and Health Education 3*(1) (1992): 21–25.

Robertson, M. Morag. "Lesbians as an Invisible Minority in the Health Services Arena." *Health Care for Women International 13*(2) (1992): 155–64.

Romm, M.E. "Sexuality and Homosexuality in Women." In *Sexual Inversion: The Multiple Roots of Homosexuality*, ed. J. Marmor. New York: Basic Books, 1965.

Saghir, M.T., and E. Robins. *Male and Female Homosexuality: A Comprehensive Investigation.* Baltimore, MD: Williams and Wilkins Co., 1973.

Saunders, J.M., J.D. Tupac, and B. MacCulloch. *A Lesbian Profile: A Survey of 1000 Lesbians.* West Hollywood, CA: Southern California Women for Understanding, 1985.

Schwanberg, Sandra L. "Changes in Labeling Homosexuality in Health Sciences Literature: A Preliminary Investigation." *Journal of Homosexuality* 12(1) (1985): 51–73.

———. "Attitudes towards Homosexuality in American Health Care Literature 1983–1987." *Journal of Homosexuality* 19(3) (1990): 117–36.

Selye, Hans. *The Stress of Life.* New York: McGraw-Hill Book Company, 1956.

Shilts, Randy. *And the Band Played On: Politics, People and the AIDS Epidemic.* New York: St. Martin's Press, 1987.

Smith, Barbara. "The Wedding." In *Home Girls: A Black Feminist Anthology,* ed. Barbara Smith, New York: Kitchen Table Press, 1983. 171–76.

Smith, Elaine, Susan Johnson, and Susan Guenther. "Healthcare Attitudes and Experiences during Gynecological Care Among Lesbians and Bisexuals." *American Journal of Public Health* 75 (1985): 1085–87.

Socarides, C.W. *The Overt Homosexual.* New York: Grune & Stratton, 1968.

Steering Committee of the Physician's Health Study Group. "Final Report on the Aspirin Component of the Ongoing Physician's Health Study." *New England Journal of Medicine* 321 (1989): 129–35.

Stevens, Patricia E. "Lesbian Health Care Research: A Review of the Literature from 1970 to 1990." *Health Care for Women International* 13(2) (1992): 91–120.

Stevens, Patricia E., and Joanne M. Hall. "Stigma, Health Beliefs, and Experiences with Health Care in Lesbian Women." *Image: Journal of Nursing Scholarship* 10(2) (1988): 69–73.

———. "Abusive Health Care Interactions Experienced by Lesbians: A Case of Institutional Violence in the Treatment of Women." *Response: To the Victimization of Women and Children* 13(3) (1990): 23–27.

Swanson, D.W., S.D. Loomis, R.C. Lukesh, R. Cronin, and J.A. Smith. "Clinical Features of the Female Homosexual Patient." *Journal of Nervous and Mental Disease* 155(2) (1972): 119–24.

Tallen, Bette S. "Twelve-Step Programs: A Lesbian Feminist Critique." *NWSA Journal* 2(3) (1990): 390–407.

Trippet, Susan E., and Joyce Bain. "Reasons American Lesbians Fail to Seek Traditional Health Care." *Health Care for Women International* 13(2) (1992): 145–54.

Underhill, B.L., and S.E. Ostermann. "The Pain of Invisibility: Issues for Lesbians." In *Alcohol and Drugs Are Women's Issues.* Vol. I: *A Review of the Issues,* ed. P. Roth. Metuchen, NJ: Women's Action Alliance and the Scarecrow Press, 1991.

Watters, Alan T. "Heterosexual Bias in Psychological Research on Lesbianism and Male Homosexuality (1979–1983): Utilizing the Bibliographic and Taxonomic System of Morin (1977)." *Journal of Homosexuality* 13(1) (1986): 35–58.

Weathers, B. *Alcoholism and the Lesbian Community.* Washington, DC: Gay Council on Drinking Behavior, 1981.

West, C., "Lesbian Daughter." *Sage: A Scholarly Journal on Black Women* 4(2) (1987): 42–44.

White, T.A. "Attitudes of Psychiatric Nurses Toward Same Sex Orientations." *Nursing Research* 28(5) (1979): 276–81.

Wilbur, C. B. "Clinical Aspects of Female Homosexuality." In *Sexual Inversion: The Multiple Roots of Homosexuality*, ed. J. Marmor. New York: Basic Books, 1965. 268–81.

Wolff, C. *Love Between Women*. New York: Harper & Row, 1971.

Young, E.W. "Nurses' Attitudes toward Homosexuality: Analysis of Change in AIDS Workshops." *Journal of Continuing Education in Nursing 19*(1) (1988): 9–12.

Zeidenstein, Laura. "Gynecological and Childbearing Needs of Lesbians." *Journal of Nurse-Midwifery 35*(1) (1990): 10–18.

PART THREE   **Aging Women**

CHAPTER EIGHT

When Does Menopause Occur, and How Long Does It Last? Wrestling with Age- and Time-Based Conceptualizations of Reproductive Aging

HEATHER E. DILLAWAY

Biomedical and feminist researchers have documented much about menopause over the last several decades, yet there are still major gaps in our knowledge about women's experiences of reproductive aging. Indeed, we lack a comprehensive definition of what menopause is, when it occurs, how women transition through the different stages of reproductive aging, and how long the entire process lasts. Likewise, aging scholars have made strides in understanding age identities and the meanings individuals attribute to chronological age at different stages of adult life, yet we lack a full understanding of how chronological age figures into individuals' experiences, medical treatment, and academic research. The gaps in our knowledge about chronological age are particularly glaring when thinking about women's experiences, as most research on aging identities is not about women or gender directly (Calasanti 2004; Lysack and Seipke 2002; Ray 2004; Reinharz 1997; Silver 2003; Twigg 2004). That is, gerontologists have inadequately addressed gender differences and inequalities in aging, and feminist scholars have often overlooked the concerns of aging or older women (Reinharz 1997; Pearsall 1997). There is ample room for feminist research on how chronological age is experienced during reproductive aging; the importance women, doctors, and researchers attach to chronological age; and ultimately, whether connections between particular chronological ages and aging experiences make sense.

In this essay, I use data from 61 in-depth interviews with menopausal women to explore the ways in which chronological age appears in women's discussions of menopause experiences and their interactions with doctors. I also analyze how chronological age initially shaped my own conceptualizations of menopause and, therefore, how it shaped my early recruitment efforts for this study. I conclude that, despite unclear information about when women begin, experience, and exit reproductive aging and questionable equations of particular chronological ages and menopause (Deats and Lenker 1999; Greer 1993; Mansfield et al. 2004; Boston Women's Health Book Collective 1992), we still use chronological age to diagnose and operationalize women's experiences at midlife. I argue that this hinders our understandings of menopause, chronological age,

Originally published in the spring 2006 issue (vol. 18, no. 1).

women's midlife, and women's overall well being, and suggest that feminist scholars need to continue to work toward broader conceptualizations and understandings.

Before moving forward, I must make a disclaimer. In taking the stance that considerable feminist work still needs to be done as I write this essay, in no way do I seek to discount the important feminist work already done on the subject of menopause and aging. Indeed, within the last three decades, many feminist scholars (some gerontologists as well as many others in social science and the humanities) have helped us gain a broader understanding of this reproductive transition, as well as the gendered dimensions of maturation processes (see Callahan 1993; Coney 1993; Deats and Lenker 1999; Gannon 1999; Greer 1993; Grossman and Bart 1982; Jones and Estes 1997; Komesaroff, Rothfield, and Daly 1997; Lock 1993; Pearsall 1997; Sontag 1997). In emphasizing social contexts, feminist scholars present a powerful critique of the biomedical perspective and the equation of women with their reproductive capacities. They also illustrate how most women do not have an illness or disease orientation toward menopause or aging in general (Dillaway 2005; Frey 1981; Gannon and Ekstrom 1993; Grossman and Bart 1982; Kaufert and Gilbert 1986; Lock 1993; Lysack and Seipke 2002; McCrea 1983; Voda 1992; Zita 1997). Some feminist gerontologists have made inroads into showing how aging processes can vary by gender because of the social contexts of women's lives as well (see Gannon 1999; Jones and Estes 1997; Markson and Hess 1997; Reinharz 1997; Sontag 1997). Nonetheless, most feminist scholars have not yet researched women's apprehensions about menopause or faced the definitional issues surrounding menopause and aging head on. The result is that little feminist research exists on when menopause occurs, how long it lasts, and whether medical definitions of menopause affect individual women (Mansfield et al. 2004). Further, the feminist research that does exist on the topic does not meet with a wide audience (or, alternatively, does not have a significant public impact outside feminist academic circles) and therefore biomedical definitions and doctors' diagnoses are not directly challenged.[1] In this essay, I use empirical data to reaffirm what some feminists already have found—that equations of chronological age and menopause are problematic—and highlight age- and time-based definitions of menopause that some feminist scholars already know are faulty. I argue, however, that in light of my data and previous feminist research, we must challenge existing definitions of menopause more directly, gather more empirical data on the problematic nature of existing definitions as they affect individual women, and work toward a wider dissemination of findings from feminist research so that the health needs of midlife women are met.

As Koeske warned two decades ago, "feminists must be clear about their role. Their perspective is not a simple adjunct to biomedicine. Neither should it be a repudiation of the role of biological factors in women's experiences or an exclusive focus on psychological and sociocultural factors as these have been traditionally defined" (1983, 12). Scholars have not fully responded to Koeske's and others' calls for more complex biosocial analyses of menopause (McCrea 1983; Oakley 1998). While this critique could be made about almost any topic (because most research topics are not fully explored), the study of menopause (and aging in general) will not go deep enough until we empirically recognize that a portion of the menopause experience is based purely on established age- and time-based definitions and that these definitions may affect how women feel about and experience menopause and how doctors respond to them. I review these definitions and their problems in the following section.

Literature Review

Menopause refers to the cessation of menstruation, and it is caused by the fluctuation of hormone levels within the ovaries and within women's bloodstreams (Fausto-Sterling 1992). Clinical studies suggest that the average age of cessation is around 48–52 years of age, although women in Western countries end menstruation between their early 40s and late 50s (Roberts 1991, 421; McKinlay, Brambilla, and Posner 1992; Brett and Madans 1997; McElmurry and Huddleston 1991; Kaufert, Gilbert, and Tate 1987; Mansfield et al. 2004). Thus, despite the average, there is considerable variation and heterogeneity (Deats and Lenker 1999; Boston Women's Health Book Collective 1992). Further, regardless of popular belief, the decrease of estrogen hormones is not the sole cause of menstrual cessation; rather, many hormones fluctuate to cause this reproductive transition, or "climacteric" (Fausto-Sterling 1992, 116–17). Some hormone levels increase while others decrease. These hormone fluctuations can occur anywhere from eight to ten years prior to cessation to several years afterward (116–17). What women experience is not just menopause, then, but a complex reproductive transition that can span multiple decades. Because of the often long-term nature of this transition, current definitions of menopause are "notoriously problematic" (Hunt 1988, 398; Kaufert, Gilbert, and Tate 1987; Mansfield et al. 2004; Boston Women's Health Book Collective 1992). Some contemporary scholars have adopted the term *reproductive aging* as the best conceptualization of this long-term process, illustrating its similarity to other gradual aging processes as well as its ties to previous, gendered reproductive experiences (Dillaway 2005; Mansfield et al. 2004).

Nonetheless, it is still difficult to know what experiences actually fall within this process, when it starts and ends, and how long it lasts. No definition of this process seems complete or clear, and no term can fully explain to women what they should expect to experience during this transition.

Most commonly, doctors and researchers use a three-part clinical definition of menopause to make sense of women's experience of reproductive aging (Mansfield et al. 2004). According to clinical research and medical diagnosis guidelines, *menopause* is defined by the lack of menstruation for 12 consecutive months (McElmurry and Huddleston 1991; Rostosky and Travis 1996; McKinlay, Brambilla, and Posner 1992; Im, Meleis, and Park 1999; Mansfield et al. 2004). *Perimenopause* refers to the period leading up to actual menopause, and this is usually the time when symptoms such as hot flashes, dry or less elastic skin, weight gain, irregular bleeding, and others begin (McElmurry and Huddleston 1991; Rostosky and Travis 1996; McKinlay, Brambilla, and Posner 1992; Im, Meleis, and Park 1999; Mansfield et al. 2004). This stage is sometimes referred to as a menopausal stage simply because it precedes the time when a woman will become menopausal (McElmurry and Huddleston 1991). But at this stage women are not actually *going through menopause. Postmenopause* is the point after which a woman has not had a period for 12 months (Im, Meleis, and Park 1999; Mansfield et al. 2004; McElmurry and Huddleston 1991; McKinlay, Brambilla, and Posner 1992; Rostosky and Travis 1996); often this stage is not diagnosed until approximately two years after the cessation of periods (Boston Women's Health Book Collective 1992).

The notion that there are clear transitions from one menopausal stage or status to another is faulty, however (Fausto-Sterling 1992; Mansfield et al. 2004). For example, a woman who is perimenopausal may still be having periods or may have stopped menstruating temporarily. Second, a woman who has not had a period for almost a year may still be considered perimenopausal or menopausal when in fact she feels postmenopausal (i.e., despite having bled within the past year, she may feel that most of her other symptoms have dissipated). Third, a woman with a history of irregular periods may not know what stage she represents until she is diagnosed as postmenopausal.[2] Fourth, Mansfield et al. (2004, 225) suggest that, despite the official definitions of these three categories, postmenopausal women can sometimes bleed.

Mansfield et al. (2004) explain that there is considerable variation in women's movement across menopausal status categories, so much so that researchers have to be ready to reject the notion of a regular progression from perimenopause to menopause to postmenopause or a regular menopausal age or duration, and to search for a broader conceptualization of menopause in future studies. In one longitudinal study of 100 women that took place over the span of 3–12 years, some women lasted in one stage for numerous years and then moved on quickly, some flip-flopped between stages over many years, and some progressed quickly through all three stages as they are clinically defined (Mansfield et al. 2004, 225). This study and other definitional critiques (see Fausto-Sterling 1992; Greer 1993; Kaufert Gilbert, and Tate 1987; Boston Women's Health Book Collective 1992) suggest that not only is the length of reproductive aging variable, but also that the clinical definitions of menopause are somewhat faulty as they stand. Fausto-Sterling notes that since we have little "baseline data" on menopausal women, we do not even have a way of knowing whether a symptom is actually "normal" or not at any given time (1992, 118).[3] There is no symptom we can use to diagnose the true onset of any menopausal stage.

Fifth, researchers have attempted to predict the age onset of menopause. Some studies have suggested that determinants for age at natural menopause are established at birth (or at least in early childhood) and are carried throughout life (Lawlor, Ebrahim, and Smith 2003). Others suggest that age at menopause is determined over the lifespan by a combination of physiological and social factors (Gold et al. 2001; Lawlor, Ebrahim, and Smith 2003; Reynolds and Obermeyer 2003). There is little agreement about when or why the onset of menopause occurs at particular times. Based on existing research, we know that birth weight, educational attainment, marital status, employment status, childhood and adult economic circumstances, childhood nutrition, race and ethnicity, demographic location, national origin, being bottle-fed or breastfed as an infant, smoking, certain types of contraceptive use, age at menarche, and body mass index can all affect the onset on menopause (Gold et al. 2001; Lawlor, Ebrahim, and Smith 2003; Reynolds and Obermeyer 2003). Yet, no specific chronological age can be pinpointed as the "normal" age for perimenopause or menopause, especially since women can flip-flop between the three stages defined above (Mansfield et al. 2004). Further, with the exception of studies about contraceptive use (e.g., the birth control pill), most research has looked at factors that may contribute to "early" menopause rather than "late" menopause. In addition, if these factors do indeed affect age at onset, we still lack knowledge about the extent of the effect. Clinical research has not studied the connections between chronological age and reproductive aging in full. Considerable research must be done on the potential links between chronological age and the onset of the various stages of reproductive aging, for there are still more questions than answers. Mansfield et al. (2004) suggest that, with the current state of knowledge on menopause, the fact that women may take considerable time to make it through all three stages of this transition, and the unclear age at onset, researchers should make sure to include broad age ranges of women in their studies if they wish to truly understand the experience.[4]

Finally, if we think more critically about the actual definition of menopause, this definition illustrates the fact that, as a whole, researchers have trouble identifying the actual time frame or event of reproductive aging. Defining women as having gone through menopause after 12 months without menstruation means that doctors and researchers rely on women's retrospective accounts; that is, women must be able to remember exactly when they began to miss menstrual periods—something that is extremely difficult if irregular periods come first (Im, Meleis, and Park 1999; Mansfield et al. 2004; Rostosky and Travis 1996; Boston Women's Health Book Collective 1992). Theoretically, then, no woman is ever in menopause because it is literally a nonevent by definition and is diagnosed afterward. Women are perimenopausal or postmenopausal.

Perhaps because we have had considerable difficulty defining menopause and its stages, the onset of menopause, and the length of this reproductive transition, researchers, doctors, and women sometimes fall back on chronological age as a proxy for reproductive aging, using it to diagnose or operationalize menopause. That is, we still rely on questionable links between chronological age and reproductive aging. Specifically, chronological age figures prominently in women's thoughts about their own menopause experiences, doctors' treatment decisions, and researchers' attempts to define menopausal women as they study them. In this essay, I attempt to outline how chronological age is woven through women's discussions of menopause, doctors' diagnosis and treatment of menopause, and my own initial recruitment of a sample of menopausal women. I aim to show that the use of chronological age as a means of defining menopause leads to uncertainty and frustration among menopausal women, potentially incomplete medical treatment, and a narrow conceptualization of the reproductive aging experience. I argue that we must conceptualize menopause and connections between age and menopause more broadly if we are ever to understand what women experience at midlife or how chronological age and menopause are linked. And unless we are willing to wrestle with the age- and time-based constructions of reproductive aging, we will not arrive at a fuller understanding of chronological age or reproductive aging.

While there has been little work on the importance of chronological age in women's midlife or reproductive aging experiences, there is contemporary work that begins to distinguish chronological age from aging experience and aging identity. Thus, feminist scholars need to pick up where other aging scholars have left off. Aging scholars, including a few feminist gerontologists, have begun to analyze the differences between chronological age, how old individuals feel (i.e. what age they identify with), and their bodily or experiential age. One's experiential age refers to the status of one's physical health; whether or not, for instance, one is still able to engage in a daily routine, whether or not one can do the same activities as they did when younger, or how "old" one's body "feels" (Calasanti 2004; Cremin 1992; Deats and Lenker 1999; Dillaway 2005; Featherstone and Hepworth 1991; Kaufman and Elder 2002; Laz 2003; Lysack and Seipke 2002; Morell 2003; Reinharz 1997; Silver 2003; Twigg 2004). These scholars illustrate how people can feel much younger or older than their chronological age depending on their physical well being and regular involvement in daily activities; in fact, some scholars suggest that chronological age and "feel age" rarely match (Cremin 1992; Deats and Lenker 1999; Kaufman and Elder 2002; Laz 2003; Lysack and Seipke 2002). Until individuals "embody" their construction of their own age, they do not identify with their chronological age (Kaufman and Elder 2002; Laz 2003; Lysack and Seipke 2002; Morell 2003); thus, chronological age and bodily or experiential age can be quite separate. In most of these studies, however, scholars discuss elderly individuals as they reflect on current or future physical incapacity (Cremin 1992; Kaufman and Elder 2002). These scholars steer away from examining how chronological age figures into specific aging processes (e.g., menopause), and therefore cannot trace how individuals think about chronological age, how doctors use chronological age in treatment decisions, or how chronological age might hinder researchers in their efforts to study specific aging processes. In addition, aging scholars rarely look at how chronological age is experienced in midlife. Finally, few scholars concentrate on how women think about and experience chronological age over their life spans, and whether/how chronological age may affect women and men differently.[5]

To fill gaps in our knowledge about chronological age and reproductive aging experiences, I use this essay to discuss how women's experiences illustrate yet also demystify the equation of particular chronological ages and menopause. While some feminist scholars have covered the problematic equation of chronological age and menopause in previous research, I also suggest that when chronological age appears in doctor-patient interactions, women's health concerns are not legitimated and their treatment options are limited. Thus my data suggest that age- and time-based definitions are seemingly still used in medical diagnoses and affect some women in unique ways as a result. Last, I discuss how my own initial equation of menopause and chronological age led me to limit early recruitment of women for my study even though I should have known better; thus I show how feminist researchers can still be affected by these faulty equations as well. Before moving on to my findings, I describe the methodology used in this study.

Methods

Between January and September 2001, I interviewed 61 women, age 38 to 60, in a midwestern state about their menopausal experiences. Before engaging in one-on-one interviews, I organized two focus groups to ensure that I was asking relevant, straightforward questions and to see how women conversed about menopause. Eight women participated in focus groups and 53 interviewed separately.

I developed my sample through snowball and purposive sampling procedures. Participants were recruited via women's organizations, targeted businesses (a real estate office and a school), doctors' offices and women's health clinics, churches, advertisements in newsletters/listservs/magazines, sports leagues, fitness clubs, community centers, word of mouth, and well-placed flyers. Following Morell (1994), I also used "network sampling" in an attempt to create a heterogeneous sample. After interviews, I asked women for a list of others who might participate. Individuals with distant emotional and/or social connections to the interviewees were contacted first. If these contacts did not elicit interviews, I moved up the lists, successively approaching those closest to original interviewees.

All procedures undertaken followed the ethical standards of the university's review board, including the securing of human subjects' approval for focus groups and individual interviews for the 2001 year. Participation in the study was voluntary, and therefore, interviewees were self-selected. In addition to an interview, participation in my research included a questionnaire that elicited demographic information as well as reproductive history.[6]

Table 8.1 depicts the demographic profile of my sample. The fact that a solid three-quarters of my sample identified as European American and white means that it is racially biased. Moreover, the majority of women of color are self-reportedly African American. Second, most women were financially stable at the time of the interview. The majority (53 women, or 87 percent) worked outside the home and had some sort of autonomy and authority in paid work (based on their job titles) as well. Almost two-thirds had graduated with an undergraduate degree and many held a graduate or professional degree. Given the income and education distributions in Table 8.1 as well as my assessment of their job authority, I designated 54 women (88.5 percent) as middle class and only seven women (11.5 percent) as working class.

The third significant bias in my sample is the fact that 57 of the 61 women I interviewed (93 percent) identified themselves as heterosexual. Because of this bias, I do not analyze sexual identities or orientations in this essay, and my findings primarily represent the thoughts and experiences of heterosexual women. This does not discount the

Table 8.1
Demographic Characteristics

Women's Age		Individual Income (N=52)	
35–39	1 (1.6%)	$0–9,999	7 (13.5%)
40–44	4 (6.6%)	$10,000–19,999	5 (9.6%)
45–49	16 (26.2%)	$20,000–29,999	6 (11.5%)
50–54	23 (37.7%)	$30,000–39,999	10 (19.2%)
55–59	14 (23.0%)	$40,000–49,999	8 (15.4%)
60 and over	3 (4.9%)	$50,000–59,999	7 (13.5%)
		$60,000–69,999	3 (5.8%)
		$70,000 and over	6 (11.5%)

Race		Marital Status	
African American	11 (18.0%)	Never Married	2 (3.3%)
Chicana	3 (4.9%)	Married[1]	34 (55.7%)
Asian American[2]	2 (3.3%)	Divorced	19 (31.1%)
European American	43 (70.5%)	Widowed[3]	2 (1.6%)
Other[4]	2 (3.3%)	Domestic Partner[5]	3 (4.8%)
		Separated	1 (1.6%)

Education (N=53)		Parental Status	
Some High School	1 (1.9%)	Biological Parent	52 (85.2%)
High School Diploma	5 (9.4%)	Adoptive Parent	4 (6.6%)
Some College	15 (28.3%)	Foster Parent	1 (1.6%)
College Diploma	11 (20.8%)	Step Parent	4 (6.6%)
Some Graduate Work	7 (13.2%)		
Graduate Degree	14 (26.4%)		

Family Income (N=48)		Stage of Process[6]	
$0–9,999	1 (2.1%)	Perimenopausal	31 (50.8%)
$10,000–19,999	2 (4.2%)	Menopausal	2 (3.3%)
$20,000–29,999	4 (8.3%)	Postmenopausal	15 (24.6%)
$30,000–39,999	5 (10.4%)	Hysterectomy	8 (13.1%)
$40,000–49,999	1 (2.1%)	Unclear[7]	5 (8.2%)
$50,000–59,999	5 (10.4%)		
$60,000–69,999	5 (10.4%)		
$70,000 and over	25 (52.1%)		

Note: I do not include dichotomous variables in this table and, rather, talk about them in the text. Unless noted, n=61 women.
1. Includes two women who reported they were in their second marriages. I suspect a few other women were also in their second and third marriages (based on the prevalence of divorce and remarriage in the U.S. population at large), but I did not explore this. I also did not ask how many times women had been divorced.
2. Both were South Asian in descent.
3. Includes one woman who was also formerly divorced.

(Continued)

Table 8.1 (continued)

4. Includes one multiracial woman and one West Indian woman. Both women were careful to distinguish themselves from African American individuals, since usually they are characterized based on the color of their skin. The multiracial women reported Native American as well as African American descent. The West Indian woman was from Jamaica.
5. Includes one woman formerly divorced and one woman formerly widowed.
6. Based on my understanding of the medical definitions of the three stages of this reproductive process.
7. Because some women have been on some form of hormone replacement therapy (HRT) since the beginning of perimenopausal symptoms (or even before), it is impossible for them or me to tell which stage of the process they exemplify.

need to reach scholarly conclusions about the different experiences that heterosexual and nonheterosexual women have during menopause (Winterich 2003).

Fourth, in early recruitment I had difficulty finding women of color and working-class women who would volunteer for my research. As a result, all eight participants in my focus groups are European American and middle class. While this may have affected the questions I used during data collection (in that I might have varied the questions more if I had interviewed women of color or working-class women early on), similar data on chronological age and definitions of menopause came out of focus group conversations and individual interviews. For the purposes of this essay, then, I consider my focus group and interview data to be comparable and include all 61 women in my analyses. This does not discount the possibility of serious differences between the focus groups and interviews, however, especially because the purposes of each data collection method are different as well.

Despite its biases, my sample includes women with a variety of family and reproductive experiences. Slightly more than half of the women I interviewed (56 percent) were married and slightly more than one-third (38 percent) were divorced from at least one marriage. Twenty-three (38 percent) were self-reportedly "single," often actively looking for a romantic partner. The vast majority (85 percent) had biological children. Of those who were parents, almost half (46 percent) still had children under the age of 18 living in their homes at the time of the interview.

Almost all interviewees (87 percent) were between 45 and 59 years of age, yet were at varied stages of reproductive aging based on their reports of symptoms. About half of the women I interviewed reported that they started menopause well before age 48—the typical age cited in clinical literature as the point at which women reach menopause; what they were referring to, however, was the time when their perimenopause began (I discuss this more in my findings). Based on standard medical definitions of the process, however, my sample included 51 percent (31) perimeno-pausal, 3 percent (2) menopausal, and almost 25 percent (15) postmeno-pausal women (see Table 8.1). Nonetheless, most women reported contin-ual or chronic symptoms of some sort and all 61 women in my sample referred to themselves as menopausal or "going through menopause" rather than denoting a particular menopausal stage; therefore, transitions between categories did not make much difference in women's perspectives or bodily experiences (Mansfield et al. 2004). Additionally, many also were unsure into which category they fell; thus these are my characterizations of women's menopausal stages. About 56 percent of my sample (33 women) were taking doctor-prescribed hormone replacement therapies (HRT) to al-leviate symptoms of menopause at the time of the interview.[7]

I conducted the focus groups on a university campus and scheduled them on weekends for women's convenience. Each focus group lasted ap-proximately three hours. Individual interviews took place in private set-tings (e.g., a woman's home, a workplace, a university conference room, a library study room, or a secluded corner of a coffee shop or bookstore). Individual interviews varied in length, as some women had more infor-mation to share (or felt more comfortable sharing information) than oth-ers. On average, individual interviews lasted one and a half hours. My interview schedule followed a focused interview format (Rubin and Ru-bin 1995).

The purpose of this research project was to explore the social meanings and experiences of menopause, broadly defined. Therefore, I tried to main-tain an inductive, rather than deductive, approach throughout data collec-tion, coding, and analysis. Especially during early interviewing, I did not know what answers to expect. While I included specific categories of ques-tions on my interview schedule (based on my reviews of literature on menopause and other women's health experiences), questions purpose-fully were general enough to elicit a variety of responses. Rubin and Rubin suggest that this semi-structured interview format allows a researcher to "keep on target while hanging loose" (1995, 42).

Findings and Discussion

I use this section to present both empirical and methodological evidence for my argument that chronological age is used as a way to think about and even operationalize menopause, even though it may be fairly well known as a questionable measure of how/when women really experi-ence reproductive aging. Thus, even though feminist scholars have done research on the variability in menopause experiences (Deats and Lenker

1999; Fausto-Sterling 1992; Greer 1993; Mansfield et al. 2004; Boston Women's Health Book Collective 1992), medical providers and popular culture may still reinforce the three-part biomedical definition as well as an equation of chronological age and menopause. In this section I detail my empirical data to reinforce previous feminist work on this subject and suggest why we must take on biomedical definitions of menopause more directly than we have, in order to challenge current medical treatment for menopause and meet the health needs of contemporary menopausal women.

First, I discuss women's reasons why contemporary menopause might be distinct from chronological age, or how old women are in actual years. Women's comments discredit the supposed relationship between particular chronological ages and menopause since they suggest that reproductive aging does not begin, end, or persist according to predetermined ages or time periods. Second, I suggest that when doctors link menopause to chronological age (as women in my sample report), women's treatment choices are potentially affected and their health concerns are dismissed. Third, because menopause is diagnosed via chronological age and operationalized through three stages, there are definitional issues that surface within qualitative research on menopause. Recruitment and sampling procedures depend on definitions of who is and is not experiencing this process or transition, yet women defined menopause very differently than clinical definitions allowed and reported a much broader age range for reproductive aging than originally expected. In this section, I use the term *menopause* broadly the way my interviewees do, to connote the entire reproductive transition and not just a specific stage.

When Do Women Enter, Experience, and Exit Menopause?

According to my interviewees, women actually enter into and experience menopause during a range of about 30 years. The youngest woman I interviewed, a 38-year-old European American, middle-class woman, was in "full-blown menopause," having started the process in her early 30s. In contrast, a 56-year-old European American, middle-class woman I interviewed was still waiting for perimenopause to fully take hold; so far she had experienced only a few hot flashes and still had fairly regular periods. The majority of women reported beginning perimenopause in their early- to mid-40s, which is similar to what Mansfield et al. (2004) report, but it was not uncommon to hear women report starting it earlier or later. Of the women in my sample, 14 (23 percent) believed they started perimenopause by age 40, 18 (30 percent) believed they started between ages 41 and 45, 14 (23 percent) believed they started between ages 46 and 50, and nine (15 percent) thought they started perimenopause after age 50. Six women (approximately 10 percent) could not remember their age at the onset of perimenopause. The following quotes further illustrate how chronological age does not always dictate the onset of perimenopause or any particular menopausal stage.

> I was looking forward to [perimenopause] at 45 but then that changed to 50 and then 55. And [my body] kept putting it off, and it meant I had to wait longer and longer. [European American, middle class, age 59]

> I'll be 49 this year. Actually, my blood work showed that I was postmenopausal like two years ago. It's rather amazing to me, but the doctor said that's not all that unusual. It could be even earlier, in your 40s. I was shocked. I didn't expect it until in my 50s, really. [European American, middle class, age 48]

> When I started, [I was] 39 because that's when the hot flashes and the mood swings and all that hit me at one time and my doctor said it was probably an onset of menopause and I had asked him how long, you know, it would go on, because I thought I was kind of young for that and he said, "Oh, it can go on for years. Everybody is different in that." So basically I told him, I said, "Well, give me something before I croak," [laughs] and it was rough at first [and] my periods, they didn't stop until about, um, oh, probably ten months ago. [European American, working class, age 49]

> I started having periods at a young age, so I think I've gotten thrown into this pretty early too. Like I'm 47 now and I bet it's been seven years, but I even have sisters younger than me who are done [with menopause] like 42, 40.
> *HD:* So were you surprised to get it that early or not?
> Not really. I kind of do everything early; I married early, [had] kids early. [African American, working class, age 47]

The comments of these four women depict how varied menopausal experience is by chronological age and menopausal stage. Chronological age and menopause do not align in the way medical definitions or lay expectations might suggest. In fact, after completing my interviews, I conclude that we cannot link the onset, duration, or end of menopause to any particular chronological age and expect to be accurate, at least for my sample of menopausal women. Other feminist scholars have hinted at the same finding (e.g., Fausto-Sterling 1992; Greer 1993; Mansfield et al. 2004; Boston Women's Health Book Collective 1992).

Not only does the age for onset of perimenopause and cessation of menstrual periods appear questionable based on women's reports, but also reproductive aging seems like an indefinite and ever-lasting process. It is not a time-defined event for most women I interviewed. Of the women I interviewed, five women (8 percent) reported experiencing this transition for 15 or more years. Twelve (20 percent) had been experiencing menopause for ten or more years. Thirty-two women (52 percent) had been experiencing reproductive aging for five or more years. None of these women expected the symptoms of reproductive aging (e.g., hot flashes, dry skin, mood swings, or irregular bleeding) to end any time soon. For some, menopause was something that essentially would last indefinitely because of their use of HRT, but others opting not to take HRT also reported the indefinite nature of reproductive aging. Thus, the notion of menopause being a single event or a confined moment in time runs contradictory to the actual experience of my interviewees. Any discussion of "pre-" or "peri-" and "post-" menopause seemed suspect to most women as well, in that there are no clear beginnings, ends, or transitions in between "stages." Many questioned whether some symptoms (e.g., hot flashes or dry skin) ever ceased (since some of their elderly mothers still had these symptoms), and they also could not pinpoint when these symptoms began. In fact, no woman in my sample knew what symptoms signified the "beginning" or "end" of this transition. Mansfield et al. (2004, 221) suggest that the "vagueness" of perimenopause in particular is often a problem for women and doctors. Fausto-Sterling (1992), too, suggests the inability to pinpoint the onset and duration of symptoms.

According to my interviewees, nothing about menopause was certain and nothing about the experience as a whole was age- or time-defined. This uncertainty about when menopause started and how long it would continue was one of the biggest concerns for most women, especially when they compared it to other, more finite, reproductive processes (e.g., pregnancy, birth, or "normal" menstruation).

I'd rather have a baby, because at the end of nine months, I know it's over and done with. Menopause can go on and on. Your periods stop, but you still have hot flashes and all that other stuff. That, to me, is what makes it harder, because you go through such a long period of not knowing when one [period] is going to cease, and when it's not. Any other illness, unless it's cancer, once you got it and you take your medicine or whatever, it's through. [African American, working class, age 52]

I'm thinking I'm either in the middle of this or I'm getting close to the end of this. I don't know, and they say it is different for everyone, so I don't know. [African American, middle class, age 42]

All the other things [i.e., other reproductive experiences] were much easier, you know? You knew when they [i.e., menstrual periods] were coming, and that was going to be the end of it. With menopause, you don't know. Even the periods coming and going, little and big.
HD: So it's the uncertainty that really makes it harder?
Yeah. I think that's true of anything in life. If you know where you're going and you know what you want. But if you're just sort of window shopping it can be a lot harder, because you don't know. The uncertainty of it is the challenge, I think. [European American, working class, age 55]

I guess "indifferent" would be a good word [to describe how I feel about menopause] because I'm in the position where I'm not quite sure when I began or ended and I guess my experience has been, "Well, gee, I wonder if this was it (laugh) or not," you know? I never was quite sure about that. [European American, middle class, age 51]

A focus group conversation with five interviewees also illustrates the indefinite nature of menopause and shows how frustrating the "never-ending" process can be, in comparison to other gendered health experiences.

Woman #1: That's one of the things that struck me is that, [with] all that's written about menopause right now, it's still all a mystery, in terms of what's really happening. "Is this really [menopause]?" And [doctors] don't know a lot, and you're left sort of hanging out there. So, it's just sort of waiting to see what will happen. I think I have a fairly good OB/GYN, and she will talk you through it and she'll give you the options, but the last thing she said to me this last time was, "Well, let's see what happens this year, and you know, maybe the research, hopefully by the time you need it, will catch up and we will be able to figure it out." So it's quite an unknown.

Woman #2: Well, and pregnancy has an end, you know.

Woman #1: It's definable, right? [laughs] Yeah, like my son was two weeks late and I thought I was going in the *Guinness Book of World Records*! [laughs] I thought I was going to be pregnant forever, but it does end. And this [menopause] is just, it's so amorphous!
[Everyone says, "Right." "Right."]

Woman #3: Right, that's exactly right. And it [pregnancy] ends with a peak experience; I think of birth as a peak experience. It's just exciting; it's a miracle. And this is like never-ending.
[Others say, "It goes on and on," "Yeah," or "Yes," interrupting the speaker.]

Woman #1: That's actually something that I am going to have to deal with. Because I know for me, I want to have an end in sight. [I know when I have] twelve months [of no periods, my OB/GYN said] I can go off birth control. When that, whenever that happens [a small laugh] I'm sort of looking at it as this ending point. [But] I'm not sure it's going to be.

Woman #2: [I]t's a long-term process. And it's a natural process, I mean, so it's finally kind of out at least in the open, certainly more than it was for our mothers' generation. But it's still this big amorphous thing, you know, that doesn't get taken maybe as seriously as, you know, men having heart attacks. But it's not an illness, it's not an illness though. It's just a natural progression that you have to go through.

Woman #3: And it doesn't happen like a birth. There's not an ending like that. It probably makes us more patient. I don't know what it does! [Laughing] There's not a real end! All of a sudden, it's gone!

[All five women in this conversation were European American, middle class, and in their early 50s but were at varying stages of menopause.]

These tensions over the timing and length of menopause seemed to be an emotional issue for women, especially as they compared what they are going through to other reproductive events in their lives. Menopause is unnerving to women specifically because it is not a clearly defined, straightforward, or age- or time-restricted transition, and because it seems less defined than other gendered health experiences they have had in the past. In interviewees' conversations, we can see that women use other time-defined events in their gendered lives to make sense of menopause, which ultimately makes menopause seem more indefinite and confusing. In contrast to menopause, most health-related and/or bodily experiences, especially earlier reproductive events, appear to be defined by some sort of time clock. Menopause, according to women I interviewed, was the only "condition" or life process they could think of that is not experientially marked by time.[8] As quoted above, the only analogy one woman could come up with was "window shopping." No matter how hard women tried to confine or define it via a time schedule, menopause could not be bounded in such a way. They repeatedly gave me examples of how menopause was unpredictable and not defined by their age in years or the passage of time. While most interviewees felt positively about reproductive aging and sometimes aging in general (Dillaway 2005), the negativity they did express was often a result of the uncertainty they felt about the lack of age and time boundaries for this reproductive transition.

Am I Experiencing Menopause or Not?
Women's versus Doctors' Diagnoses

Experiences with doctors also highlight an imperfect equation of chronological age, time, and menopause, even though I did not ask interviewees directly to talk about these aspects of their experience. When I asked them to describe their experience of menopause and when it began and/or whether they had been to the doctor for the treatment of symptoms, woman after woman in my sample reported going to their doctors in their late 30s and early 40s with menopausal symptoms that their provider would not legitimate and label for years.[9] They reported frustration with doctors who told them they were way too "young" to be entering into menopause when a few years later they would be told they were now going into perimenopause with the same symptoms they had years before. According to interviewees' reports, medical diagnosis and treatment still are dictated by particular chronological ages, despite feminist researchers and women themselves reporting broader variations. One woman hinted that an old definition of menopause might be prevailing over a new experience of menopause.

> [N]ine times out of ten the doctors are going to have probably been practicing for ten or more years [and they] are not thinking the way that we are thinking

now . . . Their practice was in the books a long time ago and they are thinking what the books are telling them. [Thus, to them,] menopause starts in the 50s [or] early 60s. [African American, middle class, age 42]

Those "books," however, may have never held an accurate description of menopause experience. There is little reason to believe doctors' definitions of menopause ever matched women's accounts. Feminist scholars suggest that medical authorities have defined women's biological processes narrowly over time, specifically because they misunderstand them (Fausto-Sterling 1992; Martin 1992; Riessman 1983).

Consequently, doctors and women disagree about where women are in the menopausal experience. While doctors attempt to restrict menopausal meanings by defining this transition in terms of chronological age, interviewees experientially recognize a more comprehensive reproductive transition. As a result, they report struggling with doctors about menopausal diagnoses.

[At age 38] I went to the doctor at the beginning of the summer, and she said, "Oh, no. We don't even need to see you. You're too young. You just don't start menopause this early. Maybe in the fall we'll check again." [European American, middle class, age 55]

[M]y doctor, whom I have been going to for twelve years, she kept saying no, I'm too young, no, I'm too young . . . Yeah, I was about 34 [or] 35 when I started noticing symptoms and I would say, "But I know my body, I know something is going on." And I would give her all these signs and symptom issues and [she would say,] "No, you are too young." My physician even attached a number to it.
HD: What did she say?
["You'll be] 50, 55 when you'll start going through perimenopausal symptoms." [My doctor] concluded that I wasn't old enough to go through menopause, when, in fact, I had been going through perimenopause and she didn't recognize it. [African American, middle class, age 42]

A third woman, a middle-class African American also age 42, told me, "I've been flashing [i.e., having hot flashes] for a long time. In church they say, 'Why are you always fanning?' So I don't know. Is it possible it [menopause] could be going on, and the doctors not know it?" This particular woman supposed that her doctor might be unwilling to diagnose her because she was "so young." Similarly, a European American, middle-class woman, age 44, felt that she had started perimenopause but was not completely sure. She had asked her physician about menopausal symptoms and he told her that they "will do something about menopause soon." The physician told her she was "too young" when she came in with symptoms the year before. She too felt "too young" to be going through menopause but was convinced that her symptoms were hormonal and knew "it ha[d] to be related" somehow to the early stages of menopause. She also reported

irregularity of periods within the last year as well. Women relayed countless stories of doctors' dismissal of symptoms. These dismissals almost
always were made on the basis of women's chronological ages. Unless
women's complaints fell within an acceptable time period, they were not
addressed.

An opposite scenario also occurred, however. When women went to
physicians for other reasons, physicians were quick to tell them that everything they were experiencing was due to perimenopause. Based on
their age in years alone,[10] physicians would diagnose them as in a certain
stage of the menopausal process. One Asian American, middle-class
woman, age 51, described how she went to the doctor around age 45 simply
because her energy level seemed lower than normal. Her doctor said, "Oh,
you're just getting older," and therefore her symptoms were "simply that of
perimenopause." Her doctor directly linked her symptoms to chronological age. Another 59-year-old European American, middle-class woman
who started perimenopause at age 56 had a similar experience.

> I went to a male physician [a general practitioner] for years and whatever I was
> experiencing, [he said it] was pre-[peri-]menopausal. Now that went on for ten
> years, I was diagnosed as pre-[peri-]menopausal like that. Well, he didn't know!
> And I was convinced he didn't know. I mean, because ten years before [this]
> and all through the rest of my lifetime, this is attributable to menopause?

These women's experiences illustrate that, despite doctors' attempts to
link menopause to chronological age, the equation is not exact and perhaps partial at best. Much of the uncertainty voiced by the 59-year-old
interviewee is related to the fact that menopause was the primary diagnosis regardless of her symptoms. She mentioned later in the interview
that she could have sought care for a common cold and her doctor would
have attributed it to menopause. She became frustrated with the complete disregard of other possible diagnoses simply because of her age in
years and felt that her medical care was incomplete as a result.

According to my interviewees, more doctors than women viewed
menopause as a symptom of "getting older" and therefore linked it to
chronological age. Alternatively, women often discussed menopause as a
"life stage" or "passage into" another period in their life, reconstructing
it as broader than chronology.

> I just kept going to the doctor to get checked, and finally, just this year, they
> said, "Well, you're in menopause or peri . . . we don't know what you are. You
> could be post-menopausal based on your estrogen levels." In my family, estro-
> gen levels are high. Well, apparently my estrogen went down enough to where
> my doctor said, "I don't even know if you're post-menopausal." But like last
> year, I still had six periods. So, it wasn't that I was totally past it, and I don't
> know that I am now, but I haven't had a period in, this is my fourth month. A
> lot of the [web]sites that I read, you know, *they made me feel like maybe I re-*

ally wasn't going through [menopause] because they tie it to age, and I really think it's more of a life-stage thing than age. [European American, middle class, age 43, emphasis added]

Basing her assessment on her and her mother's experience with doctors, the woman cited above proposes that age-based definitions never represent accurate descriptions of what women are experiencing. Conceptualizing menopause as a life stage means allowing for a broader range of experiences and chronological ages than if we think of it as an age- or time-defined event. Ultimately, this woman hints that women's experiences (including her own and her mother's) would not be seen as "abnormal" if menopause was constructed broadly.

Not only do health care providers not always have time to listen to women's anxieties and concerns (and, as a result, sometimes dismiss women's concerns as unimportant), menopausal women report leaving doctors' offices still being unsure about their symptoms, what they should expect from the menopause experience, what the distinct markers of the menopause experience are, what menopausal stage they represent, and how long reproductive aging will last (Tannenbaum, Nasmith, and Mayo 2003). The doctor-patient relationship therefore leads to, rather than lessens, confusion and uncertainty for women at menopause, as doctors are at times unable to diagnose menopause exactly, provide a clear treatment plan, and/or pinpoint distinct markers of the experience in order to alleviate women's frustration (Tannenbaum, Nasmith, and Mayo 2003). As is clear in the above quotes, however, the operationalization of chronological age as menopause does not always match women's lived experience of reproductive aging. Yet, according to my sample of women, doctors sometimes rely on chronological age as a symptom of menopause in its own right, because of an absence of any other clarity about the experience; thus, a "young" chronological age can mask menopause. Or, perhaps because of the equation of women with reproductive activities over their life span, menopause is the only condition some doctors legitimate once women move beyond particular chronological ages.

Ultimately, when parallels are drawn between chronological age and menopause, women may be affected in ways that are not wholly positive. Based on the information my interviewees reported, it seems that the lack of clearly defined age and time boundaries to reproductive aging causes frustration and uncertainty for many, and often, doctors are as confused as women in terms of how to define women's menopausal status or treat their symptoms. Doctors' characterizations of women's experiences influence both women's treatment choices and their confidence in their own abilities to realize what is happening to their bodies. The end result is that women's health conditions are ignored and/or mistreated and women lose confidence in their own abilities to understand bodily transitions.

The findings above represent tentative results, in that the data about doctors' diagnoses of menopause were unprompted, and I did not fully explore this topic with my interviewees. Specifically, I should have probed more about the types of doctors they were visiting in each case, the types of treatment plans that followed different diagnoses, and the specific effects of these doctor-patient interactions on women. Moreover, the age and sex of the physician might matter in how much they understand about menopause and its variability. Nonetheless, my findings still highlight a need to continue problematizing an equation between chronological age and menopause and counter biomedical definitions of menopause more directly than we have, as menopausal women still feel constricted by age- and time-based definitions of their reproductive transitions. While feminist scholars have noted problems with the definitions of menopause in previous research, the idea that existing definitions potentially affect doctor-patient interactions and individual women's medical diagnoses is new and needs to be explored further.

Researching an Age- and Time-Defined Process or Maybe Not? Experiences in the Field

Before concluding about these findings, I suggest that researchers, including myself, also fall back on faulty equations of chronological age and reproductive aging when studying menopausal women—even when they know better. Despite reading feminist literature on the variability of menopause experiences and consciously realizing that existing clinical definitions of menopausal women and the average age of cessation reported in the literature might not coincide with interviewees' experiences, I still initially called for volunteers who considered themselves to be perimenopausal, menopausal, and postmenopausal when I began recruiting for this study in November 2000. In other words, I tried to use the three-stage medical definition of reproductive aging when looking for participants because I was uncertain as to what other language to use. I also planned to interview women between 50 and 60 years of age, since these are supposedly the years during which most women will enter and exit menopausal years (based on existing clinical literature[11]) and because I wanted to make sure that women I interviewed had been experiencing this reproductive transition long enough to answer questions about it. My adherence to medical definitions and previous literature, then, led me initially to limit the age range of my sample. I operationalized "menopausal women" partially through chronological age.

Quickly after I began recruiting, however, I confirmed that the age range I had picked for respondents did not match women's actual experiences. Early on women in their 40s contacted me, telling me that they were menopausal and, if I wanted to extend the age range in which I was recruiting, that they would volunteer for the study. Eventually, women in their late 30s requested to be interviewed as well. A few months into recruitment and interviewing I also realized that women in their late 30s and early 40s could be menopausal or postmenopausal while women in their mid-50s could still be in perimenopause (Mansfield et al. 2004). Furthermore, because I wanted women to tell me a considerable amount about their feelings and experiences, the best time[12] to interview women seemed to be when they were in the heart of perimenopausal symptoms. I realized, however, that there was no way I could predict—using chronological age as a marker—when that would be. It was difficult to secure detailed information about menopausal symptoms (and therefore a rough estimate of menopausal status) before sitting in an interview with a woman. Eventually these recruitment experiences became data in and of themselves, in that they illustrated that there is no uniform experience of reproductive aging and that the links between menopause, time, and chronological age are often hazy.

This experience did not necessarily surprise me, yet it made me realize that I had fallen into the trap of trying to standardize my recruitment efforts and create a sample of women that had uniform experiences, when I should have known this was impossible. In addition, I finally realized that, in confining study participants to those over age 50, clinicians typically aim to study only those who are postmenopausal. Despite my initial readings of biomedical and feminist literature, I did not realize that clinicians do not study women who are recently perimenopausal. Nor did I realize until well into recruitment that the women I really wanted to interview were perimenopausal. Mansfield et al. (2004) make a similar point. If researchers desired to truly understand reproductive aging, they would interview a wider range of ages and stages of menopause. During my recruitment and data collection I also learned that most interviewees did not understand the distinctions between the three stages. Even a few women's doctors told them that they were in a different category than the three-part medical definition would denote.[13] Furthermore, the use of HRT makes these distinctions fuzzy because some women start taking HRT early on in perimenopause and then do not experience the same transitions between the three stages; these women would have to rely on doctors to administer laboratory tests (blood or otherwise) to figure out their stage. The same would be true for those who take a chemical method of birth control through the early stages of menopause, as was true for six women in my sample.

During later recruitment efforts, I simply called for participants who felt they were menopausal or going through "the change." I employed a broader definition, essentially re-operationalizing reproductive aging so that if women told me they were menopausal and reported symptoms of any kind, I agreed to interview them. I did not try to continue my attempts to distinguish the stage women were experiencing before I secured the interview. And despite what symptoms they reported or what stage I felt they represented, interviewees always reported being "menopausal" (as mentioned earlier). Thus, interviewees conceptualize the boundaries of menopause experiences differently from those in medical/clinical communities. My methodological experiences suggest that, for women in my sample, menopause is a broad process that often defies existing medical definitions and any age or time prescriptions. If I started the study over again, I would forgo any operationalization of menopause and allow women to define reproductive aging themselves, as ultimately this sample of interviewees and Mansfield et al.'s (2004) work should teach us all to do. As mentioned, there is other feminist work on this subject that suggests the need to pay attention to heterogeneity and variability in menopause (e.g., Deats and Lenker 1999; Greer 1993; Boston Women's Health Book Collective 1992; Winterich 2003). Individual researchers need to be ready to respond more to previous feminist work than fall back on biomedical or cultural definitions of when menopause happens.

In retrospect, I am embarrassed and disappointed in myself that I restricted recruitment efforts so much in the beginning stages of my study; nonetheless, this was a lesson for me in that it has forced me to think about the need to pay close attention to existing feminist literature in the conceptualization and operationalization steps of the research process. I suggest that other feminist scholars need to be ready to question the boundaries and definitions they begin research projects with as well, to learn from my experience. Even the most well-intentioned qualitative researcher can be caught up in a faulty equation of chronological age and menopause.

Conclusions

I present women's discussions of the contradictions between chronological age and menopause and details of my own research experience to suggest that chronological age—any age- and time-based definition for that matter—is not the best measure of women's menopausal experiences. My analysis of women's responses shows that there is no chronological age at which menopause naturally occurs or ceases; women report varying onsets and durations. And when physicians attempt to align menopause and chronological age, women's treatment choices are limited and women's confidence in their own bodies' symptoms is undermined. Thus the equation of menopause and chronological aging eventually affects women negatively, at the very least causing uncertainty and frustration and, at worst, causing incomplete medical treatment. A description of my recruitment and interviewing experiences also illustrates that chronological age, as well as existing medical definitions, can limit rather than expand scholarly efforts to understand menopause if a researcher is not careful in the beginning stages of her research.

My findings illustrate how women, doctors, and researchers still may attempt to use chronological age to define and understand a specific reproductive experience, even though age- and time-based definitions fall short of giving us a comprehensive picture of reproductive aging. In addition, a simple, three-stage, medical definition of reproductive aging may not work to increase our understanding of women's midlife experiences either, unless we are a bit more flexible in defining these three stages (Mansfield et al. 2004). I call for feminist scholars to explore more fully the links between chronological age and reproductive aging, as well as the importance women attach to chronological age as they engage in various midlife or aging experiences. At best, we have partial understandings of the meanings and experiences of both chronological age and menopause.

I also call for feminist scholars (including myself) to take on biomedical definitions and clinical operationalizations of menopause more directly, perhaps first taking back words like *menopause* and redefining them in our own terms like Mansfield et al. (2004) have begun to do. To fully respond to Koeske's and others' calls for broader biosocial research on health experiences such as reproductive aging, however, feminist scholars also need to be ready to challenge existing medical and cultural conceptualizations head on, coming out strongly and publicly against established definitions. We also need to be ready to engage in research on menopausal topics that have typically been the domain of biomedical researchers (e.g., definitional issues, doctors' diagnoses, physiological/biological experiences, women's apprehensions). Thus far, feminist research has not had the widespread impact on menopausal women that it could, for the knowledge gained from feminist scholarship often remains within the confines of feminist, academic publications. Even within academia it still remains marginalized.

Feminist scholars have carved out a niche within menopause research all their own; that is, feminist scholars have dedicated their time to studying the social contexts for menopause (Dillaway 2005; Koeske 1983; McCrea 1983; Oakley 1998). Now that we understand a little bit about these social contexts, it is time to broaden our conceptualizations of what is "okay" for feminists to study, and wrestle with the very definitions that are still hindering women from understanding and maneuvering their own health processes. In addition, perhaps we need to be more careful about introducing our ideas to larger audiences and not stopping our efforts when we find a happy home for our articles and books. We need to make sure that our research findings make it outside our feminist circles to larger health and gerontological circles, the women we research, and medical settings in which these women receive care. Perhaps this means we also should engage in some self-research to understand better why our ideas become stagnated in our own circles and have limited effects on medical fields, individual menopausal women, or sometimes researchers like myself currently working in the field.

My study is one of the largest qualitative projects to date on the meanings and experiences of reproductive aging in the United States. Nonetheless, my sample has limitations. First, my research is based on a snowball sample, so I cannot generalize my results to any group of menopausal women. Second, I rely solely on women's self-reports of symptoms, ages at onset and durations of reproductive aging, and their interactions with doctors. In future studies, scholars should match women's and doctors' diagnoses of menopause and complete longitudinal studies with women as they engage in reproductive aging, so as to better understand confusing and questionable links between chronological age and menopause. Researchers also should ask women more about the actual doctors they visit and the effects of doctors' diagnoses on their health outcomes. Third, while I present interviewees' race and class locations to illustrate potential commonalities across women in my sample, commonalities and differences by race and class must be explored further with a more diverse sample of women. More effort should be made in the beginning of data collection to secure a diverse sample as well, so that our interview guides are not skewed toward European American, middle-class populations (see my earlier discussion of the limitations of my focus groups in the "Methods" section). Finally, the impact of other social locations should be examined more fully, such as sexuality, national origin, marital status, or bodily ability.

Despite the limitations, this study contributes to feminist literature on menopause in several ways. First, I highlight the necessity of challenging existing definitions and operationalizations of menopause, as well as the taken-for-granted equation of chronological age and menopause. As feminist scholars, we must continue to critique medical knowledge as well as lay assumptions about women's experiences, and I point to ways we can continue to do so by paying more attention to the ways in which chronological age and confusing medical definitions are used to explain menopause. Second, in focusing on reproductive and aging contexts, I begin to remedy two key oversights in feminist scholarship on menopause. For the most part, we have left (1) the study of chronological age to other aging scholars and (2) the formulation of a basic definition of menopause to medical science. By doing so we have allowed reproductive aging to be equated with chronological aging and a questionable three-stage model for menopause that limits our understanding of women's experiences. Exploring the partial, confusing, and often misleading connections between chronological age and menopause is a complicated task, but I hope this essay begins to illustrate how we can push the boundaries of feminist analyses of menopause and aging further than we already have.

Acknowledgments

The author thanks Rita Gallin, Maxine Baca Zinn, Leni Marshall, and anonymous reviewers for suggestions on early drafts of this essay. The author also thanks Sonica Rehan for her research assistance and the 61 women who volunteered for this study.

Notes

1.   Fausto-Sterling's (1992) work and Mansfield et al.'s (2004) article are important exceptions.

2.   All three of these women may be told by others she is menopausal or "going through menopause" since the colloquial definition of menopause generally refers to all three medically defined stages, despite the fact that this may go against medical characterizations.

3.   Some research shows that menopausal symptoms appear at every stage of life (Fausto-Sterling 1992; Gannon and Ekstrom 1993; McKinlay, Brambilla, and Posner 1992; Rostosky and Travis 1996), and that these symptoms are not always experienced negatively (Weed 1999; Woods 1999). Social scientists and even some clinicians therefore question the very notion of menopausal symptoms. So far only hot flashes or hot flushes are clearly linked to menopause. Some research even counters this connection (Fausto-Sterling 1992; Lock 1993; McKinlay, Brambilla, and Posner 1992; Rostosky and Travis 1996). Because clinicians draw their data from clinical samples that include a very high proportion of women who have had hysterectomies and postmenopausal women, their results are often only partial and lead to false assumptions about the incidence of menopausal symptoms, problems, and/or the effects of certain treatments (Fausto-Sterling 1992; Im, Meleis, and Park 1999; Lock 1993; Rostosky and Travis 1996). Furthermore, the definition of a symptom is complicated. In other words, is a symptom something to be worried about? Clinicians who espouse biomedical models may designate changes in women's physiology/biology as negative and/or in need of "fixing," whereas women themselves may note the changes in their bodies but characterize them as neutral or positive changes (Dillaway 2005; Fausto-Sterling 1992; Woods 1999). Thus it is what symptoms or bodily changes signify that is confusing, thereby prompting us to ask whether there are truly menopausal symptoms at all. Further, the fact that menopause coincides with other processes of chronological aging complicates this matter,

because no one knows which symptoms are strictly menopausal and which symptoms simply parallel the process (Fausto-Sterling 1992).

4. While variability in menopause experiences has been highlighted as a finding in previous feminist work (e.g., Deats and Lenker 1999; Fausto-Sterling, 1992; Greer 1993; Kaufert, Gilbert, and Tate 1987; Pearsall 1997; Boston Women's Health Book Collective 1992), Mansfield et al. (2004) are one of the first to state directly that research should include a wide age range.

5. Calasanti (2004), Lysack and Seipke (2002), Twigg (2004), Silver (2003), and Morell (2003) are some important exceptions. All of these authors suggest that gendered experiences make aging unique for women, and that women will have different experiences of aging processes as a whole because of the gendered contexts of their lives. These authors have not yet analyzed chronological age specifically, however.

6. My rationale in developing a separate questionnaire is similar to that of Morell (1994), in that demographic and reproductive history information are important background information, yet are not the subject of the interview guide (see also Creswell 2003). Because I desired this information for analytical purposes yet did not want to use interview time, I initially had women complete the questionnaire after interviews. Filling out the questionnaire while I was present, however, made some women uncomfortable due to questionnaire length (five pages) and the open-ended nature of reproductive history questions. Midway through data collection I allowed women to mail questionnaires back to me; inevitably this led to nonresponse problems. Fifty women (82 percent) completed questionnaires. In retrospect, I would shorten the questionnaire or offer incentives to mail it back.

7. This includes six women (approximately 10 percent) who were on some form of birth control pill to regulate early perimenopausal symptoms.

8. Even chronic illnesses are defined via time (chronic meaning lasting a long time). Menopause, though, is not defined as a "chronic" condition. A few women did make comparisons between other chronic conditions they faced (e.g., arthritis, back pain, multiple sclerosis) and menopause, suggesting that menopause was more frustrating than these conditions sometimes because it was supposed to be a finite process but was not. Thus they could deal with conditions defined as "chronic" better than menopause, simply because the definitions of the former seemed to match their experiences of them.

9. While I did not ask women specifically about the types of doctors they visited, I gathered from women's conversations that many of the doctors were OB/GYNs; future research should follow up on the types of doctors from which menopausal women seek care and whether the type of doctor influences the way in which a woman is treated.

10. Blood tests sometimes were done to secure diagnoses. Yet, women seemed to think that doctors' characterization of their symptoms was almost always related to their chronological age.

11. Most women are 50 years or older when they participate in clinical menopausal research (Brett and Madans 1997; Kaufert and Gilbert 1986).

12. When I say "best" here, I mean in terms of information gathering (e.g., what they can remember about their experiences, how much they know about what they're going through, and/or whether they themselves have been thinking about the process).

13. This makes sense in light of Mansfield et al.'s (2004) recent reports of women flip-flopping between menopausal stages.

References

Boston Women's Health Book Collective. 1992. *The New Our Bodies, Ourselves.* New York: Touchstone Books.

Brett, Kate, and Jennifer Madans. 1997. "Use of Postmenopausal Hormone Replacement Therapy: Estimates from a Nationally Representative Cohort Study." *American Journal of Epidemiology 145*: 536–45.

Calasanti, Toni. 2004. "New Directions in Feminist Gerontology: An Introduction." *Journal of Aging Studies 18*(1): 1–8.

Callahan, Joan C., ed. 1993. *Menopause: A Midlife Passage.* Bloomington: Indiana University Press.

Coney, Sandra. 1993. *The Menopause Industry: A Guide to Medicine's Discovery of the Mid-Life Woman.* North Melbourne, Victoria: Pinifex.

Cremin, Mary C. 1992. "Feeling Old Versus Being Old: Views of Troubled Aging." *Social Science & Medicine 34*(12): 1305–15.

Creswell, John W. 2003. *Research Design: Qualitative, Quantitative, and Mixed Methods Approaches.* Thousand Oaks, CA: Sage Publications.

Deats, Sara. M., and Lagretta T. Lenker. 1999. *Aging and Identity: A Humanities Perspective.* Westport, CT: Praeger Publishers.

Dillaway, Heather E. 2005. "Menopause is the 'Good Old': Women's Thoughts about Reproductive Aging." *Gender & Society 19*(3): 398–417.

Fausto-Sterling, Anne. 1992. *Myths of Gender.* New York: Basic Books.

Featherstone, Mike, and Mike Hepworth. 1991. "The Mask of Ageing and the Postmodern Life Course." In *The Body: Social Process and Cultural Theory,* ed. Mike Featherstone, Mike Hepworth, and Bryan Turner, 371–89. London: Sage Publications.

Frey, Karen A. 1981. "Middle-Aged Women's Experience and Perceptions of Menopause." *Women & Health 6*: 25–36.

Gannon, Linda. 1999. *Women and Aging: Transcending the Myths.* New York: Routledge.

Gannon, Linda, and Bonnie Ekstrom. 1993. "Attitudes Toward Menopause: The Influence of Sociocultural Paradigms." *Psychology of Women Quarterly 17*: 275–88.

Gold, Ellen B., Joyce Bromberger, Sybil Crawford, Steve Samuels, Gail A. Greendale, Sioban D. Harlow, and Joan Skurnick. 2001. "Factors Associated with Age at Natural Menopause in a Multiethnic Sample of Midlife Women." *American Journal of Epidemiology 153*(9): 865–75.

Greer, Germaine. 1993. *The Change: Women, Aging, and the Menopause*. New York: A. Knopf.

Grossman, Marilyn, and Pauline Bart. 1982. "Taking the Men out of Menopause." In *Biological Woman: The Convenient Myth*, ed. Ruth Hubbard, Mary Sue Henifin, and Barbara Fried, 185–206. Cambridge, MA: Schenkman.

Hunt, Kate. 1988. "Perceived Value of Treatment Among a Group of Long-Term Users of Hormone Replacement Therapy." *Journal of the Royal College of General Practitioners* (September): 398–401.

Im, Eun-Ok, Afaf Ibrahim Meleis, and Young Sook Park. 1999. "A Feminist Critique of Research on Menopausal Experience of Korean Women." *Research in Nursing and Health 22*(5): 410–20.

Jones, Vida Yvonne, and Carroll J. Estes. 1997. "Older Women: Income, Retirement and Health." In *Women's Health: Complexities and Differences*, ed. Sheryl B. Ruzek, Virginia L. Olesen, and Adele E. Clarke, 425–45. Columbus: Ohio University Press.

Kaufert, Patricia, and Penny Gilbert. 1986. "Women, Menopause, and Medicalization." *Culture, Medicine and Psychiatry 10*: 7–21.

Kaufert, Patricia, Penny Gilbert, and Robyn Tate. 1987. "Defining Menopausal Status: The Impact of Longitudinal Data." *Maturitas 9*: 217–26.

Kaufman, Gayle, and Glen Elder, Jr. 2002. "Revisiting Age Identity: A Research Note." *Journal of Aging Studies 16*: 169–76.

Koeske, Randi D. 1983. "Lifting the Curse of Menstruation: Toward a Feminist Perspective on the Menstrual Cycle." *Women & Health 8*: 1–15.

Komesaroff, Paul, Philipa Rothfield, and Jeanne Daly, eds. 1997. *Reinterpreting Menopause: Cultural and Philosophical Issues*. New York: Routledge.

Lawlor, Debbie A., Shah Ebrahim, and George Davey Smith. 2003. "The Association of Socio-Economic Position Across the Life Course and Age at Menopause: The British Women's Heart and Health Study." *BJOG: An International Journal of Obstetrics & Gynecology 110*(12): 1078.

Laz, Cheryl. 2003. "Age Embodied." *Journal of Aging Studies 17*: 503–19.

Lock, Margaret. 1993. *Encounters with Aging: Mythologies of Menopause in Japan and North America*. Berkeley: University of California Press.

Lysack, Cathy, and Heather Seipke. 2002. "Communicating the Occupational Self: A Qualitative Study of Oldest-Old American Women." *Scandinavian Journal of Occupational Therapy 9*: 130–39.

Mansfield, Phyllis K., Molly Carey, Amy Anderson, Susannah H. Barsom, and Patricia B. Koch. 2004. "Staging the Menopausal Transition: Data from the Tremin Research Program on Women's Health." *Women's Health Issues 14*: 220–26.

Markson, Elizabeth W., and Beth B. Hess. 1997. "Older Women in the City." In *The Other Within Us: Feminist Explorations of Women and Aging*, ed. Marilyn Pearsall, 57–72. Boulder, CO: Westview Press.

Martin, Emily 1992. *The Woman in the Body: A Cultural Analysis of Reproduction.* 2nd ed. Boston: Beacon Press.

McCrea, Frances B. 1983. "The Politics of Menopause: The 'Discovery' of a Deficiency Disease." *Social Problems 31:* 111–23.

McElmurry, Beverly, and Donna Huddleston. 1991. "Self-Care and Menopause: Critical Review of Research." *Health Care for Women International 12:* 15–26.

McKinlay, Sonja M., Donald J. Brambilla, and Jennifer G. Posner. 1992. "The Normal Menopause Transition." *Maturitas 14:* 103–15.

Morell, Carolyn M. 2003. "Empowerment and Long-Living Women: Return to the Rejected Body." *Journal of Aging Studies* 17(1): 69–85.

———. 1994. *Unwomanly Conduct: The Challenges of Intentional Childlessness.* New York: Routledge.

Oakley, Ann. 1998. "Science, Gender, and Women's Liberation: An Argument against Postmodernism." *Women's Studies International Forum 21:* 133–46.

Pearsall, Marilyn, ed. 1997. *The Other Within Us: Feminist Explorations of Women and Aging.* Boulder, CO: Westview Press.

Ray, Ruth. 2004. "Toward the Croning of Feminist Gerontology." *Journal of Aging Studies* 18(1): 109–21.

Reinharz, Shulamit. 1997. "Friends or Foes: Gerontological and Feminist Theory." In *The Other Within Us: Feminist Explorations of Women and Aging,* ed. Marilyn Pearsall, 73–94. Boulder, CO: Westview Press.

Reynolds, Robert F., and Carla M. Obermeyer. 2003. "Correlates of the Age at Natural Menopause in Morocco." *Annals of Human Biology* 30(1): 97–108.

Riessman, Catherine Kohler. 1983. "Women and Medicalization: A New Perspective." *Social Policy* (Summer): 3–18.

Roberts, Paula. 1991. "The Menopause and Hormone Replacement Therapy: Views of Women in General Practice Receiving Hormone Replacement Therapy." *British Journal of General Practice* (October): 421–24.

Rostosky, Sharon, and Cheryl Travis. 1996. "Menopause Research and the Dominance of the Biomedical Model 1984–1994." *Psychology of Women Quarterly* 20: 285–312.

Rubin, Herbert, and Irene Rubin. 1995. *Qualitative Interviewing: The Art of Hearing Data.* London: Sage Publications.

Silver, Catherine. 2003. "Gendered Identities in Old Age: Toward (De)Gendering?" *Journal of Aging Studies* 17(4): 379–97.

Sontag, Susan. 1997. "The Double Standard of Aging." In *The Other Within Us: Feminist Explorations of Women and Aging,* ed. Marilyn Pearsall, 19–24. Boulder, CO: Westview Press.

Tannenbaum, Cara B., Louise Nasmith, and Nancy Mayo. 2003. "Understanding Older Women's Health Care Concerns: A Qualitative Study." *Journal of Women and Aging* 15(1): 103–16.

Twigg, Julia. 2004. "The Body, Gender, and Age: Feminist Insights in Social Gerontology." *Journal of Aging Studies* 18(1): 59–73.

Voda, Ann. 1992. "Menopause: A Normal View." *Clinical Obstetrics and Gynecology* 35:923–33.

Weed, Susan. 1999. "Menopause and Beyond: The Wise Woman Way." *Journal of Nurse-Midwifery* 44(3): 267–79.

Winterich, Julie. 2003. "Sex, Menopause, and Culture: Sexual Orientation and the Meaning of Menopause for Women's Sex Lives." *Gender & Society* 17(4): 627–42.

Woods, Nancy Fugate. 1999. "Midlife Women's Health: Conflicting Perspectives of Health Care Providers and Midlife Women and Consequences for Health." In *Revisioning Women, Health and Healing: Feminist, Cultural, and Technoscience Perspectives*, ed. Adele Clarke and Virginia Olesen. 343–54. New York: Routledge.

Zita, Jacquelyn. 1997. "The Premenstrual Syndrome: 'Dis-easing' the Female Cycle." In *Feminism and Science*, ed. N. Tuana, 188–210. Bloomington: Indiana University Press.

CHAPTER NINE

What Have We Learned? An Historical View
of the Society for Menstrual Cycle Research

ALICE J. DAN

Establishing the Society for Menstrual Cycle Research

The menstrual cycle encompasses biological, psychological, social, and cultural phenomena and can provide a model for thinking about mind-body relationships. Yet its history in human experience has been largely one of avoidance. Even feminists have been leery of too much attention to menstruation. A well-known biologist, one of the founding mothers of the Association for Women in Science, refused to make a keynote presentation at the first interdisciplinary menstrual cycle research conference in 1977 because she believed it was unwise to focus on things that make us different from men. As she said, "They will use it against us." I do not dispute the accuracy of her conclusion, but I disagree with her implication that we ought not to study menstruation. Menstruation has been, and unfortunately may well continue to be, used against women, but this is not a reason for us to avoid looking at it. In fact, it is preferable that feminists develop our own menstrual cycle and women's health research, precisely because we cannot trust conclusions drawn from studies based on patriarchal assumptions about women. And this is a key theme of my exploration: how can we gain knowledge to use for women's health in an oppressive patriarchal context? Or stated differently, what is the emancipatory potential of menstrual cycle research?

When the first conference was held in 1977, ibuprofen had only recently been approved for treatment of dysmenorrhea and was not yet available over the counter. It was not acceptable to mention menstruation on TV or radio, let alone to advertise menstrual products on those media. In 2003, menstrual cramps are easier to manage, and it seems that there is greater social comfort with speaking of menstruation, although it is still usually referred to in indirect, vague, or coded ways.

The 1977 conference was an historic event, bringing together researchers and women's health advocates from many disciplines to focus on women's experiences related to menstruation (see Appendix 1). The conference embodied the energy and enthusiasm of the reemerging women's movement, representing "a gathering wave of new work" in the area

Originally published in the Fall 2004 issue (vol. 16, no. 3).

(Dan, Graham, and Beecher 1980, 2). Before the conference ended, the second and third interdisciplinary conferences had been planned for the following years; between the second conference in St. Louis (1978) and the third in Tucson (1979), the Society for Menstrual Cycle Research was incorporated.

During the St. Louis conference, a steering committee was selected to represent the broad range of constituencies interested in menstrual cycle research. Lengthy discussions resulted in the choice of a name for our Society—an important basis for legitimating our work. Although we were cognizant of our broader interests in women's health, it was clear that the Society for Menstrual Research would have a unique function. Membership in the Society was and is open to individuals who have an interest in research on the menstrual cycle or related issues and who support the purposes of the Society (see Appendix 2). Although the Society has remained relatively small (currently about 160 members), it has shown remarkable survival skills through difficult times. We have continued to offer a network of support and communication that spans disciplines, professional responsibilities, and geography to provide women-centered perspectives on menstrual experiences. Significant contributions of the Society include the 15 conferences held to date, with at least 14 published volumes of research. More information is available at the Society's Web site (www.pop.psu.edu/smcr/).

Valuing women's experiences and seeing research questions from women's perspectives have been key aspects of the feminist approach to research adopted by the Society. Early in the Society's history, a sympathetic male researcher suggested that funding would be more readily forthcoming if the Society redefined itself as concerned with reproduction, "because menstruation is just one part of the reproductive cycle." Society members replied that from a woman's perspective, reproduction could also be seen as just one aspect of the menstrual cycle. "Untangling the knot patriarchy has made of this basic life experience" (Culpepper 1992, 282), the menstrual cycle, is no easy project. If we don't recognize that the larger societal context may distort our intentions, we can end up harming as much as helping women's health. I've identified several key arenas of menstrual-related research below. Each offers a vantage point from which to learn about the interactions of feminist intentions with patriarchal systems. The arenas chosen include hormone therapy, toxic shock syndrome, perimenstrual symptoms, and menstrual suppression.

Hormone Therapy

Many of us in the Society felt vindicated by the recent release of yet another round of reports from the Women's Health Initiative (WHI) study showing that Prempro (combination estrogen/progestin hormone therapy) does not show the promised positive effects for postmenopausal women and, in fact, produces unanticipated negative risks for many women. In a paper on "The Politics of Menopause" given at the first conference in 1977, Pauline Bart and Marilyn Grossman noted, "The one fact that most frequently prevails is that we live in a capitalistic society in which there is a great deal of money to be made from the successful marketing of menopause" (Grossman and Bart 1980, 179). At that time, estrogen therapy had been widely prescribed to women at menopause, but it had also been definitively documented as a significant risk factor for endometrial cancer. As Grossman and Bart noted, the manufacturer of Premarin (then Ayerst laboratories) had launched a public relations campaign for their product, and for its reformulation, which included progestin, purported to reduce the risk of uterine cancer. Despite the lack of randomized clinical trial evidence to support many of the claims for positive effects of combination hormone therapy, most medical practitioners remained convinced of its efficacy until 2002, when the WHI first began reporting higher health risks for women taking hormone therapy. Why did it take so long (25 years) to get this evidence?

Think about what it has taken since 1977 to produce the evidence that women have needed to evaluate hormone therapy:

- It took *all* of the major feminist health groups raising questions over and over and over again to focus attention on the safety of long-term hormone therapies. In particular, the National Women's Health Network and Our Bodies, Ourselves (aka the Boston Women's Health Book Collective) were tireless advocates, but many other groups, including our Society, voiced doubts and lobbied for better evidence.
- It took women working together inside and outside of government, in corporations, at universities, and especially in communities everywhere to build a constituency for women's health.
- It took Pat Schroeder, Olympia Snowe, and all the other women in Congress to stand up for us and demand attention to women's health issues.
- It took the Medical Women's Health Movement, finally getting on board in the early 1990s, to put women's health on the public agenda (see Weisman 1998).
- It took Bernadine Healy, the first woman director of the National Institutes of Health, to make the Women's Health Initiative a top priority.
- It took the "Mother of all clinical trials"—the WHI—a study involving more than 150,000 women, and more than 50 investigators over more than thirteen years to provide sound and representative data on women.

- And let's not forget that it also took men who can listen, who are honest
  and truly curious, who are not in the pockets of medical industries, to
  take women's health concerns, research priorities, and activism seriously.

So we need to congratulate ourselves, and all who have been involved,
because it took a lot to get this research done—to get the information
that women will need to make good decisions about their health during
the menopausal and postmenopausal years.

The Society's Role in Shaping Health Information about Toxic Shock Syndrome

One of the big women's health issues in the 1970s was the alarming
"outbreak" of lethal cases of toxic shock syndrome (TSS) that sprang up
in healthy young women as a result of the introduction of synthetic fiber
materials into menstrual tampons. The Boston Women's Health Book
Collective was one of the first advocacy groups to call for government
investigations and improved safety reforms in the tampon industry. In
1980, the U.S. Food and Drug Administration (FDA) took action, based
on evidence of the link between super-absorbent tampons and the incidence of TSS. The agency worked with the tampon industry to remove
the brand that had been most associated with TSS and to place warnings
about TSS on or in the tampon boxes. Finally in 1982, the FDA began
requiring that the warning include advice to use the least absorbent tampon needed. "Unfortunately, the advice to use the least absorbent tampon necessary was meaningless because there was no way to compare
the absorbencies of different brands of tampons in the absence of uniform absorbency labeling" (Rome and Wolhandler 1992, 261). Considerable pressure was needed to produce further action, but finally in 1982, a
voluntary task force was convened to consider the issue of tampon
standards.

Society members Nancy Reame, a nurse and reproductive physiologist
at the University of Michigan, and Esther Rome, of the Boston Women's
Health Book Collective, collaborated as nonindustry members of the FDA
task force to set new tampon safety and labeling guidelines. As part of that
effort, Dr. Reame replicated tampon absorbency studies in her lab and
compared her findings to those of each of the tampon companies (Reame,
Delonis, and Lewis 1987). A series of scientific and policy publications
emanated from this FDA initiative, which eventually transformed industry labeling standards. Some of this work is summarized in Chapter 12 of
the now classic women's health "bible," *Our Bodies, Ourselves*. Esther
Rome reported back to the Society on these developments at the 1985 conference (Rome and Wolhandler 1992).

The task force experience was frustrating because there was a serious power imbalance between consumers and manufacturers, whose respective interests were polarized. There were more industry than consumer representatives, and the industry representatives were paid for their time, had all expenses covered, and were provided with other forms of assistance and support by their employers. In the end, the manufacturers agreed to provide funds to the convening agency to cover travel and limited other expenses for the nonindustry reps, but the consumers were never paid for their time.

The major issues for consumers were: (1) standard absorbency labels, so women could judge the relative absorbency of different products for themselves; (2) product safety testing, so new materials or designs would not prove more harmful than products already on the market; and (3) independent research with publicly available results, to hold manufacturers accountable for safety and effectiveness. Manufacturers, on the other hand, wanted: (1) the freedom to label products in whatever ways their market research suggested would sell more products; (2) the ability to change products at will, using new materials, new designs, or new production methods without subjecting them to safety testing; and (3) protection of their "trade secrets" from competitors (see Rome and Wolhandler 1992 for more details). The task force deadlocked over these differences. After further petitions, letters, a congressional report, and demands from the consumer representatives on the task force, the FDA agreed in 1985 to issue a mandatory absorbency disclosure rule. It was not until 1989, however, that labeling regulations were finally issued, following a series of successful lawsuits and letter-writing campaigns by consumer groups.

These experiences illustrate the political nature of protecting women's health in the current marketplace. Manufacturers have powerful advantages that consumer groups often lack, such as access to lobbyists, technical and legal advice, and financial resources. Even so, and despite many obstacles, advocates for women's health were able to achieve some of their objectives by becoming part of the political process. Most important, consumers gained familiarity with the perspectives of all parties, in both government and industry. They became acquainted with the individuals involved and came to understand their respective motivations. In addition, they learned about the routes of action available to them as consumers, including the FDA's Device Experience Network, which maintains complaint records accessible to the public (Rome and Wolhandler 1992). Letter-writing campaigns and legal action also proved to be important tools: consumer representatives' familiarity with the situation enabled them to maximize their timing and take advantage of opportunities for collaboration among advocate groups. Their perseverance paid off, resulting in the establishment of a rational system of labeling requirements, nearly ten years after the FDA's recognition of the need for action.

Perimenstrual Symptoms

I don't menstruate anymore. As a student of the menstrual cycle, I recall my last menstrual period with vividness. In May of 1993 I gave a paper as part of a panel on Premenstrual Symptoms at the Annual Meeting of the American Psychiatric Association (APA). I wondered what the audience would think if I told them I was menstruating. I considered that kind of openness way too scary to be tempting and knew it would be perceived as very unprofessional. I needed to retire in order to even write about this!

The 1993 Premenstrual Symptoms symposium at APA in San Francisco proved to be very interesting (see Gold and Severino 1994 for papers). It included women who had brought the best science available to the crafting of the then-newly formulated psychiatric diagnosis of Pre-Menstrual Dysphoric Disorder (PMDD).[1] These women, including Judith Gold, Nada Stotland, Barbara Parry, and Sally Severino, carefully outlined the required and optional symptoms of PMDD. They differentiated it from premenstrual exacerbation of depression and from the physical symptoms referred to as Premenstrual Syndrome, or PMS. They specifically emphasized the relative rarity of true PMDD, which is incapacitating by definition. They elaborated the concern of women's health advocates regarding over-diagnosis. During the discussion, the first comment, offered by a young male psychiatrist, was that he saw women with PMDD all the time in his practice, and thought that the symposium presenters were under-estimating its incidence. Hmmm, I thought; I wonder what this means about how the diagnosis will be used in practice? It apparently fills a need that is different from the one intended by its framers.

This example teaches us what often happens to women's work, and women's experience, in a patriarchal context that disregards or reinterprets women's knowledge. The men "know" about menstruation; they know that it is incapacitating, on the basis of their personal or clinical experiences. The thoughtful analysis, circumscribed meanings, or careful research put forth by feminists may not survive such recycling.

Society members like Diana Taylor, whose recent book (Taylor and Colino 2003) is an important resource on premenstrual symptoms, and Nancy Woods (Woods, Most, and Dery 1982; Woods, Mitchell, and Lentz 1995), to mention only two, have pioneered approaches that both validate women's experiences of symptoms *and* refuse to over-medicalize women's bodies. Symptoms are viewed in holistic perspective rather than as manifestations of disease; they are understood as outcomes of multiple factors in women's lives, rather than as directly "caused" by the hormonal changes of the menstrual cycle. In addition, these feminist researchers have studied large numbers of diverse women in the community over many cycles, rather than depending exclusively on clinical populations of women who seek treatment at health care facilities. They have emphasized the context of women's lives, with attention to stress, for example, and its impact on premenstrual symptoms. And they promote awareness of one's own body and the development of coping skills as treatment options rather than over-reliance on powerful medications like Sarafem, a repackaged version of the antidepressant Prozac being marketed for PMDD.

Menstruation Suppression

The latest challenge to our efforts to understand the menstrual cycle in ways that will support women's health is emerging as we speak. The new medication, Seasonale, has recently been approved by the FDA for use as a menstrual suppressant. Young women are being encouraged to take this oral contraceptive-like formulation as a way of avoiding about two-thirds of their menstrual bleeding episodes. As reported in the *Washington Post*, 3 March 2003:

> Experimental Pill Puts Menstruation on Hold
> Seasonale Expects FDA Approval Soon
>
> "I love it," said one young woman. "My friends all know all about it because I rant and rave about it" (A.01).

As discussed by a Society member, menstrual suppression is also "all the rage" in Brazil, where the developer of Depo Provera has declared that "menstruation is obsolete" (Elson 2003).

What are we to make of this development, which might lead large numbers of young women to take hormones continuously through most of their adult lives? Negative views of menstruation in society have been widely accepted, by both men and women. Now there are "scientific" claims that today's women menstruate "too much": based on studies of hunter-gatherer societies in which women were frequently pregnant, lactating, or insufficiently nourished to menstruate, it has been suggested that menstruating each month throughout adulthood is "unnatural." Pro-suppression authors also say that menstruation represents "reproductive failure" and that repeated exposure to high estrogen levels during the cycle is unhealthy, contributing to cancer.

The pro-suppression literature contradicts the view that menstruation is a sign of health and fertility. Clearly this issue is one that requires feminist investigation and critique. We need to point out the essentialist error of assuming that what was true for women in a long-ago context is somehow more "natural" than what contemporary women experience (see the Society Web site for an informative position paper). And we need to counter the negative views that make menstruation an easy target for new drugs and an ever-widening medicalization of women's bodies. By learning from past experiences we can use tools like the FDA reporting system to record recurring problems. We should remember that woman-centered menstrual health research need not take place only in universities. It begins when women start to validate their own experiences, or when determined feminists challenge the medical and drug industry's "business as usual."

What Have We Learned?

Despite the endurance of male domination in medicine, business, and politics, women's health researchers and advocates have accomplished some key successes contributing to women's well-being. The significance of research has certainly been demonstrated: that providing clear evidence to support our case can change minds. This is the importance of the Women's Health Initiative study, which has had a tremendous impact on women's lives and on doctors' prescribing practices. From the magnitude of the efforts required to achieve this major victory, over a period of more than 25 years, we also learn how important it is to collaborate across disciplinary, class, and gender boundaries and to persist in the face of setbacks. While research has a key role to play, without broad support from many sectors of society, the resources to undertake studies may not be available. This underlines the need to support advocacy groups, like the National Women's Health Network, whose mission is to organize and lobby for women's health.

The Society's experience in helping to put in place regulations for tampon manufacturing and labeling was instructive in additional ways, showing us some of the processes at work in the agencies whose support we need to hold industries accountable for their impact on women's health. The value of knowing how regulatory and legislative efforts work and how to influence them is clear. Perhaps most impressive is the courage and determination of those who volunteer to represent us in this difficult arena.

Perimenstrual symptoms remain a complex and controversial area of practice. In February 2002, together with other groups, the Society presented a congressional briefing questioning the evidence for PMDD and recommending against direct-to-consumer marketing for Sarafem (see the Society's Web site for a newsletter report of the briefing). As reported in the *British Medical Journal* recently (Moynihan 2004). European regulators have forced the removal of PMDD as an indication for prescription of fluoxitine (Prozac). The need for balanced, women-empowering perspectives remains critical. The difficulties that women have with perimenstrual symptoms are not unrelated to the issues surrounding the new menstrual suppression drugs. In this instance as well, the negative social views of menstruation are likely to influence healthy women's use of powerful medications over potentially many years. In both instances, we know that for some women, these medications can be helpful. However, as with homone therapy at menopause, we don't want to see marketing efforts to extend the usage far beyond the groups that will truly benefit. Women must continue to demand the evidence to judge the benefits and risks for themselves.

As a support structure for researchers and others interested in women's health, the Society for Menstrual Cycle Research has provided leadership and a forum for feminist intellectual community. Our commitment to providing evidence to enhance women's well-being brings many different individuals together around the table. The examples here represent only a small sampling of the ways that women's health research is generated and used by feminists, as well as how feminists can critique the larger health research establishment and demand accountability. Clearly this is a continuing conversation, and I invite you to be a participant.

Appendix 1

A Sampling of Participants in the First Interdisciplinary Research Conference on the Menstrual Cycle

Chronobiologists: Franz Halberg, Michael Smolensky

Nurse researchers: Effie Graham (co-director of 1977 conference), Pauline Komnenich (director of 1978 conference), Ann Voda (co-director of 1979 conference), Harriet Werley (provided seed funding for 1977 conference), Margaret Williams, Nancy Woods (co-director of 1983 and 1991 conferences)

Psychologists: Jeanne Brooks-Gunn, Sharon Golub (director of 1981 conference), Randi Koeske, Perry Nicassio, Mary Parlee, Anne Petersen, Diane Ruble, Barbara Sommer

Sociologists: Pauline Bart, Alice Rossi

Women's health activists: Suzann Gage, Francie Hornstein, Lorraine Rothman

Appendix 2
Purposes of the Society for Menstrual Cycle Research

- to identify research priorities, to recommend research strategies, and to promote interdisciplinary woman-centered research on the menstrual cycle.
- to provide a formal communication network to facilitate interdisciplinary dialogue about menstrual cycle events in the context of women's health over the life span.
- to examine the practical, ethical, and policy issues surrounding menstrual cycle research.
- to generate and exchange information and to promote public discussion of issues related to the menstrual cycle.
- to influence public policy for the enhancement of women's health.

Note

1. This experimental diagnosis had previously been called Late Luteal Dysphoric Disorder, or L2D2, but nobody could figure out what or when that was supposed to be!

References

Boston Women's Health Collective. 1998. *Our Bodies, Ourselves: For the New Millennium*. New York: Touchstone.

Culpepper, Emily E. 1992. "Menstruation Consciousness Raising: A Personal and Pedagogical Process." In *Menstrual Health in Women's Lives*, ed. Alice J. Dan and Linda L. Lewis, 274–84. Champaign: University of Illinois Press.

Dan, Alice J., Effie A. Graham, and Carol P. Beecher. 1980. *The Menstrual Cycle: A Synthesis of Interdisciplinary Research*. New York: Springer.

Elson, Jean. 2003. "Manipulating Menstruation Is Misguided." *Society for Menstrual Cycle Research Newsletter*, Winter issue, 4–5.

Gold, Judith H., and Sally K. Severino. eds. 1994. *Premenstrual Dysphorias: Myths and Realities*. Washington, DC: American Psychiatric Press.

Greer, Germaine. 1999. *The Whole Woman*. London: Doubleday.

Grossman, Pauline, and Pauline Bart. 1980. "The Politics of Menopause." In *The Menstrual Cycle*: Volume 1—*A Synthesis of Interdisciplinary Research*, ed. Alice J. Dan, Effie A. Graham, and Carol P. Beecher, 179–85. New York: Springer.

Moynihan, Ray. 2004. "Controversial Disease Dropped from Prozac Product Information." *British Medical Journal*, *328*, 365.

Reame, Nancy E., Susan Delonis, and Ruth Lewis. 1987. "Menstrual Tampons: Changes in Absorbency and Styles since 1982." Paper presented at the Seventh Conference of the Society for Menstrual Cycle Research, Ann Arbor, MI.

Rome, Esther, and Jill Wolhandler. 1992. "Can Tampon Safety Be Regulated?" In *Menstrual Health in Women's Lives*, ed. Alice J. Dan and Linda L. Lewis, 261–73. Champaign. University of Illinois Press.

Taylor, Diana, and Stacey Colino. 2003. *Taking Back the Month: A Personalized Solution for Managing PMS and Enhancing Your Health*. Perigee/Putnam Penguin.

Weisman, Carol. 1998. *Women's Health Care: Activist Traditions and Institutional Change*. Baltimore: Johns Hopkins University Press.

Woods, Nancy, Ada Most, and Gretchen Dery. 1982. "Prevalence of Perimenstrual Symptoms." *American Journal of Public Health*, 72, 1257–64.

Woods, Nancy, Ellen Mitchell, and Martha Lentz. 1995. "Social Pathways to Premenstrual Symptoms." *Research in Nursing and Health*, 18, 225–37.

CHAPTER TEN

Hormone Replacement Therapy (HRT): Getting to the Heart of the Politics of Women's Health?

NANCY WORCESTER

> *The widespread popularity of hormone replacement therapy in the United States is a triumph of marketing over science and advertising over common sense.*
>
> —NATIONAL WOMEN'S HEALTH NETWORK (2002, XII)

On July 9, 2002, the National Institutes of Health announced that the hormone replacement therapy (HRT), estrogen/progestin portion, of the largest hormone study to ever be done on healthy women was being stopped. Approximately three years before any results were expected, scientific investigators for the Women's Health Initiative (WHI) already had information they knew they had to share with the participants in the study and the public: the risks of estrogen plus progestin outweighed the benefits. Specifically, the study had shown that women taking HRT had a 26 percent increase in breast cancer, a 41 percent increase in strokes, and a 200 percent increase in the rates of blood clots in legs and lungs (National Women's Health Network [NWHN], 2002). Later analysis of the studies also showed that HRT does not improve "quality of life" issues or memory. The "good news" often highlighted by reporters who had sung the praises of HRT for years was that women taking HRT had 37 percent less colon cancer and 34 percent fewer hip fractures.

The Personal Is Political

Approximately six million women in the United States were taking HRT that day when headlines everywhere announced that, instead of preventing heart disease, this most important study had shown that hormone "replacement" therapy increased a healthy woman's risk of heart disease (Spake 2002). What were women to do with this news? What did women do with this news? One crucial question this essay asks is whether the HRT story was one where women saw that "the personal is political," or did six million women simply feel that "the personal is personal"? Instead of feeling a sense of outrage that once again women had been sold unsafe products, how many women felt alone and worried about their own individual, individualistic decision-making as they were bombarded

---

Originally published in the fall 2004 issue (vol. 16, no. 3).

with messages about how shocking this news was and new products they could try? Using this as a time for self-reflection within the Women's Health Movement, I challenge us to think about how we can use the HRT story to politicize women and their health care providers about "the triumph of marketing over science" in women's health. Instead of letting the HRT news get framed as being about one particular product at one particular moment in time, it is more important than ever that women's health activists, researchers, teachers, and policymakers identify that HRT is not a unique story. HRT is symbolic of the pattern of untested, unneeded products being marketed to healthy women for pharmaceutical-company inspired "medical conditions."

Responses to the July 2002 Announcement

The post-study reality represents one of the biggest disconnects that has ever occurred in medicine.
  —(Peter Wilson, Framingham Heart Study, quoted in Spake 2002, 42)

No one should have been surprised by the news that HRT did not prevent heart disease and that its long-term safety was questioned. Many researchers and activists have been saying this for over a decade. The Society for Menstrual Cycle Research conferences and publications have for many years brought together researchers, clinicians, and activists asking important questions about the medicalization of menopause and the safety of products marketed to midlife women. How many times has Cindy Pearson, executive director of the National Women's Health Network, asked an audience, "Does estrogen make women healthy, or do healthy women take estrogen?" Since 1989, the NWHN has been publishing *Taking Hormones and Women's Health,* an accessible summary and critique of all the (midlife) hormone studies. This regularly updated publication continually warned that the benefits of hormones had not been proven and the long-term risks were not fully understood.

Arguing that every heart disease prevention drug used by men has been tested in a large randomized trial, the NWHN played a key role in the early 1990s in advocating and lobbying for a large randomized trial (which eventually became the Women's Health Initiative) to study the risks and benefits of estrogen (Estrogen "Replacement" Therapy [ERT]), and estrogen plus progestin (Hormone "Replacement" Therapy [HRT]) in healthy women. As we now recognize the importance of this study, it is important to remember that it almost did not happen: "At various times, the trial is opposed by members of Congress, who think it is too expensive, by epidemiologists, who think the design is too complicated, and by leading gynecologists, who think the heart disease benefit is so well proven that it is unethical to ask women to accept the possibility that they might be randomized to a placebo" (NWHN 2002, 180).

Published a few months before the July 2002 announcement, *The Truth About Hormone Replacement Therapy* contained the NWHN's version of a "center-page spread," a two-page fact sheet for women to give to their health practitioners in case "your health care provider may still be under the 'impression' that HRT may somehow be good for your heart." This fact sheet reminded practitioners that both the safety and effectiveness (in relation to heart disease) of ERT and HRT have been questioned continually: in 1990, the FDA denied approval to Wyeth-Ayerst, manufacturer of Premarin, to market Premarin for heart disease prevention (neither ERT nor HRT was ever given FDA approval for heart disease); in 1998, the Heart and Estrogen/Progestin Replacement Study (HERS), the first randomized study to look at heart disease outcome, demonstrated that HRT did not help women who already had heart disease, and in March 2000, participants in the Women's Health Initiative study were sent letters letting them know that, in the earliest stages of the study, women on ERT and HRT were showing more heart attacks, blood clots, and strokes than women in the placebo group. (Interestingly, these were downplayed as "early findings," but some researchers felt they would be useful for keeping women motivated to stay in the study. In a climate where women and their physicians were constantly bombarded with "information" saying ERT and HRT prevented heart disease, it was challenging to find women who were willing to be a part of a study where they might be randomized to what they viewed as the "wrong" group.)

Precisely because the July 2002 Women's Health Initiative results were not surprising to any of us who had been evaluating the studies and critiquing the marketing of hormones, reaction to the announcement proved to be a useful barometer for measuring people's understanding of the politics of women's health. A great teaching project would be to have students assigned to read and contrast the actual results reported from the Women's Health Initiative (Writing Group for WHI 2002) and comment on how that information was covered in a wide range of popular media (Whatley, personal communication). While there were some delightful cartoons and refreshing commentaries that captured the real meaning of the HRT news story, I found the following reactions I encountered in the media, among students and colleagues, to be the most thought-provoking in exploring the challenges of building a more sophisticated consumer awareness of the recurring pattern of the marketing of unsafe and unneeded products to healthy women:

> From a middle-aged woman doctor appearing on the evening news: In a great example of internalized sexism and ageism, this doctor appeared on July 9th news shows to discuss the WHI findings. She stated confidently that it was

urgent that physicians have *something* to prescribe to mid-life women. She actually said that without some sort of medication mid-life women were going to have all sorts of problems and their husbands would leave them! With absolutely no analysis of how menopause has been medicalized, here was a physician simply looking for one more product to prescribe for her patients.

From an undergraduate in a women's health course: In the spirit of this article, my teaching team was eager to use the HRT headline story as a teaching theme in the fall 2002 semester to demonstrate the ongoing problem of the medicalization of women's health. In October (only three months after the HRT study was stopped), an undergraduate criticized our dwelling on "old news," saying there was no reason to keep talking about the risks of HRT because people had known since July that it was dangerous so no one should be using it anymore. Despite our attempts to use HRT as one example among many unsafe products marketed to women, this undergraduate (who had enthusiastically chosen to take this Women's Studies women's health course) served as an example of someone who very much wanted as much information as possible for her own personal decision-making, but was not interested (yet!) in looking at the bigger picture of the politics of information.

From science graduate students applying to teach a women's health course: Asking applicants how they would handle the above HRT discussion situation (where an undergraduate fails to look beyond an individual issue to develop a broader analysis) proved to be a most useful interview question in selecting teaching assistants for my women's health course. Many feminist graduate students, particularly the social scientists, quickly realized they were being asked to describe how they would teach the politics of women's health and gave exciting answers. Interestingly, some more scientifically confident applicants totally missed the point of the question and immediately demonstrated how up to date they were on scientific issues by describing the Women's Health Initiative in much detail and saying that they would be able to share the scientific details of the study with students and that they would emphasize that the ERT part of the study continues and that there is still much potential for what will be learned about ERT.

From a male university colleague who works on communications: This colleague was intrigued with my quick "good-bye" the evening before the WHI results were to be announced. I had simply said to think of me as he listened to the next day's news and to remember that, "I told you so!" As someone who has read my work (as we are required to do for each other for annual peer reviews in a department where our research and teaching interests do not overlap), he had no trouble matching my good-bye comment to the HRT headlines. He was the person who most understood the significance of the HRT announcement: he immediately went on-line to watch the effect this would have on the stock market. In conversations since that day, it is obvious that he has developed a great appreciation for the politics of women's health by seeing the financial implications of that one announcement.

There is nothing scientific about my sample, but it certainly is thought-provoking. It is probably not a coincidence that the triumph of marketing over science or the triumph of wealth (of pharmaceutical companies) over (consumers') health was more apparent to someone who understands the stock market than to an undergraduate wanting information for personal decision-making, graduate students immersed in studying the details of health science, or a busy physician who has undoubtedly been greatly influenced by pharmaceutical industry-influenced "physician education."

Lessons from the Past Should Be Informing Present Debates

The HRT news was not just about one particular product at one particular moment in time. There is an incredible amount of money to be made any time a company can find a product to market to healthy women. Why are the companies that produce menstruation-related products willing to spend so much money on middle-school education resources or give so many free samples to girls starting their periods? Think of the money they can make if they hook someone into buying their particular brand for most of her reproductive years. My students love to calculate the amount of money an average woman spends in her lifetime on menstruation-related products.

Women of all ages should be aware that HRT is only the most recent addition to an ever-growing list of products sold to healthy women that turned out to be dangerous or lethal. Any consumer or clinician who will be involved in decision making about women's health products deserves to have, or has the responsibility to have, information on the recurring history of unsafe products hurting healthy women. The safety-monitoring committee of the Women's Health Initiative knew that it was important ethically to let participants know in March 2000 that early findings indicated some increased risks with hormones. Similarly, all consumers have the right to know much more about the risks they may be taking when they make the decision to use a product that has not been proven safe in large, long-term, double-blind, randomized studies.

Here are a couple examples of women's health history lessons that are important for safety-conscious consumers to know:

DES (Diethylstilbestrol)—This drug was widely used in the United States from 1941 to 1960. In the 1950s, 4 to 7 percent of all pregnant women took this drug. Although it was originally prescribed specifically for the treatment and prevention of miscarriage, both pregnant women and their clinicians liked the effect of the drug so it started to be used routinely in healthy women to promote healthy pregnancies. Two decades after the drug had become popular, it was discovered that some of the daughters who had been fetuses in pregnant women taking DES developed a very rare, potentially lethal, form of vaginal cancer when they were in their late teens or twenties. By the time the FDA withdrew DES from the market in 1971, approximately four million women had taken it. Today, *six decades* after this drug became available, researchers and consumers groups like DES Action are still trying to understand the long-term impact of this drug as it keeps unfolding in the daughters, sons, and grandchildren of women who took DES and in the women themselves. *The DES story should be the only one we need to remind us that we will never really know the long-term safety of a product until the long-term safety of that product has been proven* (Sloane 2002).

The Dalkon Shield—A crab-shaped intrauterine contraceptive device with a multi-filament tail became very popular in the 1970s due to a very aggressive marketing campaign where the manufacturer falsified safety studies and pregnancy prevention rates. The product was associated with a high rate of Pelvic Inflammatory Disease, a much-increased rate of infertility, and was blamed for causing at least fourteen deaths before it was withdrawn from the U.S. market in 1974. By that time the manufacturer had "dumped" many thousands of Dalkon Shields on unsuspecting consumers around the world where they might never hear of its dangers. Even in the United States, it was controversial as to whether it was safer to leave the device in place or risk damage to the uterus in having it removed. In speaking to executive officers of the company that marketed the Dalkon Shield, Chief Judge Miles Lord of the U.S. District Court in Minnesota summarized the irresponsibility of selling women dangerous products:

> If one poor young man were by some act of his—without authority or consent—to inflict such damage upon one woman, he would be jailed for a good portion of the rest of his life. And yet your company, without warning to women, invaded their bodies by the millions and caused them injuries by the thousand . . . Your company has, in fact, continued to allow women, tens of thousands of them, to wear a device—a deadly depth charge in their wombs, ready to explode at any time. The only conceivable reasons you have not recalled this product are that it would hurt your balance sheet and alert women who have already been harmed that you may be liable for their injuries . . . This is corporate irresponsibility at its meanest. (Engelmeyer and Wagman 1985, 254–56)

Similarly, consumers need to know how certain menstrual products had to be removed from the market after their association with more than 100 toxic shock syndrome deaths (Riley 1986), how 1.2- to 2.4-million women were affected the day it was announced that the popular diet drug combination Fen-Phen was being removed from the market because of the deaths that it had caused and the fact that approximately 30 percent of people who had used the drug had heart valve abnormalities (Mundy 2001); that debates still continue about the long-term safety of Depo-Provera, oral contraceptives, and silicone breast implants; and that debates *should* be taking place about every new product (Sathyamala 2000; Sloane 2002; Zuckerman 1998; Worcester and Whatley 2000).

In 1986, Joan Rachlin wrote an excellent review of four books on the Dalkon Shield, Rely tampons, and toxic shock syndrome for the *Women's Review of Books*. She concluded:

> These books are important from both a historical and women's health per-
> spective; they remind us that other substances, such as Depo-Provera, could
> well provide the material for the next set of books to be reviewed in these
> pages, if we don't learn well enough the lessons from the past. We have to ex-
> ercise our rights and responsibilities as empowered consumers of health care
> services and products. We have to demand safe and effective pharmaceuticals,
> produced and marketed by honest and competent organizations and adminis-
> tered by caring and capable physicians. We can only, after all, really *rely* on
> ourselves; we need to be as informed and as involved as possible if we are to
> navigate the medical-corporate complex. These books show us what the alter-
> natives will continue to be. (Rachlin, 1986, 7–8)

Increased Medicalization of Women's Health

Nearly two decades later, now with the HRT story added to the DES, Dalkon Shield, Rely tampons, and Fen-Phen stories, and the increasingly powerful partnership of the pharmaceutical industry, the FDA, the adver-tising industry, and industry-influenced medical education, Joan Rachlin's words are more important than ever. Consumer literacy and action related to demanding safe, effective products, marketed by ethical corporations and administered by physicians who have accurate, science-based infor-mation, is urgent. Important new trends in the 1990s in how drugs get to the market and how products can be marketed come together in a way that makes it more likely than ever that women will end up using products that are not necessary, are not effective, and may not be safe.

In the political climate of the late 1980s and early 1990s, there were major changes in the Food and Drug Administration's (FDA) relationship with the pharmaceutical industry, which affected the speed at which new drugs can get to the market. The FDA, the "watchdog" organization re-sponsible for ensuring that only safe products are allowed on the market, was accused of being too cautious, so that it was said that it took too long for good drugs to be available to Americans. Primarily, conservatives in Congress and "friends of industry" pushed for a more industry-friendly FDA, but it is important to note that consumer activists, particularly AIDS activists and later breast cancer activists, were also instrumental in demanding that promising drugs be made available to patients sooner. The contradictions in claiming this as a consumer victory are obvious and serve to highlight a consequence of the Women's Health Movement's shift from broader, grassroots organizing for a more holistic, health-promoting approach to women's health to the more recent emphasis on specific disease-focused campaigns (Ruzek and Becker 1998). There are extremely different ramifications of demanding speedy access to life (quality or quantity) enhancing drugs for terminally ill patients than of setting the safety standards for a drug that will be marketed to healthy woman to be consumed for many years. When drug companies started promoting ERT and HRT for heart disease and osteoporosis, they hoped to hook women into a product they would stay on for the rest of their lives; such products must be extremely safe.

The Prescription Drug User Fee Act (PDUFA) of 1992 requires that the FDA and pharmaceutical companies work together now in somewhat of a "partnership" so that "good" drugs get to the market sooner. PDUFA requires industry to pay a user fee to the FDA; in exchange the FDA works with the company to help the process of drug approval go more quickly. Everyone acknowledges that there is a tension between ensuring the safety of products and speeding patient access to new drugs. There is certainly no doubt that more drugs are reaching the market faster as a result of PDUFA. While some media attention has focused on the number of drugs that have had to be withdrawn from the market (often with much public attention as in the Fen-Phen case) since the approval process has been speeded up, the FDA emphasizes that the rate of drug withdrawals has not changed significantly. (Approximately 2.8% of drugs are withdrawn after they have been on the market and problems emerge.) What matters to consumers wanting safe drugs is that the number of people impacted by taking drugs that later are recalled is much higher if the volume of drug approvals is higher, even if the rate of withdrawals is not increasing. Another major change for U.S. consumers is that approximately 80 percent of new drugs now go on the market in the United States before they are available elsewhere. In contrast, it used to be that most drugs were used and tested first in other countries so Americans had often heard about risks and undesirable side effects before new products reached the U.S. market (FDA 2002).

The importance of the FDA maintaining its role as our "watchdog" without too much influence from industry is well documented and discussed in Philip J. Hilts's *Protecting America's Health: The FDA, Business, and One Hundred Years of Regulation*. In responding to New Right groups in Washington that continued to criticize the FDA as being too cautious so as to "filter out almost all harm," even after the PDUFA mandated the new FDA-industry collaborations and drug-approval processes had been speeded up, Hilts explained:

With the present FDA system (described as overcautious), drugs that are *reviewed and approved* kill about 100,000 people annually and seriously injure more than a million in the United States. The system has not filtered out all risk, apparently. No other cause of accidents approaches the level of injury attributed to pharmaceuticals. (A table of risk put together by Thomas Moore of George Washington University estimates the lifetime chance of being put in the hospital by accidents: severe injury by prescription drugs, 26 in 100; auto accident, 2 in 100; murder, 1 in 100; commercial air crash, 1 in 35,000.) And the vast majority of deaths occur not among people knowingly taking a risk, but among the innocent. We accept this high level of risk because we are seeking greater benefit—saving lives and preventing or minimizing illness. The FDA is not an overcautious agency by nature. (2003, 307–8)

In the weeks and months following the announcements about the risks of HRT, the media has been full of feature stories focusing on a number of new products that women could try to "replace" their "replacement hormones." The obvious irony is that HRT has been widely available since the early 1980s, but the important questions about its safety and effectiveness have only started to be answered. The important thing to remember about these new products is that they are new: some may prove to be wonder drugs, some may be less effective than promised, some may be dangerous. To have the kind of useful information we now have about HRT will require large, long-term randomized controlled studies.

In addition to its new influence on the FDA, the drug industry also has increasing influence on both consumers and health care providers. The drug industry speaks directly to women these days, coming into their minds and conversations through their televisions and radios and in their magazines and newspapers. The industry-sponsored ads, industry-spokespeople, and industry-prepared ready-to-use health segments (which 100% of surveyed television news stations admit they use) not only powerfully influence the purchase of particular products, but also influence more broadly what women identify as health issues and fears, and what needs medication. Even before Merck had a product approved for osteoporosis (Fosamax was still going through FDA-approval processes at that stage), many women's magazines ran a two-page ad paid for by Merck. The very eye-catching image showed a young woman riding a bicycle, casting a large shadow of a wheelchair. The words "The shadow of osteoporosis doesn't have to influence future independence" effectively sold women the fear of osteoporosis and the feeling that they should start taking *something* to prevent it. Advertising is so effective that many women enroll for menopause classes feeling they have to get more information on which medicine to take: inevitably they have been so influenced by the industry-promoted medicalization of menopause that they have forgotten there is a choice not to take *any* medication.

Television ads have been an especially powerful source of drug pushing since guidelines for direct-to-consumer ads were liberalized in 1997. By 1999, the pharmaceutical industry spent more than $1.8 billion on direct-to-consumer advertising. Because the ads often give misinformation, their power can be dangerous. The FDA does not pre-approve ads, so ads containing misinformation get pulled only after they have already been seen and it is too late to undo the message they gave. Although most consumers underestimate how much they personally are affected by advertising, studies consistently show that drug ads are incredibly influential in manipulating what consumers want. One-third of consumers have spoken to their health care providers about a product they saw advertised, and 15 percent of consumers admit they might switch doctors if their doctor would not prescribe a medication they saw advertised and requested (NWHN 2002, 14).

The power of advertising may be the most detrimental to women's health when the advertising is geared toward her physician. In today's world where the FDA is pressured to get more drugs onto the market faster and where consumers are trained to ask for specific medications, the way-too-busy physicians, whose health maintenance organizations (HMOs) demand they see an almost impossible number of patients per hour, have ever-increasing responsibilities as the gatekeepers to the smorgasbord of medications available. Philip Hilts emphasizes the importance of this role in stating: "Drug approvals are in the hands of the FDA, but medicine is in the hands of doctors" (2003, 235). He identifies that the most common system failure in terms of the safety of medicine is in getting the appropriate knowledge to physicians:

> By the mid-1990s, the FDA, under pressure, was pinning its hopes on warning labels and doctors' care in prescribing. The burden of dangerous drugs thus shifted away from the agency. Good, but worrisome drugs are sent to market, and worries are often expressed on the label, rather than waiting for more data or proof of safety.
>
> That system may work if doctors read and heed the labels. Reviewers (at FDA) say the crafting of the label and related information is one of the chief satisfactions of the job—it amounts to giving the official word on what science knows about a drug. But as one reviewer said, "Doctors aren't often paying attention. We may put crucial information in a label and have it end up as a dead letter." Studies confirm it: the labels are largely unheeded and often completely unread. At the same time, pharmaceutical manufacturers effectively use the full arsenal of advertising and promotion to tout a drug's good qualities and downplay its problems. (2003, 234–35)

"Manufacturing Need, Manufacturing Knowledge" in *The Truth about Hormone Replacement Therapy* provides page after page of examples of how physicians' knowledge and prescribing practices are very carefully influenced by pharmaceutical companies. We all know about those mugs, pens, prescription pads, free lunches, and industry-supported conferences in Hawaii, but how many of us have thought about how much our physicians' knowledge about our health is manipulated by the drug industry that has just managed—or not managed—to get a new product on the market? How many of the millions of women who have had prescriptions for ERT or HRT for the prevention of heart disease know that neither ERT nor HRT was ever given FDA approval for the prevention of heart disease? In one of the most important examples of the physicians' ultimate control of medicine, physicians have the right to prescribe a medication for a condition even if the FDA has never approved the medication for that condition, as long as the medication has had FDA approval for some condition. Because ERT and HRT have been approved for osteoporosis prevention, it is perfectly legal—and obviously was even considered "good medicine"—for a physician to prescribe it "off label" for heart disease. Keeping that in mind, it becomes even more obvious how influential a fast-talking drug rep, a slick PowerPoint presentation (designed and paid for by the drug company but actually delivered by a respected colleague), a study demonstrating the effectiveness of a particular drug (who reads the fine print to see that the drug company influenced the study design and funded the study; who knows how many industry-funded studies do not get published if they don't find the "right" answer?), or free samples of medications can be in helping that busy physician know what to prescribe. Drug companies know that money spent influencing physicians is money well spent. In 2001, they spent more than $16 billion on this line item. In other words, pharmaceutical companies pay $8,000–$13,000 per year to influence each physician's drug-prescribing practices (NWHN 2002, 3–18).

Using the HRT Story to Get to the Heart of the Politics of Women's Health

"Millions of healthy women were taking long-term hormone therapy for a preventative benefit not yet proven because medical practice was determined under the influence of industry rather than under the influence of (scientific) evidence" (Pearson 2003, 3). This was a statement made by NWHN executive director Cindy Pearson at an October 24, 2003, National Institutes of Health meeting organized for the purpose of discussing the implications of the Women's Health Initiative. Emphasizing the lessons that must be learned from the fact that "drug companies, professional societies, women's groups, policymakers, and government agencies had all been complicit in creating a 'climate of enthusiasm for hormone therapy' and allowing the needless suffering of tens of thousands of women," Pearson identified the following steps that must be taken:

- Get drug company money out of medical education.
- Give the FDA the authority to pre-approve direct-to-consumer advertisements for prescription medications.
- End industry payments to physicians for writing papers that appear in medical journals.
- Stop quoting medical experts in media reports on health without reporting on their financial relationship with industry.
- Clean up consumer groups' health education so that the all-too-common and dangerous influence of drug company money is replaced with healthy skepticism.
- Bar anyone with significant financial ties to industry from involvement in the development of professional guidelines. (2003, 3)

The role of the Women's Health Movement is as important as ever. We must

- Insist that large, long-term, randomized studies are done on all products that are marketed to healthy women. Science must triumph over marketing. Safety must be seen to be more important than money.
- Shift the emphasis to lifelong health-promoting practices. We must constantly ask whether the availability or overuse of drugs and other products distracts attention from looking at safer ways of taking care of women's health.
- Organize around the fact that consumer activism and consumer medical literacy are more important than ever so that common sense and health promotion triumph over marketing.

Acknowledgments

While I take full responsibility for ideas expressed in this essay, I give much credit to the other members of the writing group of *The Truth About Hormone Replacement Therapy* (National Women's Health Network, 2002) and to the book for some of the ideas and information shared here.

References

Engelmeyer, Sheldon, and Robert Wagman. 1985. *Lord's Justice*. New York: Anchor Press/Doubleday.

Food and Drug Administration (FDA). 2002. Center for Drug Evaluation and Research Orientation for New Advisory Committee Members, January 22.

Hilts, Philip J. 2003. *Protecting America's Health: The FDA, Business, and One Hundred Years of Regulation*. New York: Alfred A. Knopf.

Mundy, Alicia. 2001. *Dispensing with the Truth: The Victims, the Drug Companies, and the Dramatic Story Behind the Battle over Fen-Phen*. New York: St. Martin's Press.

National Women's Health Network (NWHN). 2002. *The Truth About Hormone Replacement Therapy: How to Break Free from the Medical Myths of Menopause*. Roseville, CA: Prima Publishing.

National Women's Health Network (NWHN). 2000. *Taking Hormones and Women's Health: Choices. Risks and Benefits*. National Women's Health Network, 514 10th Street, N.W., Suite 400, Washington, DC 20004, 202/347-1140, from http://www.womenshealthnetwork.org.

Pearson, Cindy. 2003. "Hormone Therapy: Six Steps Toward a Better Future." *Network News*, January–February: 3.

Rachlin, Joan. 1986. "Business as Usual." *The Women's Review of Books* 4(2): 7–8.

Riley, Tom. 1986. *The Price of a Life: One Woman's Death from Toxic Shock*. Bethesda, MD: Adler & Adler.

Ruzek, Sheryl Burt, and Julie Becker. 1998. "The Women's Health Movement in the United States: From Grass-roots Activism to Professional Agendas." *Journal of the American Medical Women's Association*, January 30: 4–8.

Sathyamala, C. 2000. *An Epidemiological Review of the Injectable Contraceptive, Depo-Provera*. Pune, India: Medico Friend Circle and Forum for Women's Health (11 Archana Apartments, 163 Solapur Road, Hadapsar, Pune 411028).

Sloane, Ethel. 2002. "DES Mothers and Children." *Biology of Women*. 4th ed., 287–92. Albany, NY: Delmar.

Spake, Amanda. 2002. "The Menopausal Marketplace." *U.S. News and World Report*, November 18: 42–50.

Worcester, Nancy, and Mariamne Whatley, eds. 2000. *Women's Health: Readings on Social, Economic, and Political Issues*. 3rd ed. Dubuque, IA: Kendall/Hunt.

Writing Group for the Women's Health Initiative Investigators. 2002. "Risks and Benefits of Estrogen Plus Progestin in Healthy Postmenopausal Women: Principal Results from the Women's Health Initiative Randomized Controlled Trial." *Journal of the American Medical Association* 288(3): 321–33.

Zuckerman, Diana. 1998. Briefing Paper: *The Safety of Silicone Breast Implants*. Washington, DC: Institute for Women's Policy Research.

Aged Mothers, Aging Daughters

SONDRA M. BRANDLER

*I retired from teaching six months before my mother started to lose her vi-
sion and had to come to live with us. She was 85-years-old then, and I was
62, retiring early for health reasons. My brothers, who live in other states,
provided no support financially or emotionally for either my mother or for
me, not that we ever thought to ask for their help. My mother lived with us
for eight years before she died. At one point, both she and my husband were
in the hospital at the same time. I had accidents, once falling down a whole
flight of stairs, and on several occasions was unable to even manage my own
care. At least twice, we three stayed for extended periods at my daughter's
house because I was ill or injured. My mother also stayed with my daughter
and her family when my husband and I went away for a rare week-end trip.
At first, when my mother came to live with us, she was able to join us when
my husband and I went out socially; she was never the sort to give up going
or doing anything, and she didn't feel that she was intruding either. She
loved music, so we would take her to every concert. Afterward, my husband
would go to get our car, and my mother and I would wait for him together,
with her leaning heavily on me. I tried not to let her know how hard it was
for me, and I still don't think she ever realized. In the last few years, as she
became more disabled, we gave up trying to take her to the concerts and had
to hire help if we were going out for an evening because she was not safe stay-
ing alone. She began to lose her hearing as well as her eyesight and needed
more and more attention. Near the end of her life, it became too difficult for
her to come downstairs to the kitchen for her meals, so I tried to bring them
upstairs to her bedroom. I have a severe tremor. In order to carry a tray of
food to her when my husband was at work, I placed the tray two or three
steps ahead of me on the stairs, advanced a few steps, and repeated the process. It was very difficult, but I felt that there was no choice.*

—B.R., study interviewee

A significant new population of women 65 and older are involved in caregiving responsibilities as they simultaneously confront their own aging.
These women may be providing care to adult children, grandchildren,
spouses, or siblings, or to their own parents. Caregivers are likely to be
struggling with their own health and economic difficulties and with various competing demands on their time, energy, and attention. Also, the
nature of the relationship between generations is often problematic and
increasingly stressful as bad relationships age and the difficulties for both
the caregiver and care recipient are exacerbated by issues of dependency
(Albert, Litvin, Kleban, and Brody 1991 476–82).

Originally published in the spring 1998 issue (vol. 10, no. 1).

The costs associated with caregiving belong primarily, and in many families exclusively, to women (Montgomery and Datwyler 1992; Horowitz 1978; Walker and Allen 1991). While modern life often includes men in child-rearing chores, household responsibilities, and other areas once chiefly the realm of women, there is no evidence of men sharing equally in caregiving responsibilities for aged relatives. In particular, the affective component that is the emotional rather than the instrumental caring falls to daughters. Clearly, caregiving to an aged parent, even when the caregiver herself is aged, is part of the fabric of our culture and is regarded by women as an obligation and responsibility consistent with their gender role and one that they will not forsake (Walker 1996, 269–85).

Demographic information highlights the enormity of the problem. Approximately 31 million people in the United States are over 65, but census projections suggest that this figure will double by the year 2025 to 62 million people, almost one in five Americans. In addition, 60 percent of women over age 55 have at least one living parent, and it is estimated that 20 percent of a woman's lifetime will be spent with a parent over age 65 (Boyd and Treas 1996, 262–68). Ten percent of older Americans have adult children over age 65, and this figure is growing steadily (Atchley 1996). Most important, the population over age 85 is growing at a faster rate than the total elderly population, and since women live longer than men, most of the oldest old are widows, with 2.6 women for every man over age 85 (Longino 1996). Disability inevitably increases with age, with women more commonly than men suffering chronic illnesses (Moody 1996). Researchers have also found a significant increase in the prevalence of chronic diseases in the "young-old" though not among the rest of the aged population. Only 9 percent of people age 65 and older require help with eating, bathing, toileting, or dressing, but 45 percent of people over age 85 require such assistance. The ultimate feminist issue is that caregivers, many of whom are frail, elderly, impoverished (Ozawa 1995; Meyer 1996), chronically ill, and widowed themselves, are likely to remain in service to their parents and other relatives until they have outlived all those who need them. Dying, like living, has been prolonged and the length of interaction between the aged generations has been extended (Watt and Soifer 1992).

While recent studies explore the relationships between caregivers and their elderly parents (Quadagno and street 1996; Walker 1996; Boyd and Treas 1996; Atchley 1996; Merrill and Dill 1990; Noelker and Townsend 1987; Miller and Montgomery 1990; Walker and Allen 1991; Horowitz 1978), few focus on the aging of caregivers and its impact on both mothers and daughters. Policymakers and feminists in particular must address the issues of aging and caregiving simultaneously, for without support for women caregivers and their dependents, far too many will be denied a productive old age. When daughters and other female relatives (daughters-in-law, sisters, and nieces) are overburdened to the point where they can no longer bear the responsibility alone for aged family members, they are likely to seek more public support through costly and not necessarily desirable institutional care. Less expensive and extensive family support services (respite programs, supportive housing, shopping services, transportation to appointments, meals on wheels, etc.) might result in families better able to maintain their loved ones in the community rather than in institutional settings.

This research focused on 100 Jewish women, 50 elderly, widowed mothers and 50 of their daughters over age 65 who identified themselves as their mothers' primary caregivers. Half of the mothers resided in the community (some living with their daughters) and half resided in an institutional setting, under Jewish auspices, with skilled nursing facilities available. Ethnic background is a strong determinant of attitudes concerning filial responsibility (Savishinsky 1990; Merrill and Dill 1990; Gelfand 1994). The study should be replicated with other ethnic populations to ascertain which of the findings can be generalized to other groups.

While other studies of caregiving focus primarily on the caregivers, this research includes both mothers and daughters as they faced the shared concern of their mutual aging and its influence on their relationship. Since both mothers and daughters needed to respond to questionnaires and to an interview, both parties in all mother-daughter pairs chosen were sufficiently mentally intact to participate. However, many respondents exhibited signs of significant impairment in cognitive function, a factor that certainly created additional stress for families. Since the most severely mentally impaired older adults could not be included in the study, the impact of severe mental disability on the filial relationship could only be inferred from the findings of this study.

Two purposes of the research were: (1) to see how filial expectations were perceived by each generation (Seelbach Filial Expectation Scale, 1978); and (2) to understand the concerns of the two generations regarding the performance of the filial role, identifying the biological, economic, psychological, and social strains experienced by the aged caregivers.

Perceptions of Filial Expectations

Earlier literature (Streib 1972; Seelbach 1978) suggested that mothers would have higher expectations about the filial role than would their daughters, but this study found quite the opposite. In general, daughters had higher expectations for themselves regarding their filial responsibilities than did their mothers. Several factors may explain this. Although the mothers were more likely familiar with extended family living, they may not have had positive associations with the experience. Providing all of the physical, financial, and emotional care to infirm parents, without any assistance from other sources, must have been extraordinarily burdensome for struggling immigrant families in the earlier part of the twentieth century (Schorr 1980). As they themselves indicate, mothers do not want this burden for their own children (Hess and Waring 1975). Some of the foreign-born mothers (47 percent of the mothers sampled were foreign-born) left their own parents in Europe, which was the ultimate step in asserting independence from parents, suggesting that filial ties may not have been that strong (Mindel 1979). Aside from sending money home, these adult children provided none of the care for their parents. Visiting and telephoning were not options. It should not be surprising that now, in very old age themselves, these mothers might not have high expectations for daughters' filial responsibilities.

Research indicates that older people prefer to maintain close ties but to live apart from their families. While they may still hold traditional values, mothers also have been exposed to modern ideas and are impressed by the notion that generations benefit from living apart from one another. Financial and social independence seem to be as important for mothers as they are for daughters, a view expressed repeatedly by both mothers and daughters throughout this study.

Another explanation for mothers' lower filial expectations is that mothers retain perceptions of themselves as nurturers and protectors of their children, even when they have become physically dependent upon daughters as caregivers. The role of a daughter of an aged parent is enhanced rather than reversed as she attains what Blenkner (1965) called "filial maturity"; the mother holds on to her role as parent even when she cannot fully care for herself. This factor may be more significant for Jewish mothers and daughters among whom parents are often comfortable with giving support to adult children but uncomfortable in accepting support.

Mothers in the study often expressed concern about the strains of caregiving on their adult children. Some said that they could do without various forms of attention and so "spare" their children difficulty. Surely some of these mothers feared that too great a demand on their children might result in resentment and a lack of attention, but most often their desire to be helpful and self-sacrificing, in at least some small measure, appeared genuinely unselfish. Apparently, as Cantor found in the Inner-city Elderly Project (1975), whenever possible relationships between children and their aged parents are reciprocal rather than dependent. In this study, even infirm persons 90 years old still consider themselves to be in a reciprocal relationship with their daughters so that both parties in the relationship give and take. Daughters, in addition to expressing love for their mothers, spoke of intense feelings of obligation and duty in the care of their mothers.

Filial expectations differed between the responses of mothers who were living in institutions and mothers who were living in the community. Institutionalized mothers had lower filial expectations than did community mothers; daughters of institutionalized mothers had lower filial expectations than daughters whose mothers lived in the community. The interviews helped to explain some of this difference. A number of mothers in the institutionalized sample indicated that they had elected placement because they did not think that children should have to care for them (Hess and Waring 1975). Several of these mothers said that they recognized that they were ill and might someday become more ill and thought that they would prefer to be cared for in an institution of their choice rather than to become a burden on children. One mother even told how she planned an elaborate dinner party for her family where she announced that she was planning to enter an institution. The children and the mother both confirmed that the family opposed the placement, but the mother had decided and would not reconsider.

Of course, circumstances surrounding the institutionalization of the mothers varied a great deal, and it is unclear how many of the mothers, in reality opposed to placement, merely said that they opted for placement. In expressing lower filial expectations than do community mothers, many mothers in the institutionalized sample may be adjusting to the disappointment of placement. The finding that daughters whose mothers were in the community had higher filial expectations than did the daughters of the institutionalized mothers is reflected in the fact that several of the mothers living in the community resided with their daughters. Crediting the sharing of one's home as an indicator of high filial expectations is perhaps an oversimplification of the issues. Nevertheless, by sharing their households, the daughters do demonstrate a certain level of involvement and commitment to their parents.

Performance of the Filial Role

Clearly, physical, emotional, social, and financial stressors contribute to difficulties in the performance of the filial role as caregivers and their mothers age; this study focused on each generation's perception of these. In both the institutional and the community samples, daughters identified more areas related to the mutual aging of the mothers and daughters as potentially problematic in the performance of the filial role than did their mothers. Both institutionalized mothers and their daughters identified more problems than did the community mothers and their daughters, which is not surprising since all placements relate to some problem in functioning in the community setting. The difference in numbers of problems cited by the institutional sample and the community sample is entirely in the areas of mental and physical health. Data from the Health Scale indicate that the institutionalized mothers perceived themselves to be more ill and disabled than the community mothers perceived themselves to be.

The most frequently cited problem for the institutionalized group was that the mother was unable to live alone; all 25 daughters in this group and 23 of their mothers agreed that this was so. Although this problem ranked lower for the community sample, 15 daughters and 13 mothers in the community believed that their mothers could not live alone. The most frequently cited problem for the community sample daughters was that their mothers needed emotional support. Their mothers' most frequently cited problem was that they had grown more feeble.

In general, nearly all of the mothers had a somewhat more positive view of their health, both physical and mental, and their ability to function independently than did their daughters. Sometimes this may have reflected the fear, concern, or pessimism of the daughter, but observation suggests that more often mothers failed to recognize or admit their difficulties. Again, this may be related to the aged mother's perception of herself in the nurturing role even when in reality she needs the nurturing herself. This too may be related to Jewish ethnicity in so far as Jewish mothers value their independence from the assistance of children (Zborowski and Herzog 1952). The mothers' more positive perceptions about their health and independence were seen most markedly in one item concerning the daughter's inability to attend to the mother's physical care. Thirty-one of the daughters found this to be problematic while only 23 of their mothers perceived this to be true.

By far, respondents' most pressing problems were health related. The very old were obviously in constant physical peril. Four times the researcher arrived for a scheduled interview to find the mother in a health crisis. For example, a 94-year-old mother suffered a gall bladder attack. Her daughter, familiar with the symptoms, was debating whether this was the time for an operation that had been put off repeatedly because of the mother's general debility. This mother and working daughter shared their home, and the daughter had to save up her own sick leave to be at home whenever the mother had a health emergency. When the daughter was at work, the mother was cared for by home attendants, some of whom arrived late or were absent without notice. The daughter's work schedule had to accommodate the homemakers. There was an ongoing danger that the daughter, the sole support for both herself and her mother, would lose her job. Community daughters more frequently than institutional daughters said problems in having aged parents were that the daughters were not feeling well physically or were busy with their work. The institutionalization of the parent clearly reduced the physical strain of caregiving, and the daughter's health became less of an issue once her mother was placed (Spark and Brody 1970). Also, it seems apparent that the conflict between work obligations and responsibility for an aged or infirm older person can be extraordinary. With round-the-clock care provided in the institution, part of that conflict was reduced (Spark and Brody 1970).

It is not enough to say that old people get sick and die. The impact of health emergencies and chronic illnesses on family life is immeasurable. The strains are greater when the caregiver's health is also perilous, when she too is aged. As an example of a mother and a daughter with special problems, on the day of their interview the mother had started to hemorrhage, as reported to the daughter by a home attendant. The home care providers had to be especially vigilant in this situation because both mother and daughter were blind. Although the majority of daughters did not report severe health problems, some were seriously ill. Others were hampered in their daily activities by various impairments and chronic health problems. One daughter, living with her wheelchair-bound centenarian mother, broke an ankle a few weeks before the scheduled interview. The daughter needed someone to accompany her to the doctor, do the shopping, and manage household chores, but the homemaker, assigned through Medicaid to the mother, was not permitted to provide services to other members of the household. When the daughter/caregiver fell ill, both mother and daughter were in jeopardy (Streib 1972).

The health situation of several daughters led directly to institutional placement of their mothers. In one case, the mother had been living with her daughter and son-in-law for over 20 years. When the son-in-law suffered a heart attack and was hospitalized, his mother-in-law refused to believe that he was really ill, insisting that it was just a bad flu. Simultaneously, the daughter learned that she needed major surgery and that the outcome of this procedure was very uncertain. In the midst of her own and her husband's health problems, the daughter had the worry of her mother remaining in the house alone. The mother was not accepting of any home care plan, denying her own and her daughter's limitations. The daughter felt that institutional care for the mother was the only option.

On several occasions it appeared that daughters were neglecting their own health in order to provide care to their mothers. When it was physically impossible for them to provide the care themselves, some felt that they were forced to accept placement for their mothers. A daughter who was seriously ill with diabetes and could barely walk spoke of the frustration of having her disabled mother dependent on paid companions, some of whom were unreliable and provided poor or undependable care. The mother and daughter came to a mutual decision that the supervised setting of an institution was safer for the mother and less worrisome for the daughter.

In short, daughters who were aged themselves suffered many of the health problems that occurred in a more exaggerated form in extreme old age. This did not seem to prevent them from involvement in their mothers' care, but surely it made everything more difficult for them.

As with health issues, mothers and daughters differed over whether the mothers' need for emotional support was problematic. Although this was the problem most often cited by community sample daughters, it was not perceived to be a problem by most of their mothers. This finding is consonant with other research on caregiving (Horowitz 1978, Zimmer and Mellor 1981). During interviews, emotional factors were constantly mentioned, and their impact on the relationships between mothers and daughters was profound. Daughters' interviews included words like *guilt, fear, frustration, annoyance, conflict, and worry.* A number of daughters felt physically and emotionally drained and tired of trying to prove their devotion to their mothers. When asked about her greatest concern in being an older person with a very aged parent, one daughter answered, "My psychological needs are trampled. Her physical needs are met by the institution. It was the only alternative, and it's a terrible one." Another daughter said she was "choked" by her mother's total dependence on her and feared that someday she would be unable to provide for her mother. Many asked, "What will happen to my mother if I am not around? Who would care about her?"

Some daughters said they saw their own futures in their mothers. It was especially difficult when mothers had deteriorated mentally. "I only wish that she should be peaceful, end her days quietly, not upset or disturbed, and her memory shouldn't deteriorate further. I worry that it will repeat in my generation." And, "I'm fearful of being like my mother. I hope that I won't be a problem to my kids." One woman commented, "I think of myself in terms of her. You'll probably be the same as her, only worse."

Intergenerational conflict was, in most mother-daughter relationships, exacerbated by the increased dependence of the aged mother. "I hope that I'll be able to care for her if she needs me. I'm concerned about her maintaining herself alone. I hope that she will come to live with me. I want to provide for this, but she hangs on to me, she needs me for constant reassurance, and it is sometimes so annoying." Both mothers and daughters were often on emotional tenterhooks. One mother confided that since her daughter became widowed, the daughter "flies off the handle at the least thing." A daughter talked about her concern that she and her mother "not get on each other's nerves. I must stay cool at all times."

Many daughters spoke about needing the strength and the patience to cope with the pressures and the demands of their own children, husbands, social lives, jobs, and, of course, mothers. When one daughter discussed the idea of having her mother come to live with her, her college-age sons threatened to move. After years of devotion to her mother, another daughter realized that her time away from home was jeopardizing her marriage. In some instances, the mother overrode everything and everyone else: "As a daughter with a very aged mother, I am not reaching my old age gracefully. Every day goes by, it is like losing a day. She resents my talking to anybody. I love activities, and I had to give up everything. Worries about her have tied my hands and feet. I'm at an age I want to live a little."

Daughters said that money, fatigue, care for themselves, and responsibilities to children all created difficulties in being the aging daughter of a very old parent. Mothers were either unaware or unwilling to acknowledge these difficulties to the same degree. In this and other research (Simos 1973; Silverman, Kahn, and Anderson 1977), the differences in perceptions were sources of friction in some relationships. Again, some mothers deny these are problems because they find it difficult to believe that they are a source of difficulty for their daughter. Some mothers continued to assert that daughters were capable of doing anything, that they had not aged, that they were well and strong, and that they were without flaws. The mother's perception that her daughter had the ability to take charge of the situation and, in a sense, to act as protector for her mother seemed to be both a source of pride and an assistance in survival.

Several questions addressed the relationships rather than the difficulties between mothers and daughters. For example, one item noted that a problem for a daughter is that she sometimes feels as if she is relating to a child rather than to her aged mother. The item was posed somewhat differently in the mother's questionnaire and suggested that a problem in being an aged parent was that she felt lately as if she were treated like a child. Four mothers and 14 daughters agreed with the statement. Many mothers who were emphatic that daughters knew that the mother was boss and would not dare to treat the mother like a child were the same mothers whose daughters said that lately they were relating to their mothers as if the mothers were children.

Some women were troubled by the fact that mothers refused to admit that the daughters were adults. One woman said, "Can you imagine this? I'm nearly 70 years old, and every time I visit with my mother, she reminds me to comb my hair." There are similar illustrations but none quite so dramatic as one potential 70-year-old study respondent whose mother forbade her involvement in the research project and would not permit her to even speak to the researcher on the telephone. The daughter requested that the research packet be mailed to her at the address where both mother and daughter resided. Several days later, the unopened packet was returned "to sender." Daughters in the institutional sample were more than twice as likely as their community counterparts to say that a problem for them was that mothers were demanding; they were nearly twice as likely to feel, in dealing with their mothers, that they were relating to a child. It is possible that some of the mothers were placed because daughters found them to be demanding and felt that relating to them was like relating to a child. Also, the institutional mothers were more often mentally impaired than were the community mothers.

Another finding that touched on the relationship between mother and daughter proved equally interesting. In responding to an item that said a problem was that the daughter grew impatient easily, 25 daughters agreed with the statement while only 13 mothers agreed. This may have been another case of the mother refusing to acknowledge the weakness of her daughter. It also may simply be that the daughter did not communicate the impatience that she felt; instead, she controlled behavior while defining her internal struggle as impatience.

Mothers and daughters agree on other issues raised in this study. For example, they agreed that living far apart was a hardship, that the daughter's income could be problematic, and that health was a problem. Mothers usually felt that daughters had their own worries and were concerned about their daughter's difficulties.

An important difference between mothers in the community sample and mothers in the institutional sample was their perception that a problem in being an aged parent was that the mother had used up her resources. Ten institutional mothers agreed that this was a problem but only five community mothers perceived this as a problem. Although this research did not investigate respondents' assets, findings suggest that the community sample mothers were financially more secure than the institutional sample mothers. This factor may have accounted for the choice of institutionalization rather than other alternatives for care in which private forms of payment might be required. Both groups of daughters identified, with less frequency than their mothers, the mothers' loss of economic resources as a problem. It is interesting that the institutionalized mothers, who had all of their needs met in the institution, still saw finances as a problem to which their daughters were not attuned. Whether status, security, or independence was the issue was not apparent, but mothers attached great importance to having their own assets, even when their needs were met fully by the institution.

Financial issues were sometimes quite subtle. Most of the daughters sampled were not impoverished, although several characterized their situations as "struggling" financially. Nearly every daughter provided for her mother's needs for clothing and toiletries. Since the majority of the daughters were working, the issue of reaching retirement and experiencing a precipitous decline in income had not yet been met. For those who had retired, the daily expenses related to their mothers was usually not a problem, but the unexpected health crises could be financially disastrous.

A severely ill, widowed daughter remarked, "My mother used up all her savings. I couldn't afford to keep up the companions myself, but I was afraid to leave her alone. She didn't qualify for enough hours. We decided she would have to go to the Home." Another daughter, recently divorced after a long and unhappy marriage and struggling just to support herself, found that she could not afford a private telephone in her mother's room in the institution. This had become a terrible issue between them. There were other special costs for an older person with an aged mother. One woman, crippled by arthritis, could not use public transportation to travel to her mother's home and found the cost of car service prohibitive. This necessarily limited contact between mother and daughter. Another daughter was worried that she might not be able to keep a promise she had made to her institutionalized mother that the mother would be provided with paid companions should it be necessary for her to enter the hospital division of the institution. The promise had been made when the daughter had had more resources and the expenses in hiring companions had been less.

A major financial concern of mothers and daughters in the community sample was finding affordable housing with support services for the aged. A daughter commented, "I am working and am very concerned about her living alone. She does not see well. For someone as alert and concerned as my mother, there should be good low-cost housing with services. My mother wants her independence and would prefer to live on her own and do her 'thing'—clubs, trips, and other activities." Strikingly, 10 daughters of institutional mothers noted that the availability of supportive housing might have delayed or eliminated the need for placement for their mothers.

In general, the discussions of filial expectations and of problem identification in the filial role complement each other. The picture generated by these findings is one in which very old women said that they did not think much should be expected of adult children but communicated a different reality to their daughters. Daughters contended that their mothers' needs for emotional support were a source of ongoing difficulty; 60- to 75-year-old daughters perceived a need for their continued and sometimes increased social engagement, and both mothers and daughters identified the daughter's social life as a problem for her performing her filial role. While mothers perceived fewer problems generally in their daughters' performance of the filial roles than did daughters and claimed to expect little of their daughters, daughters believed that much should be expected of them and regarded their mothers as needy both physically and emotionally. Health factors, emotional and social factors, and, to a lesser degree, financial factors were perceived as sources of difficulty for daughters in the performance of their filial roles as they faced their own aging and that of their mothers.

This project naturally created an intimacy between respondents and researcher that this report cannot always communicate. Participants in this study willingly and openly shared their most deeply felt frustrations, anxieties, and concerns. Many interviews were conducted in participants' homes in the midst of all of the daily crises, the photographs and remembrances chronicling a lifetime. Some described with great sadness how life had been for them in years past and what it had become for them now. Others expressed tremendous pride in how well they and their families were managing despite the difficulties in their situations. Pictures told a thousand stories: "This is how Mother used to look. Wasn't she a beautiful woman?"

The warmth, candor, and perceptiveness of the women eased the data collection process. Their stresses, pain, and conflicts were apparent but so too were their joys, shared reminiscences, strengths, and, above all, their enduring spirit.

References

Albert, Steven M., Litvin, Sandra J., Kleban, Morton H., and Brody, Elaine M. (1991). Caregiving daughters' perceptions of their own and their mothers' personalities. *The Gerontologist 31*(4): 476–82.

Atchley, Robert C. (1996). *Social forces and aging.* 8th ed. Belmont, CA: Wadsworth Publishing Company.

Blenkner, Margaret (1965). Social work and family relationships in later life with some thoughts on filial maturity. In Ethel Shanas and Gordon Streib (Eds.), *Social structure and the family* (pp. 46–59). Englewood Cliffs, NJ: Prentice-Hall.

Boyd, Sandra L., and Treas, Judith (1996). Family care of the frail elderly: A new look at "women in the middle." In Jill Quadagno and Debra Street (Eds.), *Aging for the twenty-first century* (pp. 262–68). New York: St. Martin's Press.

Butler, Robert N., and Lewis, Myrna I. (1983). *Aging and mental health.* New York: C. V. Mosby Co.

Cantor, Marjorie (1975, February). Life-space and the social support system of the inner-city elderly of New York. *The Gerontologist 15*: 23–27.

Donnelly, Harrison (1981, November 28). Special report: The aging of America. *Congressional Quarterly*, pp. 2329–32.

Gelfand, Donald E. (1994). *Aging and ethnicity.* New York: Springer Publishing Company.

Hess, Beth B. (1992). Gender and aging: The demographic parameters. In Lou Glasse and Jon Hendricks (Eds.), *Gender and aging* (pp. 15–24). Amityville, NY: Baywood Publishing Company, Inc.

Hess, Beth B., and Waring, Joan B. (1975, October). Changing patterns of aging and family bonds in later life. *The Family Coordinator*: 303–6.

Horowitz, Amy (1978, November). *Families who care: A study of natural support systems of the elderly.* Paper presented at the 31st annual meeting of the Gerontological Society, Dallas, TX.

Lammers, William W. (1983). *Public policy and the aging.* Washington, DC: Congressional Quarterly Press.

Longino Jr., Charles F. (1996). An aging population may not be harmful to America. In Charles P. Cozic (Ed.), *An aging population: Opposing viewpoints* (pp. 25–31). San Diego, CA: Greenhaven Press, Inc.

Merrill, Deborah, and Dill, Ann (1990). Ethnic differences in older mother-daughter co-residence. *Ethnic Groups 8*: 201–13.

Meyer, Madonna Harrington (1996). Family status and poverty among older women: The gendered distribution of retirement income. In Jill Quadagno and Debra Street (Eds.), *Aging for the twenty-first century* (pp. 464–82). New York: St. Martin's Press.

Miller, Baila, and Montgomery, Andrew (1990). Family caregivers and limitations in social activities. *Research on Aging 12*(1): 72–93.

Mindel, Charles H. (1979). Multigenerational family households: Recent trends and implications for the future. *The Gerontologist 19*: 456–63.

Montgomery, Rhonda J. V., and Datwyler, Mary McGlinn (1992). Women and men in the caregiving role. In Lou Glasse and Jon Hendricks (Eds.), *Gender and aging* (pp. 59–68). Amityville, NY: Baywood Publishing Company, Inc.

Moody, Harry R. (1996). Quality of life for the elderly: Four scenarios. In Charles P. Cozic (Ed.), *An aging population: Opposing viewpoints* (pp. 125–32). San Diego, CA: Greenhaven Press, Inc.

Neugarten, Bernice L. (1974). Age groups in American society and the rise of the young-old. *Annals of the American academy of political and social science*, 187–98.

Noelker, Linda S., and Townsend, Aloen (1987). Perceived caregiving effectiveness. In T. H. Brubaker (Ed.), *Aging, health and family* (pp. 58–79). Newbury Park, CA: Sage.

Ozawa, Martha N. (1995, May). The economic status of older women. *Social Work 40*(3): 323–33.

Quadagno, Jill, and Street, Debra (Eds.). (1996). *Aging for the twenty-first century.* New York: St. Martin's Press.

Savishinsky, Joel (1990). To grow old in a foreign land: Issues in ethnicity and aging. *Ethnic Groups 8*: 143–46.

Schorr, Alvin (1980). ". . . Thy father and thy mother . . .": A second look at filial responsibility and family policy. U.S. Department of Health and Human Services, Social Security Administration, Office of Policy, July 1980.

Seelbach, Wayne C. (1978, October). Correlates of aged parents' filial responsibility expectations and realizations. *The Family Coordinator*: 341–50.

Shanas, Ethel (1979). Social myth as hypothesis: The case of the family relations of old people. *The Gerontologist 19*: 3–9.

Silverman, Alida G., Kahn, Beatrice H., and Anderson, Gary (1977, March). A model for working with multigenerational families. *Social Casework*: 131–35.

Simos, Bertha (1973, May). Adult children and their aging parents. *Social Work*, 78–85.

Spark, Geraldine M., & Brody, Elaine M. (1970, June). The aged are family members. *Family Process*: 195–210.

Streib, Gordon (1972, January). Older families and their troubles: Familial and social responses. *The Family Coordinator*: 5–19.

Turner, Francis J. (1992). The elderly: A biopsychosocial overview. In Francis J. Turner (Ed.), *Mental health and the elderly*. New York: The Free Press.

Walker, Alan (1996). The relationship between the family and the state in the care of older people. In Jill Quadagno and Debra Street (Eds.), *Aging for the twenty-first century* (pp. 269–85). New York: St. Martin's Press.

Walker, Alexis J., and Allen, Katherine R. (1991). Relationships between caregiving daughters and their elderly mothers. *The Gerontologist 31*(3): 389–95.

Watt, Susan, and Soifer, Ahuva (1992). Family issues and the elderly. In Francis J. Turner (Ed.), *Mental Health and the Elderly*. New York: The Free Press, 1992.

Zborowski, Mark, and Herzog, Elizabeth (1952). *Life Is With People*. New York: Schocken Books.

Zimmer, Anna H., and Mellor, M. Joanna (1981, September). Caregivers Make The Difference: Group Services For Those Caring For Older Persons in the Community. A report on the Natural Supports Program of the Community Service Society of New York.

PART FOUR   **Women with Disabilities**

CHAPTER TWELVE

Old Age and Ageism, Impairment and Ableism:
Exploring the Conceptual and Material Connections

CHRISTINE OVERALL

Among most philosophers and theorists, it is now a truism that identities, or at least some identities, are socially constructed. These identities include gender identity, racial identity, and what we might call ability identity, as a disabled or non-disabled person. To this list I also want to add age identity, in particular, age identity as an elderly or aged person.[1]

To regard these identities as socially constructed is to say, first, that they are not "natural"; that is, they are not entities that exist in "nature" independent of human agency. As the work of Simone de Beauvoir revealed (1952), one is not born, let alone conceived, a woman, an Aboriginal, a disabled person, or an elderly person, but rather becomes a woman, an Aboriginal, a disabled person, or an elderly person. Second, to regard these identities as socially constructed is to say that they are created, reinforced, and sustained, although not necessarily with intention or full consciousness, through normative conventions, relations, and practices.

On this much there is fairly general agreement. However, many theorists are willing to take the social constructionist thesis only so far. Usually they insist that there is a biological "foundation" or "substratum" on which the social identity rests. In the case of disability, the biological substratum is said to be impairment, an organic injury to, defect in, or absence of a limb, organ, or physiological system. So, while being a disabled person is an identity that is socially acquired, people are thought to be born with, or at some point become the victim of, mutilating or injurious diseases and accidents whose results—impairments—are part of our biological condition. And in the case of aging, the biological substratum is almost universally thought to be the actual old age of the individual. So, while being an elderly person is an identity that is socially acquired, on a material level it is thought to be the actual number of years lived that provides the material foundation for this identity. Thus, in this analysis, impairment is the supposed biological foundation for disability, for the sake of which individuals may, unfortunately, experience ableism, and old age is the supposed biological foundation for aging, for the sake of which individuals may, unfortunately, experience ageism.

Yet, philosophers ranging from Alison Jaggar (1983) to Judith Butler (1990) have shown that this analysis, the idea of a social identity built

Originally published in the spring 2006 issue (vol. 18, no. 1).

upon a biological substratum, seriously underestimates and misconstrues the role of culture. For the so-called biological substratum in each case is, itself, socially constructed. It is not a natural entity, pre-existing human intervention and possessing an existence independent of human intervention. Instead, the so-called biological substratum is itself a product of social construction; that is, it is created, reinforced, and sustained, not necessarily with intention or full consciousness, through human relations and practices.

In her paper, "On the Government of Disability," Shelley Tremain clearly identifies and describes the social construction of impairment. She points out that the social model of disability, which is the standard view of disability and impairment, claims that disability is the social disadvantage imposed upon the "objective, transhistorical and transcultural" (2001, 617) impairment, which is biologically given. But as Tremain argues,

> allegedly "real" impairments must now be identified as constructs of disciplinary knowledge/power that are incorporated into the self-understandings of some subjects . . . [I]mpairments are materialized as universal attributes (properties) of subjects through the iteration and reiteration of rather culturally specific regulatory norms and ideals about (for example) human function and structure, competency, intelligence, and ability. (2001, 632)[2]

I suggest that there are two main ways in which the social construction of impairment occurs. First, the term *impairment* itself is given a definition by extension, by picking out certain states of physical features—limbs, organs, and systems—and attributing significance to them as fundamentally defining particular individuals and groups of individuals as abnormal or defective in ways that are believed to be "biological." Impairment also can be redefined or expanded, by picking out new arrays of features thought to be abnormal or defective. This is not to deny that real suffering—physical and/or psychological—may attach to the possession of features that are also picked out as defects. My intention here is not to deny the reality of the body or the immediacy of discomfort, pain, fatigue, depression, and weakness. But within any given social context, features that involve suffering may or may not be recognized as impairments (as opposed, say, to normal variations, sources of spiritual insight and divine inspiration, or stigmata). Moreover, in some cases, it is the identification of a feature as a defect that actually *causes* the suffering—for example, in the case of so-called birthmarks.

We also can see that a characteristic designated as an impairment, and considered to be a biological given, might not be an impairment within a different cultural environment. For example, Sophia Isako Wong imagines a situation where a characteristic currently considered an impairment is instead regarded as just another human difference (Wong 2002).

She imagines a world in which half the people have Down syndrome, and persuasively suggests that in it, "there would be integrated households, educational resources, public facilities, and political structures." In this world, "the interaction between people with DS [Down syndrome] and those without it would . . . be seen as essential to the flourishing of the human species" (Wong 2002, 102). Down syndrome is an impairment only within a particular social environment, the environment in which we happen to live.

So far, I have argued that impairment is conceptually constructed; that is, the term *impairment* itself is given a definition by extension, by picking out certain states of certain physical features and attributing significance to them as fundamentally defining particular individuals and groups of individuals as atypical, abnormal, or defective. I also want to argue that impairment is socially constructed in a second way, that is, materially. Impairment is constructed materially first, by means of maternal malnutrition, fetal alcohol syndrome, or the ingestion of teratogenic drugs, all of which cause harm to fetuses before birth, and second, by means of workplace injuries, environmental hazards and contaminants, or simple deliberate human aggression, which cause harm to the limbs, organs, and physiological systems in children and adults. Notice that there is both an individual and a societal component to this material construction of impairment. On the one hand, individuals can be individually injured or "disfigured," but also the creation of impairments across an entire population can result from broader social forces, including poverty, classism, pollution of the home and workplace contexts, and environmental degradation, as well as sexism and racism.

I now want to propose a comparable social constructionist argument, this time with respect to the identity of elderly people. Age theorists have assumed that elderly persons suffer from a social disadvantage that is superimposed upon a biologically given old age.[3] This idea is, however, mistaken, for the supposedly biologically given old age is, itself, socially constructed.

How is it possible for old age itself to be socially constructed? If old age identity is founded upon the number of years lived, isn't the number of years lived an immutable material given? Most theorists seem willing to grant that aging is at least a culturally-*imbued* process, in which age identities such as young adult, middle-aged person, young-old, and old-old are generated. The rate at which one ages, how one ages, and the ways in which aging persons are regarded and regard themselves are accepted as being at least partly socially generated. Yet, it is almost always taken for granted that the cultural process of aging is founded upon the immutable and objective biological foundation of years lived and life stage attained.

I believe that assumption is mistaken. Years lived and life stages attained are also socially constructed and interpreted, and there is no definite, biologically given number of years lived that, by itself, constitutes being old or that provides an immutable and inevitable foundation on the basis of which social aging processes are built. Years lived do not, of themselves, constitute one's age—whether young age, middle age, or old age. Aging is not a "natural" process; that is, it is in no way outside of culture. This is not to deny that, like impairment, the process of aging may entail real suffering, physical and/or psychological. My intention here is not to deny the reality of the body or the immediacy of changing capacities that may accompany the process of aging for some, though not all, persons. But within different social contexts, characteristics of the aging person may or may not be recognized as liabilities and defects—rather than, for example, reserves of wisdom.

Of course, this is not to say that one can change the number of years one has lived. Nothing will make a person who is 75 years old 40 again, for the simple reason that we cannot unmake and remake the past. Nonetheless, as baby boomers and their immediate predecessors are fond of saying, "50 is the new 40" and "60 is the new 50." They are describing a social change, namely, that what was picked out and defined as being "middle-aged" in earlier times is now taken to be pre-middle-aged.

There is a lot of cultural flexibility in the designation of the number of years that constitutes old age—and, for that matter, youth and middle age. Just as cultures pick out certain bodily features and attribute significance to them as fundamentally defining certain groups of people as atypical, abnormal, or impaired in ways that are regarded as "biological," so also cultures pick out a certain number of years and *attribute* biological and cultural significance to that number as constituting the state of being old, physically and mentally worn out, no longer in one's prime, and near the end of one's life. And, like "impairment," "old age" also can be *redefined* or expanded, by picking out different numbers of years lived and/or new arrays of features and defining them as constituting oldness (or as youth, middle age, and so on).

To take just one example of the conceptual constructedness of aging and life stages, the state that was regarded as being "old" came much earlier a century or even half a century ago than it does now. Sixty-five, 60, or even 55 was once considered definitively, inevitably, and unavoidably old, even though there were always some individuals who lived much longer than these ages, into their 80s and 90s. But over the past century, with improvements in health, nutrition, and education, and as more people work, both with and without pay, well after the normative date for retirement, none of these ages is considered as "old" as it once was. Oldness has gotten older, so to speak, and is probably now around 75 or even 80. Moreover, life stage concepts—such as youth, middle age, and elderliness—are not just empirical reflections of the actual duration of objectively given human life stages, but also incorporate and reduplicate normative judgments about how long both the parts and the whole of human life *ought* to be.

A skeptic might argue that even if there is an element of social construction in the creation of old age, there are limits to how far that construction can go. Not every human age can, for example, be defined as "old." But I'm not convinced that there are such limits. Any age, whether it is considered a young age or an old age, is young or old *with respect to* some human environment or some human purpose. Thus, for example, the age of 18 is considered too old *with respect to* learning to be a competitive skater, gymnast, or dancer. Age 30 is considered too old *with respect to* acquiring fluency in a language that will enable the individual to pass as a native speaker. The age of 50, however, is too young *with respect to* taking early retirement and benefiting from government- or corporation-sponsored pensions.

In addition to being, like impairment, socially constructed by means of a (changing) conceptual definition, old age and stage of life, like impairment, are materially constructed at both the individual and the social levels. People do not acquire the physical, psychological, and intellectual markers of aging at the same rates, and the rate of aging is strongly reflective of social context. On an individual level, a person can be "old" at 50 rather than 70 or 80 because of disease or self-destructive habits such as high alcohol consumption, or because of inactivity, both mental and physical. People also can learn, be pressured, or even decide to act "old" or to live the life of a stereotypical "old" person. But there is also a strong societal component to the social construction of old age: social factors such as poverty (along with poor working conditions and inadequate or nonexistent health care and education), racism, sexism, and environmental degradation contribute to shaping the biological reality of being 60, 70, or 80. So a class of poor persons may be considered old at 40 because of the deprived conditions in which they have lived and worked, whereas wealthy persons would have to be 70 before reaching a comparable condition. This material construction of old age is exemplified in the wide variations in life expectancies between first-world and third-world citizens; it is also evident within different socioeconomic classes in Western society.

My general point, then, is that for both disability and aging, the supposedly fixed biological foundation for each—namely impairment and old age—is, itself, socially created, sustained, and elaborated. In comparable ways the biological foundation for impairment and old age is created conceptually, through picking out particular features and defining them as constituting impairment or as constituting oldness, and materially, through the shaping and manipulation of material human features or groups of features.[4] I will turn, now, to a comparison of the two related systems of oppression, ableism and ageism, in order to highlight the ways in which they are similar and connected.

The social practices and institutions that identify and constitute so-called impaired features as individual and social problems comprise the system of oppression that is ableism. And the social practices and institutions that identify and constitute a certain numbers of years lived as individual and social problems comprise the system of oppression that is ageism. In both cases, social practices and institutions establish and reinforce negative values that make rather ordinary characteristics of some human beings into liabilities and stigmata. The systems of ableism and ageism function to make, respectively, certain bodily features (limbs, organs, or systems) and certain numbers of years lived into social liabilities, rationalizations for subordination, and sources of shame. In Western societies, thanks to ableism and ageism, it is taken to be self-evident that lives with so-called impairments, and lives that are elderly, are of lesser value than lives without so-called impairments or lives that are youthful. These lives are even considered, in some cases, not worth living.

Moreover, ableism and ageism are intertwined in malignantly effective ways that result in disrespect, reduction of autonomy, and the disregard of the rights of those targeted. First, those who are rendered disabled may be inappropriately treated as if they were either significantly older or significantly younger than is the norm for behavior toward non-disabled people with the same number of years lived. That is, they are treated as if they were in a state of decline stereotypically associated with aging, or they are treated paternalistically, as if having a disability necessarily reduces the person's competence and autonomy to the level of a child (see Paterson and Hughes 1999, 606). Cultural reactions either age them or infantilize them. Second, people who are "getting on in years" are subjected to explicitly disabling behavior, practices, and policies in cultures that are set up primarily to serve the goals and plans of those with a relatively lower number of years lived and whose features have not been picked out as impaired.[5] Thus, for example, the increasing speed of modern culture, the multiple demands of communication technologies, and the pressure to be competitive, to get ahead, and to earn more money are features of Western society in the twenty-first century that have the effect of adding to the social disablement that older people experience. Another common socially disabling practice in some jurisdictions is mandatory retirement, which makes an arbitrary number of years lived, unrelated to the specific demands of the job, the age at which individuals are forced to give up their jobs, independent of their socioeconomic needs or of any desire they may have to keep working.

There is a real (though quite imperfect) correlation between years lived and certain bodily features designated as impaired. For example, as the number of years lived increases, an individual is more likely to experience arthritis. Nonetheless, there is no one-to-one correspondence between old age and arthritis, since some who are very young may have it and others who are long lived may not. Yet, because of imperfect correlations such as these, ageism and ableism are strongly linked and even reinforce each other. A large number of years lived is stigmatized at least partly because people associate it with the supposedly inevitable development of features regarded as impairments. On the other hand, the features regarded as impairments are stigmatized because, I would argue, they are associated, stereotypically, with the loss of what is seen as youthful vigor and capacity.[6]

Both ableism and ageism incorporate normative ideas of uniformity. Every body should be similar, with similar abilities and energies, and, among other requirements, the ideal human body is a body that has not lived a long time and does not have any of the features designated as impairments. Those individuals with bodies that for one reason or another fail to conform are expected, nonetheless, and despite the difficulties or even impossibilities, to attempt to fit in or assimilate. One attempts to assimilate by minimizing or disguising one's years lived and by minimizing or disguising any of one's features that are designated as impaired. Because disability and aging are considered shameful, weak, and low in value, those who are disabled and/or aged by culture experience pressures to pass as non-disabled or non-aged, to engage in various sorts of pretense that they are as much as possible like the so-called young and healthy social norm (Paterson and Hughes 1999, 608). In other words, they are expected to try to "pass for normal"—where "normal" means "not subject to disablement or aging" (Overall 1998, 151–71). People of all ages internalize the negative valuations of impairment and old age and, as a result, almost everyone participates in the social conspiracy to pretend that there are no impaired or aged people. Assimilationist pressures are among the key tools of oppressive systems such as ableism and ageism.

Using Susan Wendell's terms, I would describe these practices as being the results of the "disciplines of normality" (Wendell 1996, 88). She points out that as the pace of life increases, "[e]veryone who cannot keep up is urged to take steps (or medications) to increase their energy, and bodies that were once considered normal are pathologized" (Wendell 1996, 90). "Keeping up" is a normative requirement, and anyone who has trouble keeping up is, in effect, rendered impaired and expected to compensate as much as possible. Individuals with these socially conferred impairments are often expected to try to act so as to compensate for the impairments, to engage in substitute activities designed to reassure others that the individual is still functional,[7] or to change their appearance so as to appear unimpaired.[8] In the case of aging, older individuals are often expected to try to dress, talk, and act like someone who is younger.[9] The purpose of trying to assimilate is, in part, to reassure others and spare them any feelings of vulnerability or anxiety about their own prospects that the perception of "oldness" or "impairments" may incite. Thereby one also reduces the likelihood of being the target of ageist or ableist prejudice.

The professional agents of ageism and ableism alike include physicians, psychologists, gerontologists, politicians, and journalists. They seize upon and reinforce ableist and ageist tendencies already present in the culture. One way they do this is by promoting the almost-ubiquitous concept of "burdensomeness," a significant negative value that is incorporated into both ageism and ableism. People who have lived many years, along with people with features deemed to be impairments, are regarded as being nonfunctional and nonproductive, hence burdensome. Such individuals can try to compensate for their putative burdensomeness by being patient, submissive, cheerful, eager to please, non-complaining, and willing to listen to others, but the possession of this constellation of virtues is usually insufficient to compensate for the ways in which they are considered to be an economic, social, and psychological problem for other people who have not lived as long or do not have impaired features. Even bioethicists contribute to making human years lived and certain human features a problem through their creation and promotion of the concept of burdensomeness as an allegedly inherent feature of aging and impairment. Key examples include John Hardwig (1997, 2000) and Daniel Callahan (1998). Hardwig, for instance, argues that one has a duty to die— even if one does not want to die—"when continuing to live will impose significant burdens—emotional burdens, extensive caregiving, destruction of life plans, and . . . financial hardship—on [one's] family and loved ones" (Hardwig 1997, 38). From this conservative biomedical ethical standpoint, prolonging human life, whether individually or collectively, and supporting individual people with features deemed to be impairments, become problematic and even morally unjustified.

In conclusion, I have argued that there are significant conceptual parallels as well as cultural connections between old age and impairment and between ageism and ableism. This comparison reveals the extent of social construction within age identity and ability identity, both of which are ordinarily believed to be biologically based. The comparison also helps to reveal the connections between two forms of oppression that are ordinarily so seemingly normal that they are nearly imperceptible. Old age, like impairment, is not a biological given but is socially constructed, both conceptually and materially. That disability and aging both rest upon a biological given is a fiction that functions to excuse and enable the very social mechanisms that perpetuate ableist and ageist oppression.

However, the societal implications of the social construction of aging are not all negative. By recognizing that old age is socially constructed we could create a truly radical transformation of prevailing cultural ideas about age and being "old." If old age is a social product, not a biological given, then aging is a potential site not only for oppression but also for liberation. Social and political reforms in the areas of employment, education, housing, health care, family structures, social welfare, and architecture could redefine the societal context of aging, eliminate or at least reduce ageism, and support increasing rights, opportunities, and freedoms for people who have lived many years. There is nothing inevitable about ageism or about the ways in which old age is currently constructed.

Acknowledgments

I am grateful to the editor, Leni Marshall, and to two anonymous reviewers for their helpful comments on earlier drafts of this essay.

Notes

1. In this essay I eschew the terms *the disabled* and *the elderly*. The problem with the term *the disabled* is that it implies the existence of a group of persons who are nothing but disabled and whose whole identity is taken up with being disabled; there is no other personal residuum. Similarly, the term *the elderly* or *the aged* has a reifying effect that suggests the existence of a group of persons who are nothing but old, individuals for whom being elderly subsumes their entire being and whose entire identity is taken up with being old. For these reasons, the term *disabled persons* or *persons with disabilities* is preferable to *the disabled*. And *elderly people* is preferable to *the elderly*.

2. Similar ideas are put forward by Hughes and Paterson (1997).

3. For example, Copper (1988), Bell (1992), Callahan (1998), Heilbrun (1997), and Hardwig (2000).

4. Where I disagree with Shelley Tremain and some others who defend the social construction of the purported biological foundations of identities is that they then conclude that the identity and its supposed biological base are the

same, because both are constructed. Thus Tremain says, for example, "impairment has been disability all along" (Tremain 2001, 632). Similarly, in talking of gender and sex, Butler writes, "If the immutable character of sex is contested, perhaps this construct called 'sex' is as culturally constructed as gender; indeed, perhaps it was always already gender, with the consequence that the distinction between sex and gender turns out to be no distinction at all" (Butler 1990, 7). However, I suggest that this type of conclusion is not correct. Although each one is socially produced and maintained, sex is not identical with gender; impairment is not identical with disability; and old age is not identical with aging. Each of the terms within each pair— *sex* and *gender*, *impairment* and *disability*, and *old age* and *aging*—has a different *denotation*. The words in each pair each signify something that is socially constructed, yet the words are used to pick out two different parts of the social world. Thus, *impairment* is *used to refer* to a supposedly given organic injury to, defect in, or absence of a limb, organ, or physiological system, whereas *disability* is *used to refer* to the social liability imposed on top of an impairment. Similarly, *old age* is used to refer to a supposedly given number of years lived, whereas *aging* is *used to refer* to a social process imposed on top of the supposedly given number of years lived.

5. It is worth noting that ageism is not just a problem for those who have lived many years. It is also manifest with respect to human beings who have not lived for many years, that is, children. Young children are, for example, systemically disabled through architectural features such as stairs, elevator buttons, toilets, and sinks that are difficult to use and might be dangerous. Young children are also systemically disabled through a social system that relegates them, like aging people, to their own age-segregated niche. For aging people that niche is nursing homes and "seniors" residences; for young children, the niche is school. Furthermore, children are disenfranchised and rendered vulnerable through political and social arrangements whose justification is not always well established.

6. In addition, the social creation of life stages, especially for women, generates disabilities and contributes to the interpersonal validation of the supposed independent reality of impairments. "Menopause," for example, no longer simply means the cessation of menses, and instead refers to a life stage that may extend for years, supposedly creating impairments by destabilizing a woman's memory, emotions, and physical capacities (Gullette 1997).

7. I'm thinking of the Paralympics and Special Olympics here.

8. For example, individuals who have had a breast removed because of cancer are usually expected to wear a prosthetic.

9. Here is where sexism intersects with ageism, since a youthful appearance is more highly valued in women and hence is more desperately sought by them. For example, both youthfulness and femininity alike can be achieved by means of "the knife" of cosmetic surgery (Morgan 1991).

References

Bell, Nora Kizer. 1992. "If Age Becomes a Standard for Rationing Health Care . . ." In *Feminist Perspectives in Medical Ethics*, ed. Helen Bequaert Holmes and Laura M. Purdy, 82–90. Bloomington: Indiana University Press.

Butler, Judith. 1990. *Gender Trouble: Feminism and the Subversion of Identity.* New York: Routledge.

Callahan, Daniel. 1998. *False Hopes: Why America's Quest for Perfect Health Is a Recipe for Failure.* New York: Simon & Schuster.

Copper, Baba. 1988. *Over the Hill: Reflections on Ageism Between Women.* Freedom, CA: Crossing Press.

de Beauvoir, Simone. 1952. *The Second Sex.* New York: Knopf.

Gullette, Margaret Morganroth. 1997. *Declining to Decline: Cultural Combat and the Politics of the Midlife.* Charlottesville: University Press of Virginia.

Hardwig, John. 2000. *Is There a Duty to Die? And Other Essays in Medical Ethics.* With Nat Hentoff, Dan Callahan, Larry Churchill, Felicia Cohn, and Joanne Lynn. New York: Routledge.

———. 1997. "Is There a Duty to Die?" *Hastings Center Report* 27(2): 34–42.

Heilbrun, Carolyn G. 1997. *The Last Gift of Time: Life Beyond Sixty.* New York: Dial Press.

Hughes, Bill, and Kevin Paterson. 1997. "The Social Model of Disability and The Disappearing Body: Towards a Sociology of Impairment." *Disability and Society* 12(3): 325–40.

Jaggar, Alison. 1983. "Human Biology in Feminist Theory: Sexual Equality Reconsidered." In *Beyond Domination: New Perspectives on Women and Philosophy*, ed. Carol C. Gould, 21–42. Totowa, NJ: Rowman & Allanheld.

Morgan, Kathryn Pauly. 1991. "Women and the Knife: Cosmetic Surgery and the Colonization of Women's Bodies." *Hypatia: A Journal of Feminist Philosophy* 6(3): 24–53.

Overall, Christine. 1998. *A Feminist I: Reflections From Academia.* Peterborough, Ontario: Broadview Press.

Paterson, Kevin, and Bill Hughes. 1999. "Disability Studies and Phenomenology: The Carnal Politics of Everyday Life." *Disability and Society* 14(5): 597–610.

Tremain, Shelley. 2001. "On the Government of Disability." *Social Theory and Practice* 27(4): 617–36.

Wendell, Susan. 1996. *The Rejected Body: Feminist Philosophical Reflections on Disability.* New York: Routledge.

Wong, Sophia Isako. 2002. "At Home with Down Syndrome and Gender." *Hypatia: A Journal of Feminist Philosophy* 17(3): 89–117.

CHAPTER THIRTEEN

Res(Crip)ting Feminist Theater through Disability Theater: Selections from The DisAbility Project

ANN M. FOX AND JOAN LIPKIN

> *MAN: Was I too healthy? Was that it? Did some secret-society deity decide I should be given a handicap to even up the race?*
> *WOMAN: Well, that is an interesting conjecture.*
> —Myrna Lamb (1971, 164–65)

One of the pieces in Myrna Lamb's classic, early feminist, and episodic play *Scyklon Z*, "But What Have You Done for Me Lately?" (first performed in 1969), features a man who is impregnated so that he might experience the dilemma of an unwanted pregnancy in an anti-choice culture. Here, disability metaphorically represents the female body within a patriarchal society as "handicapped" (as the above quote suggests) and looms as the potential punishment for women denied reproductive choice:

> WOMAN: There is a woman who unwittingly took a fetus-deforming drug administered by her physician for routine nausea, and a woman who caught German measles at a crucial point in her pregnancy, both of whom were denied the right to abortion, but granted the privilege of rearing hopelessly defective children. (1971, 164–65)

As Lamb's play suggests, feminist theater is in something of a curiously ambiguous position with regard to disability. For the conscientious reader, it quickly becomes apparent that disability images are as ubiquitous in the literary and theater landscapes as their live counterparts are in a society more inclined to either politely overlook their presence or mark it in highly controlled ways. Indeed, as disability and theater scholar Victoria Ann Lewis has noted, "It is not that the nondisabled theater world knows nothing about disability and is waiting to be enlightened. To the contrary, the depiction of disability is over-represented in dramatic literature" (2000, 93). This is no less true for the American feminist playwrights who have been writing women into theater for the contemporary stage. Consider many of the plays following Lamb's that are otherwise lauded for their feminist sensibilities and you will discover that they emulate, rather than challenge, that early and essentialist icon of disability in classic theater, *The Glass Menagerie*'s Laura Wingfield (Williams 1972). Prominent figures of this kind, for example,

Originally published in the fall 2002 issue (vol. 14, no. 3).

include paraplegic Julia in Maria Irene Fornes's *Fefu and Her Friends* (1990); the severely depressed MaGrath sisters in Beth Henley's *Crimes of the Heart* (1988); and paraplegic Skoolie in Kia Corthron's *Come Down Burning* (1996).[1] "Feminists today," notes disability studies scholar Rosemarie Garland Thomson, "even often invoke negative images of disability to describe the oppression of women," and that theoretical use finds its artistic corollary with great regularity in feminist playwriting (1997, 279). Lamb's example, while an early one, continues the use of disability as metaphor for female oppression that we can see in characters as early as the neurasthenic Young Woman battered by gender expectations in Sophie Treadwell's *Machinal* (1993) or as recent as brain-damaged Sara, literally beaten in a gay-bashing in Diana Son's *Stop Kiss* (1999).

It is certain that the use of physical difference as a metaphor, one that does not represent disability experience for its own sake, is deeply at play in theater. Disability and literature scholars David T. Mitchell and Sharon Snyder have labeled this process as it occurs in literary fiction "narrative prosthesis" (2000). That it is as pervasively present within feminist playwriting, which ostensibly rejects the socially constructed value systems embraced by more canonical theater (more on this in a moment), seems at first something of a paradox. Disability and theater scholar Carrie Sandahl points to several examples of this seemingly ironic state of affairs:

> Consider the use of epilepsy as unbearable stigma in Marsha Norman's *Night Mother*; or paralysis as a perverse, grotesque burden in Maria Irene Fornes's *Mud*. Even "positive" metaphors (as in Jane Wagner and Lily Tomlin's use of mental illness as inspiration in *Search for Signs of Intelligent Life in the Universe*) ignore the actual material conditions of the disabled people portrayed. (1999, 15)

Sandahl's list can easily be extended; the plays mentioned above are themselves also works in which "the use of disability as a dramaturgical device tends to erase the particularities of lived disability experiences" (15). Paraplegia, for example, operates as a metaphor for the punitive nature of patriarchal structures in *Fefu*. Each of the MaGrath sisters' depressive episodes contributes to the larger image of Southern eccentricity and repression Henley creates. And in Corthron's play, the poverty that circumscribes its women throughout is embodied in Skoolie, as she is compelled to wheel herself about in a crudely fashioned cart.

All this is not meant to negate the power and worth of these plays and the importance of their roles in challenging assumptions about class, race, gender, and sexuality. It is also not meant to imply that only feminist playwrights have invoked images of disability in this way; for example, plays ranging from Hanay Geiogamah's *Body Indian* (1999) to

August Wilson's *Fences* (1986) also use disability to embody the experience of racial and economic oppression. Furthermore, the move from the page to the stage, informed by a feminist sensibility, does not always of necessity follow old patterns; indeed, "when feminism and disability politics are taken into consideration together, they can productively inform and complicate one another" (Sandahl 1999, 12). Metaphor, which is at the heart of theatrical language, need not be rejected completely, but might likewise be enhanced in just this fashion. Cherríe Moraga's *Heroes and Saints* (1996), for example, is a feminist work that powerfully interweaves metaphor and the lived experience of disability. The play's main character, Cerezita, born only as a head because of her mother's drinking from the pesticide-ridden community water supply, embodies the outcome of the environmental racism leveled against her Latino/a community. But Moraga also creates Cerezita as a desiring, desirable human being whose disability is very much part of her identity and not merely a personal tragedy. Cerezita resists her mother's attempts to hide her from the stares of strangers, insisting on her own visibility; indeed, her disability later makes it possible for her to actively lead her community, not just passively inspire them. Still, there is no avoiding the fact that in much of feminist theater, we see reflected the tensions and questions that have already emerged from the movement to place disability studies and feminist thought in conversation with one another. Given feminist theater's relative inattention to the presence of disability beyond its more troublesome metaphorical uses, to what end might the feminist practitioner of theater concern herself with disability culture? What in feminist practice lends itself to creating theater centered on disability and to reclaiming the power of metaphor in representation? And what, in turn, does a "disability aesthetic" have to offer by way of expanding and interrogating feminist theater?[2]

But before engaging these questions, it is important to define what is meant by feminist theater and disability theater, respectively. For the purposes of this essay, feminist theater will be defined as that which also seeks to effect social change through questioning the traditional apparatus of theatrical representation, and by extension, calling attention to the social construction of identities upon which privilege is based. In other words, as feminist theater and performance scholar Jill Dolan points out, it is a theater whose theoretical perspective

> is concerned with more than just the artifact of representation—the play, film, painting, or dance. It considers the entire apparatus that frames and creates these images and their connection not just to social roles but also to the structure of culture and its divisions of power. (1993, 47)

This is a category of feminist theater typically defined as materialist. Engaging psychoanalytic, poststructuralist, and Marxist theories, it seeks not only to challenge traditional forms of spectatorship, but all elements of theatrical creation and presentation. The playwright is not assumed to be literally or figuratively the solitary producer of meaning (and presumably male), the theatrical space is not presumed to be a proscenium arch, and the representational style is not presumed to be mimetic or that of theatrical realism. Dolan also allies materialist feminism with "a postmodernist performance style that breaks with realist narrative strategies, heralds the death of unified characters, decenters the subject, and foregrounds the conventions of perception" (1996, 97). This challenges conventional uses of representation, history, and language that, conversely, place women either at the periphery or in the center as objectified and gazed-upon entities.

Because a definition of disability theater has not been as extensively theorized as that of feminist theater, to speak of disability theater is instantly to raise questions that point to the elusiveness of defining the thing itself and that have yet to be fully explored by critics. Does any work by a disabled playwright automatically count, regardless of subject matter? Should such a category include images of disability in canonical theater? Should it include long-established theatrical traditions within communities where the label of "disabled" is met with much more contention, such as deaf theater? Should it include art made with disabled populations that primarily emphasizes the therapeutic or cathartic effects on those involved as performers?

It is no more accurate to assume that all work by a disabled playwright or performer is of necessity disability theater than to surmise that all work by women playwrights is feminist. The most innovative and productive disability theater, for the purposes of this essay, does not include disability's more traditional theatrical manifestation, that is, the tokenized presence of the disabled character in isolation, as metaphor for insidiousness or innocence, or as overcomer. This does not mean that we should not look at the historical representation of disability in theater and ask questions about the kinds of cultural dialogues it alternately reflects and invokes around deviations from bodily normalcy. Because this kind of representation of disability experience is more widespread in popular literature and the mass media, to analyze these characterizations is no less monumental or important a task awaiting disability studies scholars.

To speak of disability theater as an entity is to speak of a self-conscious artistic movement of roughly the last three decades, during which time writers and performers within disability culture have moved to create art as multifaceted as the community from which it emerges. Victoria Ann Lewis's article, "The Dramaturgy of Disability," has been crucial in the process of not only identifying who some of the important writers of disability theater have been for an academic audience, but also in initially delineating the dramaturgical strategies that underpin disability writing for the stage (2000). Lewis points to artists whose approaches to theater run the gamut from writing plays (Mike Ervin, John Belluso, Susan Nussbaum) to conducting performance workshops (Lewis's own OTHER VOICES Project, a disability performance workshop based at the Mark Taper Forum in Los Angeles) to creating solo performance work (Cheryl Marie Wade). To her lists, we can add significant other forays into the performance of disability, including playwrights such as Katinka Neuhof; community-based theater workshops like The DisAbility Project (based in St. Louis, Missouri) and Actual Lives (based in Austin, Texas); and solo performers like Lynn Manning, Terry Galloway, Julia Trahan, and David Roche.

In her study, Lewis locates two prominent directions in disability theater: one focuses on exposing disability as a social construction and one "celebrates the difference of the disability experience, what is called 'disability culture' or 'disability cool' in the disability community" (2000, 102). The former emphasis might produce theater that advocates for disability rights, works to contravene familiar stereotypes, questions definitions of bodily normalcy, resists essentializing disability into one kind of physical experience, and foregrounds the ways in which disability intersects with other identity categories. The latter direction emphasizes representing the experience of disability and disability culture. Kathleen Tolan locates the work of disabled theater artists along slightly different lines: "There are artists and groups whose main interest is social/political, who perceive their main work as critiquing society, changing perceptions, forging communities . . . there are others whose greatest interest is in artistic and aesthetic exploration and expression" (2001, 17).

Useful as Lewis's and Tolan's works are, they suggest polarized categories of creation, a construction that we might begin to think beyond. How might we begin to imagine a definition of disability theater that negotiates these divisions between art and activism in a more synthesized fashion, producing something we might label a *disability aesthetic?* In the process of doing so, disability theater can not only expand its own artistry in dialogue with feminist theater, but can in turn problematize feminist theater's potential reification of the metaphorical use of disability as a sort of *dramaturgical prosthesis*. Through the interrelationship of these approaches, we might in turn contribute to the call Thomson has made for feminism and disability studies to productively inform one another. The DisAbility Project is a useful company through which to investigate the question of a disability aesthetic. As artistic director Joan Lipkin points out, "I always say to my ensemble . . . that we are equal parts art and advocacy. And the minute we fail to delight, surprise, move or mystify in *how* we say things as well as *what* we say, we've lost our focus" (Tolan 2001, 19). The Project is thus consciously at the intersection of the artistic and activist strains of disability theater.

The scripts that follow, "Facts and Figures," "Employment," and "Go Figure," exemplify how we might begin to answer the questions raised above and further the exploration of the ways in which feminist and disability theaters can inform and enhance one another. They are three of an expansive and growing repertoire of theater pieces created by feminist playwright and director Joan Lipkin and the members of The DisAbility Project, a grassroots St. Louis theater ensemble that creates and performs work centered around disability culture. Founded in 1997, the Project is made up of actors with and without disabilities, embodying a diverse (although by no means complete) representation of performing experience, age, race, class, sexuality, and disability. The disabilities that have been represented at varying times within the group include paraplegia, quadriplegia, AIDS, multiple sclerosis, cerebral palsy, stroke, blindness, bipolar disorder, cancer, spina bifida, muscular dystrophy, spinal cord injury, asthma, polio, epilepsy, amputation, depression, cognitive disability, and alcoholism. Under Lipkin's direction, the members of this community-based theater meet weekly in workshop sessions to share experiences, create, and rehearse work. Originally, the Project as conceived was to build toward a single theater event in the fall of 2000. The Project has evolved, however, into an ongoing ensemble that both continues to create theatrical work and to take their award-winning performances out into the greater St. Louis area, in venues from ballrooms to boardrooms to classrooms.[3] At any given performance, the company draws from a repertoire of approximately twenty pieces to assemble a performance tailored to the individual audience. The pieces cover a range of disability experiences, including disability history, transportation, parking, pain, employment, attendant care, sexuality, health care, architectural accessibility, and social interaction. In addition to depicting some realistic situations, there are also several pieces that are primarily visual in nature, in which the innovative movement and stage images that can be created by disabled bodies are the primary focus.

The creative process from which these scripts emerged begins to suggest how feminist theater practice and disability theater might engage one another. While the weekly workshops take place under Lipkin's direction, the resulting work resists privileging a single view; instead, it is collaborative, multiperspectival, and constructed in concert with Lipkin, the performers, guest artists, and the audience (whose feedback has given rise to new pieces). Because the ensemble cast contains a range of performers with and without disabilities, no one kind of bodily experience is reified as the disabled or non-disabled norm. Likewise, the presence of disabled actors emphasizes the importance of their performing their own stories. And while there are significant and material differences in the lived identities of non-disabled and disabled people, integrating this company underscores that there are concerns relevant to the disabled community that have real implications for non-disabled individuals as well. One can become disabled at any time, and we are all on our way to becoming disabled by virtue of the aging process; certainly our body-phobic culture includes a wide range of physical shapes, sizes, and capabilities for which we have little tolerance.

A playwright whose own principles of feminist playwriting and directing embody poststructuralist and materialist thought, Lipkin has long interrogated socially constructed categories of race, class, gender, and sexuality typically regarded as cohesive and natural. She has informed her work on the Project with similar innovations in theme and style, confounding traditional audience expectations and viewing habits. Each of the following three scripts links to concerns and methodologies advanced by feminist theater, but likewise infuses those ideas and dramaturgical strategies with a disability perspective.

For example, "Facts and Figures" extends a feminist critique of history and language; both are systems of meaning from which disability has been erased, except as a disembodied expression of derision ("You are so ADD").[4] In a personal interview, Lipkin emphasized that the company, in performing this piece, wants to "awaken the audience to attend to language differently and have their experience of the performance to be grounded in a sense of history." "Facts and Figures" at once presents an audience with the realities of the disability experience, while simultaneously exposing how that experience is co-opted and portrayed negatively within everyday language. This piece foregrounds the lived experience of those with disabilities, past ("Freak shows exhibiting the bodies of disabled men and women were common entertainment in the Victorian period") and present ("People with disabilities are the largest minority in the United States"). Through the revelation of these facts, disability is moved out of the world of the "private, generally hidden, and often neglected" (Wendell 1997, 266). The included facts link the experience of female and disabled bodies ("During witch trials, many of the women who were tried for witchcraft had disabilities"), foregrounding for an audience how female and disabled bodies have simultaneously occupied sites of marginalization.

But these facts also remind us that there is a specific disability experience to be articulated. Disability studies scholar Susan Wendell, in calling for a feminist theory of disability, confirms this necessity and suggests the opportunity arising from it:

> Emphasizing differences from the able-bodied demands that those differences be acknowledged and respected and fosters solidarity among the disabled. It challenges the able-bodied paradigm of humanity and creates the possibility

of a deeper challenge to the idealization of the body and the demand for its control. (1997, 272)

The reconsideration of social history that feminist theater seeks to re-create is therefore deepened by acknowledging other categories through which communities are Othered, including disability. The figures of speech interwoven with the piece's facts are a confirmation of this. Using disability negatively ("He gave me such a lame excuse!" "That is so retarded"), these expressions at once appropriate and reconfigure physical difference solely as lack. By questioning the dismissive assumptions behind our use of language that addresses disability ("She is psycho"), the piece invites each audience member to become aware of and thus accountable for her or his own use of metaphor and language. Incorporating such a consciousness of language can only help practitioners of feminist theater examine their own use of disability with as much care as they would language marking race, class, sexuality, and gender, for example.

One of the facts with which "Facts and Figures" presents audience members concerns disabled workers: "People with disabilities are the most under-employed population in the country. Mostly because our transportation systems make it difficult for them to get jobs, or employers won't hire them [*sic*]." More specifically, as Heather Gain and Lisa Bennett point out, disabled have "the highest unemployment rate of any group—somewhere between 72 and 90 percent" (2002, 16). The piece entitled "Employment" comically and pointedly expands on this fact by performing the assumptions about ability that underlie employer willingness, or rather, unwillingness, to consider disabled job applicants. The characters in "Employment" move to challenge the seeming impasse that results when a disabled person applies for a job but is quickly turned down on the grounds that she might "turn off the customers," not be up to the rigors of "a pretty demanding job," and is only suited for "the sheltered workshop." "Can this situation be saved?" asks the job seeker, turning to the audience for resolution. In some settings, the audience is given the opportunity to create potential solutions to the dilemma, imagining how the workplace and workers' roles could be reimagined to include the disabled person. Members of the Project have also constructed alternate endings that can be presented if an audience is less inclined to participate, endings in which they, along with the manager, are invited to open their minds. Lipkin and ensemble tweak the social assumptions about what disabled workers can and cannot do and offer a further pointed comment: in an age when disabled people are unemployed in such large numbers, and employers are in need of employable workers, ableist attitudes serve no one. Linking gender to economic inequity is not new in feminist theater, but the attention paid to the particular link between

disability and unemployment enhances that critique of economic priva-
tion based on social identity.

"Go Figure," the story of Katie Rodriguez Banister's reimagining of
her sexual identity after becoming disabled, both allies constructions of
gender and disability as well as speaks importantly to the unquestioned
assumption in our society that the disabled person is asexual, undesirable,
and undesiring. What is immediately striking about this piece is that
even as Banister revels in remembering her sexuality before her accident
("You may not be able to tell, but I used to be quite the Barbie girl"), that
memory is tinged with the recollection of worry about what people would
think of her. We, as audience members, are reminded that Banister's
change in experience underscores that the female body, in both its non-
disabled and its disabled identity, is policed as the site of potential trans-
gressions away from normalcy, whether the standard be one of beauty,
sexual propriety, or physical wholeness. Banister's life transition from
non-disabled to disabled is therefore not a shift from normalcy to abnor-
malcy so much as a movement from being the object of one kind of spec-
tatorial look to another. For as Thomson reminds us, "If the male gaze
informs the normative female self as a sexual spectacle, then the stare
sculpts the disabled subject as a grotesque spectacle" (1997, 285). In our
society, both female bodies and disabled bodies find themselves literally
and figuratively marginalized because of their supposed deviation from
an idealized norm, whether that model is a particular gender, a standard
of femininity or heterosexuality, or some illusory construction of wholeness. Thomson specifically points out the parallels:

> Both the female and the disabled body are cast within cultural discourse as
> deviant and inferior; both are excluded from full participation in public as
> well as economic life; both are defined in opposition to a valued norm which
> is assumed to possess natural corporeal superiority. (279)

This is comically, but pointedly, illustrated when Banister remembers, "I
placed a personal ad in the singles paper: 'Petite, professional, independent woman on wheels seeks male,'" and "one man," unable to imagine
a disabled woman placing a personal ad, "thought I drove around a lot."
But Banister's experiences, while distinct, are perhaps not as removed
from those of non-disabled women as might be imagined, since "female
bodies, like bodies of color, homosexual bodies, *and* disabled bodies, are
positioned culturally so as not to forget their embodiment" (Miner 1997,
292–93).

Banister powerfully reclaims her own particular sexuality, breaking
down the illusion that the "temporarily able-bodied" watching her performance are somehow removed from these issues. Equally important is her
assertion that she is having "the best sex of my life"; hers becomes not an

overcoming narrative on how to learn to do without, but an invitation to the audience to learn to do with differently. "Go figure!" she exclaims, but that expression of surprise can simultaneously be read as an invocation to the audience, disabled and non-disabled spectators alike, to figure out how to move beyond the narrow confines of how society defines sexual roles. For this reason, it is particularly fitting that Banister trades off the telling of her story with Rich Scharf, an openly gay male member of the company. This destabilizes the expectation that it is only her story and one grounded only in a presumption of heterosexuality.

As Nancy Mairs explains in *Waist-High in the World*, "Most people, in fact, deal with the discomfort and even distaste that a misshapen body arouses by disassociating that body from sexuality in reverie and practice" (1996, 51). "It was like I was a virgin again," Banister exclaims about her sexual identity after becoming disabled, and in a sense, she is "like a virgin." She, and the audience, have to reimagine her sexuality and desirability as manifested in ways beyond what society deems normal or acceptable. In this way, Banister is one of those paraplegics who, as Wendell asserts, "have revolutionary things to teach about the possibilities of sexuality" (1997, 274). The materiality of Banister's life as sexual being is acknowledged, celebrated, and also the means by which a reimagination of sexuality can occur *through* disability.

Dramaturgically, the pieces discussed here all sustain aesthetic challenges to traditional theater practice familiar to those historically adapted by feminist playwrights. The episodic nature of the performance, juxtaposing, for example, monologic pieces with more non-representational ones, makes for a nonlinear viewing experience, echoing movement within feminist theater to resist conventionally realistic representation and progressive plots.[5] A resistance to these more traditional forms can likewise inform a disability aesthetic that resists social constructions of physical evolution, progress, and normalcy by resisting Western theatrical convention. In form and content, these pieces invite the non-disabled members of the audience to consider new ways to perceive space, time, and the body, while not denying the materiality of those same bodily experiences as lived by disabled people.

More specifically, both "Go Figure" and "Employment" rely on Brechtian interventions into the theatrical viewing experience, including direct address to the audience and disrupting conventionally realistic representation. In "Go Figure," for example, two actors become a split subject to pass the single story back and forth; while it is Banister's experience, Scharf's presence suggests its connection to others. Scharf's readable physical and gender difference from Banister at once prevents us from universalizing Banister's experience and simultaneously compels us to consider how Scharf might have felt his own body similarly circumscribed by ideals of male beauty and masculinity. "Employment"'s rolling back the scenes to invite audience members to "replay" them in a different, more activist manner works to create a similar alienation of the audience from a passive viewing experience. This referencing of fast-forward and rewind is a product of the age of television and video, pointing to the manner in which the Project also uses references to popular culture. Deconstructing the assumption that theater is only high culture, these references, like the comedy of the pieces, invite audience members to link their own experience and vernacular with those used by the disabled characters, thus further establishing a connection.

One final note about the performance context for these scripts: these scripts are typically performed in concert with other pieces created by members of the Project; in a typical performance, anywhere from eight to twelve pieces get performed, depending on the audience, size of the ensemble, venue, and amount of time available. While other pieces might be performed in between them, when all three are part of a performance, the scripts included here are generally presented in the following order: "Facts and Figures," "Employment," and "Go Figure." The order is purposeful; as Lipkin observed in a personal interview, "the experience of any performance is an emotional, spiritual, intellectual, and visceral journey. The arc of that journey is crafted carefully." As a result, "Facts and Figures" and "Employment" both come early in the performance. "Facts and Figures" foregrounds a history with which audience members may be unfamiliar, while "Employment" simultaneously embodies the concrete reality of job discrimination while engaging an audience's support through humor. "Go Figure," as one of the most intimate and emotionally challenging pieces, comes later in the performance.

Rosemarie Garland Thomson has called for disability to become a "universalizing discourse," invested in

> asserting the body as a cultural text which is interpreted, inscribed with meaning, indeed made, within social relations of power. Such a perspective advocates political equality by denaturalizing disability's assumed inferiority, casting its configurations and functions as difference rather than lack. (1997, 282)

Toward that end, and as these pieces demonstrate, an emergent disability theater can simultaneously build upon and complicate the thematic and aesthetic interrogations feminist theater initiates with regard to other kinds of social identities. This might further encourage feminist theater to avoid the subtle reinscriptions of normalcy encoded in a too commonly well-intentioned, albeit superficial, use of disability in theater. Go figure: crip culture can rescript feminist theater in ways that contribute to establishing disability and feminism as powerful allies in imagining a more expansive view of reality, onstage and off.

Facts and Figures
Joan Lipkin and The DisAbility Project

Two groups of the ensemble

Odd numbers on stage left, even numbers on stage right. This piece can be done with as many as sixteen people, each taking their own line, or a smaller group with a doubling up on lines. There should be varying heights and levels among the groups. Each person has his or her factoid written on a piece of paper, preferably memorized. After the reading of the line, the paper is discarded in whatever way possible (crumbled, thrown to the floor, etc.)

Ensemble Member One: That is so retarded.

Ensemble Member Two: In medieval times, disabilities were seen as a curse from God.

Three: The industry has been crippled.

Four: During witch trials, many of the women who were tried for witchcraft had disabilities.

Five: He's a lame duck.

Six: Court jesters with physical disabilities were common entertainment through much of European history.

Seven: Those kids are such freaks.

Eight: Freak shows exhibiting the bodies of disabled men and women were common entertainment in the Victorian period.

Nine: He gave me such a lame excuse.

Ten: People with disabilities are the largest minority in the United States.

Eleven: Hey, four eyes!

Twelve: In China, many children with visible disabilities are killed or abandoned at birth.

Thirteen: He/she is psycho.

Fourteen: People with disabilities are the most under-employed population in the country. Mostly because our transportation systems make it difficult for them to get jobs, or employers won't hire them.

Fifteen: You are so ADD.

Sixteen: Most people with disabilities live below the poverty line.
   [At the word "below," the ensemble begins to bend over in whatever way possible. Then they begin to slowly rise up, with a collective hum, getting increasingly louder as they rise. When they are fully upright again, those people in the ensemble who can, begin to wave their fists in the air and emit a sustained roar. This comes to a collective stop. The ensemble takes several

moments to breathe and transition. They move slowly into a brief contact improvisation with each other, touching and connecting in various places on their bodies.]

[beat]

All: *[to audience, with outstretched hands and arms where possible]* Welcome to our world!

Employment
Joan Lipkin and The DisAbility Project

Salesperson
Manager
Job Seeker (a woman using a wheelchair)
Wild Shoppers (As few as three, as many as you like)
Wild Shopper #1
Wild Shopper #2
Wild Shopper #3 (A man using a wheelchair)

Salesperson is found amid the Wild Shoppers. The roar of the shoppers pushes the Salesperson from amongst their midst. She runs into the Manger's office excited and flustered.

Salesperson: It's a jungle out there! *[Wild Shoppers writhe, pull at various items, improvise comments and roar.]* I'm putting in for combat pay.
Manager: You're just a little tired.
Salesperson: I won't go back in there. *[Wild Shoppers roar and improvise comments again. Items of clothing go flying.]* I won't.

[She starts to sob.]

Manager: There, there . . .
Salesperson: Have you ever worked the post Christmas sale? *[More frenzy from the Wild Shoppers Perhaps more roar. Sales person sobs.]* Post Christmas. Pre-Christmas. Columbus Day?!!! I need more help.
Manager: We're doing all we can. But in this economy, it isn't easy. They're paying $8.50 an hour plus benefits at Taco Bell on Manchester. And $9.00 at Triple A Dry Cleaning.

[Salesperson continues to sob. In rolls Job Seeker in a wheelchair.]

Job Seeker: Excuse me. I'm here about the job.
Manager: Oh, you must be looking for the sheltered workshop. It's at the other end of the mall.
Job Seeker: No, I meant the job here. The one that was listed in the paper.
Manager: Oh. There must be some mistake. We sell clothes.

Job Seeker: Yes, I can see that. And I wear them. That's why I'm here. I live to accessorize.

Salesperson: Fantastic! I love what you're wearing. *[Manager pulls Salesperson aside to talk with her privately.]*

Manager: Excuse me. We can't hire her. It'll turn off the customers.

Salesperson: Oh, I don't know. She's more enthusiastic than most of the people we have working on the floor. And perky. You did say that perky was part of the job description. And she obviously loves clothes.

Job Seeker: [To audience] I love clothes. I never wear white after Labor Day.

Manager: It's not just that. The aisles are too crowded. She couldn't get through.

                                                        [Wild Shoppers roar.]

Job Seeker: I'd really like to work here. Really, I would.

Salesperson: And I'd like to do something but my hands are tied.

Job Seeker: [To audience] Can this situation be saved?

                        [Everyone hums theme song from Jeopardy. *A Wild Shopper breaks away from the group to offer an alternative scenario.]*

Wild Shopper #1: Excuse me. I have an idea. Could we roll this scene back a little?

            [*The Wild Shopper, Salesperson, and Manager mime rolling back of time with hand gestures and vocalization. The scene resumes.*]

Job Seeker: I'd really like to work here. Really, I would.

Salesperson: And I'd like to do something but my hands are tied.

Wild Shopper #1: I have been here for an hour and a half and no one has offered to help. Or even said hello. What you need around here is more friendliness. Why couldn't she work as a greeter?

Job Seeker: [To audience] Hi. Hi. How ya doing? Thank you for coming. Welcome.

Wild Shopper #1: See? She's great.

Manager: I don't know. I'm not sure that something like that is in our budget.

Wild Shopper #1: Sheesh. Even Wal-Mart has a greeter. I'm not shopping here any more!

[Wild Shopper #1 goes back to crowd. Everyone hums the Jeopardy *song again, this time a little faster. Wild Shopper #2 interrupts it before it ends.]*

Wild Shopper #2: I know! I know! You say the aisles are too crowded? I agree. It is way too crowded in here. How about if she was a cashier? *[To audience.]* How about that?!

Job Seeker: [To audience] Cha ching! Cha ching!

                                                    [The Wild Shoppers roar.]

Salesperson: We need to open up another register.

Manager: I don't know. It's a pretty demanding job. How do I know that
she is responsible?

Job Seeker: Oh, I'm very good with money. You have to be when you
love clothes as much as I do.

Manager: I'm sure you are. [To Salesperson] But we'd have to make
special arrangements for her. You know with the equipment and
all. It could be expensive.

Wild Shopper #2: How expensive could it be? She already has her own
chair!

> *[Manager is clearly noncommittal so Wild Shopper #2 goes
> back to crowd. At this point, Salesperson could ask the
> audience if they have any ideas and then bring them up to
> discuss them. Improv is involved. Job Seeker remains enthusiastic
> and Manager is uncomfortable and unconvinced.]*

Alternative Ending #1

*[Depending upon the audience's mood, a final suggestion could be taken
from Wild Shopper #3]*

Wild Shopper #3: You know, anyone who loves clothes as much as she
does (and I must say, you look mahvelous) . . .

Job Seeker: Thank you, dahling.

Wild Shopper #3: Anyone who loves clothes as much as she does should
be a personal shopper.

Job Seeker: Oh, yes. I love it! And I would love to spend somebody else's
money for them.

> *[The Wild Shoppers roar.]*

Manager: How would she get around?

Job Seeker: I got here, didn't I?

Manager: I don't know.

Wild Shopper #3: Well I do. *[To Job Seeker]* Here's my card. *[To Man-
ager]* I'm with that little department store down the street.

Manager: Not blah-blah-blah?!

Wild Shopper #3: The very one.

Manager: And are you blee-blee-blee?!

Wild Shopper #3: Indeed, I am.

Manager: Oh no!

Wild Shopper #3: And I know talent when I see it. *[To Job Seeker]* My
car is out front. Shall we discuss the details over lunch? [He leaves,
and she follows.]

Job Seeker: Cha-Ching, Cha-Ching, Cha-Ching!

> *[Wild Shoppers roar, Salesperson and Manager look at each
> other in disbelief.]*

Alternative Ending #2

Job Seeker: I could be a greeter, a cashier, a personal shopper and more. Maybe you've just never worked with someone like me before. Please think about it. You know, open your mind?

Manager: You're right. And I really will.

Salesperson: Just do it soon, please?!

[The Wild Shoppers roar.]

Salesperson: I need help fast!

Alternative Ending #3

[After the audience has come up to propose several endings, the ensemble needs to bring the scene to a strong close.]

Salesperson: [To Manager] So, what do you think?

Manager: I'm not sure.

Job Seeker: Look, I could be a greeter, a cashier. *[Mention all of the other things that have been proposed.]* Maybe you've just never worked with someone like me before. Please think about it. You know, open your mind?

Manager: You're right. And I really will.

Salesperson: Just do it soon, please?!

[The Wild Shoppers roar.]

Salesperson: I need help fast!

Go Figure
Katie Rodriguez Banister, Joan Lipkin, and Rich Scharf

Richard: a gay man
Katie: a woman using a wheelchair

Rich is alone on stage

Rich: You may not be able to tell, but I used to be quite the Barbie girl. Oh yeah, I always was a traditional little girl at heart. I enjoyed dressing up and all that went with it. From my first pair of panty-hose to my bouffant hair, shellacked in place with half a can of Aqua-Net. Remember how popular big hair was in the 80s? The bigger the hair, the closer to God. And with the make-up to match. The trick was to go to that borderline Barbie look without being sickening; I'm not sure I always succeeded. God, I can remember my college girlfriends and I dressing up to go out for the night with the boom box blaring, "no parking, no parking on the dance floor, baby."

[Rich starts to turn stage left as he says the following line.]

Rich: My favorite outfit was this gray cashmere sweater . . .

> *[Katie comes out from stage left as the following line is said in unison, the two of them facing each other.]*

Katie and Rich: With my black leather mini-skirt and four-inch gray snakeskin pumps.

Katie: That outfit said . . .

Rich: Look at me.

> *[Rich and Katie face back toward audience.]*

Katie: Why, I even won a wet t-shirt contest once at a bar, and the girl next to me dropped her drawers.

Rich: . . . and I still won!

Katie: My first kiss was in sixth grade at the Kirkwood ice rink. After the rink closed, John, this absolute doll, called me over, put his lips on mine and then ran off. It was so cool!

Rich: I was stunned! When my dad came to pick me up, I felt like throwing up because I was sure he knew what I had done, that he could read it on my face!

Katie: *[wryly]* And it's a good thing that dad didn't always know what I did as an adult. If there was a man I was attracted to . . .

Rich: *[Rich starts to move behind Katie]* with whom I wanted to be sexual . . .

Katie: I just went for it. I liked being sexual,

Rich: and I certainly didn't have any problems finding willing partners.

Katie: I figured . . .

> *[Rich is behind Katie by this time and they look at each other while saying the following in unison.]*

Katie and Rich: God gave us our sexuality to be enjoyed, right?

> *[Rich returns to Katie's right side and faces her.]*

Katie: Well, I did worry about what people thought about me . . .

> *[They face each other during the following lines.]*

Rich: Tramp.

Katie: Slut.

Rich: Hussy.

Katie: Trollop!

> *[Beat.]*

Rich: Intern!

> *[They face the audience.]*

Katie: . . . and sometimes I would feel worse afterward, after I'd had sex with someone,

Rich: even though I got what I wanted!

> *[Rich starts to kneel at Katie's side.]*

Katie: But I had fun, too, you know?

> *[Rich is kneeling at Katie's side so that their heads are level with each other as the following line is said in unison.]*

Katie and Rich: It felt powerful to be attractive!

Katie: Then an auto accident brought my life to a screeching halt. I
became a quadriplegic, and my life changed—ha—to say the least.
I remember the first time I saw myself in the mirror at the
hospital.

> *[Rich has sunk onto his knees by this point.]*

Rich: I was devastated. I didn't look like me. I didn't even look like a
female anymore. I felt more like an it.

Katie: And I fought for my womanhood. I told my occupational thera-
pist that I'm not leaving rehab until I can put on my own lipstick!

> *[Rich steps in front of Katie to face audience, as Katie turns to
> face upstage.]*

Rich: An old boyfriend from high school came to visit me in the hospital. We had been a very active couple. He walked up to the bed,
leaned over, and gave me a rose. Then we engaged in a major
lip-lock session. I was in heaven. Thank God my hormones weren't
paralyzed! But when we met again after I got out of the hospital, it
was a disaster. It just didn't work. I was devastated again. And it
was at that point that I realized that the life I had was no longer.

> *[During the following lines said in unison, Rich and Katie
> will rotate, lazy-susan style, with Katie ending up facing
> the audience and Rich behind her facing upstage by the
> end of the lines said in unison.]*

Katie and Rich: No more wet t-shirts. No more pumps. And I miss my
pumps, dammit. And no more sex.

Katie: It's funny. You think there are certain things in life that you'll
never accept. And then those things happen to you. And somehow
you accept them or bust, I guess. So I slowly accepted the fact that
this chair had become my world. My life. And a part of who I am.
And somehow, I refused to give up. That's when I placed an ad in
the singles paper: "petite, professional, outgoing, independent
woman on wheels seeks male." I got over 30 letters! Although one
man thought I drove around a lot.

> *[Again, Katie and Rich rotate as above; by the end of the
> following line said in unison, Rich will face the audience and
> Katie will be behind him, facing upstage.]*

Katie and Rich: I did date two men, but they were disasters. So I just
gave up.

Rich: So imagine my surprise, a few years later, when I met someone.
And he expressed interest in me. And I said, "Oh no. You don't
understand. I don't do that anymore. I can't date you. It's just not
possible." Well, let me tell you, this man is patient. And over the
course of a year and a half, he became my best friend, and I began
to trust him, and I could no longer fight my feelings of attraction

for him. So one day we were in the kitchen, and I said, "Pull up a chair and come sit by me." And we kissed. And kissed. For an hour and a half we kissed. Hey, I had to make up for lost time!

[By the end of the line Katie has turned to face the audience, even with Rich and to his right.]

Katie: But I still kept my guard up. I mean kissing was fine, but obviously it couldn't go any further than that. Well, about a month later, we're at a friend's wedding, our sixth of seven that summer! And the good ole preacher was preaching,

Rich: "If you love someone, and you know it, grab a hold of them, and let them know it, too!"

[During Katie's line below, Rich will step upstage away from Katie and look at her; this has now briefly become Katie's story alone.]

Katie: So I did. We didn't make the reception. Instead, we went back to my place and I let him know in no uncertain terms that I wanted to be with him. But as he was removing my tray, my foot pedals, and my shoes, I started crying,

Rich: "Oh God, what if this doesn't work? What if you're not satisfied? What if I can't do it?"

[By this time Rich has come up behind Katie.]

Katie and Rich: It was like I was a virgin again!

[The following lines will overlap slightly.]

Katie: Well, I told you this guy was patient . . .

Rich: And he lifted me to the bed . . .

Katie: And would position my legs, you know . . .

Rich: Move my leg if he needed to.

Katie: And even though I'm paralyzed from the chest down . . .

Rich: I could feel the pressure of his hands on my breasts.

Katie: And I could feel him inside me . . .

Rich: Kind of like a distant pressure.

Katie: I could feel it in my head . . .

Rich: Like the tingling of a limb that has fallen asleep.

Katie: And it was the same . . .

Katie and Rich: "Oh my God, oh my God, oh my God!"

Katie: Just in different places now.

[Rich comes out from behind Katie and stands to her left.]

Rich: It's funny. Don't get me wrong—I'm still pissed to be in this chair. But instead of becoming a permanent wall, this chair has helped to teach me about true love.

Katie: And I'm having the best sex of my life.

[Katie and Rich look at each other, then look at the audience.]

Katie and Rich: Go figure!

Notes

1. The plays mentioned here cover a wide range of feminist playwriting. Understandably, not all scholars would agree on their being classified as such. However, what is suggested by their use is that across the spectrum of feminist theater, however that enterprise is defined, there exists a pervasive use of disability images.

2. Daniel J. Wilson articulated this definition of a "disability aesthetic" during the National Endowment for the Humanities Summer Institute on Disability Studies at San Francisco State University in the summer of 2000.

3. Lipkin and her company have received numerous awards, including a Missouri Arts Award, the Arts for Life Special Lifetime Achievement in Progress Award, and a Community Enhancement Award from the Governor's Council on Disability.

4. "Facts and Figures" was originally developed by students at Davidson College working with Lipkin during a week-long residency, in March 2001.

5. We might think here of plays ranging from *Fefu and Her Friends* (Fornes 1990) to Ntozake Shange's *Spell #7* (1979).

References

Banister, Katie Rodriguez, Joan Lipkin, and Rich Scharf. 1999. "Go Figure." Unpublished manuscript.

Corthron, Kia. 1996. *Come Down Burning.* In *Contemporary Plays by Women of Color: An Anthology,* ed. Kathy A. Perkins, 90–105. New York: Routledge.

Dolan, Jill. 1996. "In Defense of the Discourse: Materialist Feminism, Postmodernism, Poststructuralism . . . and Theory." In *A Sourcebook of Feminist Theatre and Performance,* ed. Carol Martin, 94–107. New York: Routledge.

———. 1993. *Presence and Desire: Essays on Gender, Sexuality, Performance.* Ann Arbor: University of Michigan Press.

Fornes, Maria Irene. 1990. *Fefu and Her Friends.* New York: PAJ Publications.

Gain, Heather, and Lisa Bennett. 2002. "The Faces of Social Security." *The NOW Times* 34(1): 16.

Geiogamah, Hanay. 1999. *Body Indian: A Play in Five Scenes.* In *Seventh Generation: An Anthology of Native American Plays,* ed. Mimi Gisolfi D'Aponte, 1–38. New York: Theatre Communications Group.

Henley, Beth. 1979. *Crimes of the Heart.* In *Plays from the Contemporary American Theater,* ed. Brooks McNamara, 227–91. New York: Mentor.

Lamb, Myrna. 1971. *What Have You Done for Me Lately?* In her *The Mod Donna and Scyklon Z: Plays of Women's Liberation,* 143–66. New York: Pathfinder Press.

Lewis, Victoria Ann. 2000. "The Dramaturgy of Disability." In *Points of Contact: Disability, Art, and Culture,* ed. Susan Crutchfield and Marcy Epstein, 93–108. Ann Arbor: University of Michigan Press.

Lipkin, Joan, and The DisAbility Project. 2001. "Employment." Unpublished manuscript.

———. 2001. "Facts and Figures." Unpublished manuscript.

Mairs, Nancy. 1996. Waist-High in the World: A Life Among the Nondisabled. Boston: Beacon Press.

Miner, Madonne. 1997. " 'Making up the Stories as We Go Along': Men, Women, and Narratives of Disability." In *The Body and Physical Difference: Discourses of Disability,* ed. David T. Mitchell and Sharon Snyder, 283–95. Ann Arbor: University of Michigan Press.

Mitchell, David T., and Sharon Snyder. 2000. *Narrative Prosthesis: Disability and the Dependencies of Discourse.* Ann Arbor: University of Michigan Press.

Moraga, Cherríe. 1996. *Heroes and Saints.* In *Contemporary Plays By Women of Color: An Anthology,* ed. Kathy A. Perkins, 230–61. New York: Routledge.

Sandahl, Carrie. 1999. "Ahhhh Freak Out! Metaphors of Disability and Femaleness in Performance." *Theatre Topics* 9(1): 11–30.

Shange, Ntozake. 1978. *Spell #7.* In *Nine Plays by Black Women,* ed. Margaret B. Wilkerson, 243–91. New York: Mentor.

Son, Diana. 1999. *Stop Kiss.* Woodstock, NY: Overlook Press.

Thomson, Rosemarie Garland. 1997. "Feminist Theory, the Body, and the Disabled Figure." In *The Disability Studies Reader,* ed. Lennard J. Davis, 279–92. New York: Routledge.

Tolan, Kathleen. 2001. "We Are Not a Metaphor." *American Theatre* (April): 17–21, 57–59.

Treadwell, Sophie. 1993. *Machinal.* London: Nick Hern Books.

Wendell, Susan. 1997. "Toward a Feminist Theory of Disability." In *The Disability Studies Reader,* ed. Lennard J. Davis, 260–78. New York: Routledge.

Williams, Tennessee. 1972. *The Glass Menagerie.* New York: Signet.

Wilson, August. 1986. *Fences.* New York: Plume.

PART FIVE

**Women's Studies Methods to Transform
Health Research and Care**

CHAPTER FOURTEEN

Breasts, Blood, and the Royal V: Challenges of Revising Anatomy and Periods for the 2005 Edition of *Our Bodies, Ourselves*

MARIANNE MCPHERSON

Has our anatomy changed since 1998? What is new and different about menstruation? These are some of the challenging questions I faced as I set out last year to revise a chapter in the classic women's health book, *Our Bodies, Ourselves* (*OBOS*). Roughly 500 people, most of them women, participated in the revision of the book. Our roles ranged from writers, to editors, to photographers. My role was to be the primary reviser for the sexual anatomy, reproduction, and menstruation chapter. With the help of comments from pre-readers (who evaluated the 1998 chapter with an eye toward what should get rewritten or cut), my task was to update material from the 1998 edition of *OBOS*, to add new topics where relevant, and to cut out-of-date discussions. I received input from other women on many aspects of the chapter, including content and structure, topics, photographs, and references. Although I was its primary reviser, the finished chapter is a product of many women's work.

OBOS and Feminism for a Younger Generation

Always in my mind was one of the explicitly stated goals of the new edition of *Our Bodies, Ourselves:* to attract a younger audience while continuing to appeal to the readers loyal to OBOS across its previous editions. I immediately questioned the term *young women*, wondering what it might mean to different people in different contexts. (I often wonder the same about the word *diversity*.) The original generation of *OBOS* authors, now in their fifties and older, considers me a young women (I am 25), but when I think of "young women," I often think of women in their late teens and early twenties. How could my work appeal to this broader audience when I could not even define who that audience was?

One practical solution to the challenge of being completely overwhelmed was to take the chapter piece by piece. For example, I recognized that women may first approach the chapter for one section (such as menstruation). Thus, one goal of the revision was to attract readers to parts of the chapter that they might not originally have intended to visit. Another was to include first-person anecdotes (a defining characteristic of *OBOS*

Originally published in the spring 2005 issue (vol. 17, no. 1).

across all of its editions) from a variety of women. One comfort in this process was the recognition that I was not working alone. A team of pre-readers, post-readers, and editors was aware of these challenges and available to help. In the end, I did the best job I could with the skills, resources, advice, data, and people available to me.

Making the Cut

Some of the challenges in updating the book were common across many chapters, while other issues were topic- or chapter-specific. One over-arching concern was to keep the chapter length relatively short, as the new book is smaller in both dimensions and number of pages compared to the 1998 edition. An accompanying web-based companion to the book accommodates extended discussions of material that were not included in-text, as well as longer lists of resources. Determining what to include in the book itself and what to post on the online companion was a particular challenge of the revising process. Pre-reader comments were especially helpful in pointing to material from the 1998 edition that might be cut from the book (and put online) in 2005. In the anatomy section of the chapter, an extended narrative of the self-guided tour (described below) is in the online companion rather than in-text. From the menstruation section, more detailed descriptions of the roles of the hormones involved in the menstrual cycle are in the online piece. In the 1998 edition, there was a long section on how to conduct menstrual massage. This now will appear online.

Restructuring Sexual Anatomy

A first addition to the female sexual anatomy chapter is an acknowledgment that the term *female sexual anatomy* is not clear-cut or unambiguous. I note that people who have the anatomy described in the chapter may or may not call themselves "female" or "women." (I recognize that it could be the topic of another paper—or an entire doctoral dissertation—to deconstruct the terms *female* and *women*.) Likewise, people who label themselves "women" may or may not have the described anatomy. Additionally, people may have parts of "female" sexual anatomy and parts of "male" sexual anatomy.

For me, one of the most helpful steps in the *OBOS* revisions process was receiving comments from pre-readers. Before I started revising the chapter, several experts (including one of the authors of the 1998 version of the same chapter) commented on aspects of the chapter that remained relevant, aspects that did not, and areas that would benefit from updating. In the case of this chapter, a nearly universal comment was the need to transition away from its "textbook feel," particularly in the sexual anatomy section. The pre-readers acknowledged that the biological information covered was important but said that the presentation was dry.

Self-Guided Tour

In the 1998 edition of *OBOS*, the format of the anatomy section is blocks of narrative describing what a woman would see if she were conducting her own vulvovaginal self-exam with a speculum, flashlight, and hand mirror. There are pictures interspersed throughout the section, but it is not always instantly clear how and where they line up with the narrative text. I continue to embrace the concept of the self-exam and brought that idea forward into this edition through the metaphor of a self-guided tour. Indeed, the idea of a self-guided tour is representative of the *OBOS* tradition of encouraging women to learn about our bodies "firsthand." The goal of the update process was to overhaul the style of the self-guided anatomy tour while preserving its spirit. In so doing I hoped to encourage more women to take the tour of their own bodies and aimed to provide a helpful tour guide.

With its long sections of narrative text, the 1998 anatomy section seemed analogous to a driving tour with a continuous soundtrack describing the attractions along the road. It was strong in its detailed descriptions of anatomy but weaker in its ability to highlight particularly important areas or to allow the reader to enter the self-exam "tour" at any point along the way. Instead of the soundtrack constantly narrating a tour, I decided to rethink the 2005 sexual anatomy section as a self-guided tour with easy-to-read maps, clear couplings of text with diagrams, and special points-of-interest highlighted along the way. With my new version, I hoped readers would find it easier to find each destination.

In the 2005 *OBOS*, the sexual anatomy section is this self-guided tour and is explicitly described as such. The major sections of sexual anatomy are subdivided into six categories, as described in Table 14.1. Each body part has its own row in the table, and each table has column headings corresponding to the following categories: "Common name of the body part," "Anatomical name," "Function/role," and "Can you see it?" For example, in the "On the Outside" table, the common name for the *labia majora* is outer lips; their function/role is to protect the *labia minora*; and yes, you can see them. Near the table there is an illustration that corresponds to the name of the table and clearly labels each part described in that table. The hope is that readers can pick up any section of the anatomy chapter, easily find a particular piece or section of anatomy,

Table 14.1
Section in the OBOS 2005 Self-Guided Tour of Female Sexual Anatomy

Table Heading	Area of Anatomy	Parts Described
Exits, entrances	Openings to inside the body	Introitus, urinary opening, and anus
On the outside (and just beneath)	Vulva and neighboring parts	Vulva, pubic hair, mons, pubis symphysis, labia majora, labia minora, perineum, and vestibule
The vagina and its neighbors	Vagina and neighboring parts inside the body	Vagina, hymen, urethral sponge, pomix (part of vagina), cervix, os (part of cervix), and pubococcygeus (PC) muscle
Find your orgasm here!	The parts of the clitoris	Clitoris (as a whole), hood of clitoris, glans of clitoris, shaft of clitoris, suspensory ligament, crura, bulbs of the vestibule, and vestibular glands
All the way in	Internal sexual anatomy	Uterus, fundus, fallopian tubes, and ovaries
Our breasts	Breast anatomy	Areola, nipple, sebaceous glands, pat connective tissue, and milk-producing glands

learn something about its location and role, and see a drawing. More detailed descriptions of anatomy appear in the online companion to the book.

Another feature of the self-guided tour is a section of notes following each table. These notes highlight particular points about anatomy. One example is a note that tampons cannot get lost inside a vagina; another is the caveat that people often confuse the words *vulva* and *vagina*. In addition to the short notes, there are longer text boxes that highlight topics including labial piercing and pelvic floor exercises. In redesigning the sexual anatomy portion of the chapter, I hoped to draw more readers into learning about the look, feel, and role of the different parts of sexual anatomy. I tried to introduce the self-guided tour as an open invitation, something a woman can conduct alone or with other trusted people, something she can read about or physically experience.

Illustrations

In addition to the new format of the sexual anatomy section, the chapter has updated photographs and illustrations throughout. Each table in the "self-guided tour" section is paired with an illustration of the anatomy it describes. We worked with an artist with the specific goals of making the illustrations both accurate and realistic looking. The vulva is pictured with a woman holding a mirror up to her vulva, as if she were conducting a self-exam. In updating the illustrations, we hoped to avoid the phenomenon of the "disembodied uterus," a picture with body parts that don't seem to correspond to an actual body.

"Hot" Topics

General Challenges

In any edition of *OBOS*, one great challenge is to address "hot" topics of the moment. We aim to address those topics comprehensively and also avoid outdating the book before it even hits the shelves. As I wrote the *OBOS* chapter in 2004, I was ever mindful that the book would be published more than a year later in 2005, and that, if the *OBOS* revisions timeline stays roughly the same, it may stay on shelves until at least 2010. I thus tried to address current "hot" issues in a way that they would appeal to today's readers but still remain relevant to readers five years from now. One solution to this, as I will discuss in an example, was to use arguments that might remain current even if the key players or specific data points change. In addition to the issue of relevance, there was a constant tension between trying to address the full scope of an issue and trying to fit within the allotted page length of the chapter. All revisers had to balance gathering new information with cutting old text. This was another area where the online companion was helpful, as it allows for longer discussions than the book itself.

Example of Menstrual Suppression

In this chapter, one of the current hot-button issues is menstrual suppression. A topic of scientific and public debate, menstrual suppression is the practice of healthy women taking drugs to regulate and/or stop menstruation. Approaching the issue of suppression, I appreciated that there are myriad stakeholders in the debate. They include women and girls, health professionals, researchers, insurance companies, and the pharmaceutical industry. I myself am no expert on menstrual suppression. Since my knowledge about menstrual issues primarily concerns menarche and women's qualitative experiences with their periods, it was particularly intimidating for me to tackle this complex and hotly debated topic.

Drug companies are at the center of the debate, as they currently market oral contraceptives specifically for menstrual suppression. In my discussion of the issue, I wanted to acknowledge that one important piece of the debate centers around the safety and desirability of having drugs specifically marketed for menstrual suppression. However, I did not want to focus attention on any particular drug company or any particular product. There were a few reasons for this: (1) the drug at the center of attention now may or may not be there in six months or two years, based on factors including research and market economics; (2) focusing attention on one particular drug would obscure the larger debate around the safety and desirability of menstrual suppression in general; (3) many other public spheres give attention to menstrual suppression drugs. I thought that *OBOS* could be a space for a broader debate about suppression in a feminist voice, in terms of both safety and desirability. An overriding challenge in the menstrual suppression case was trying to accomplish these goals—keeping the relevant themes of the controversy without outdating any one specific debate—in less than 400 words.

What Does Feminism Mean: Past, Present, and Future?

Embarking on this project and continuing through each step of it, I have been overwhelmed by my place in women's health history. My mother shared her copy of *Our Bodies, Ourselves* with me when I was a young girl, and it was and is one of my primary resources for information about my body and health. I hope that girls continue to seek out and trust *Our Bodies, Ourselves* as they grow and learn about their bodies. One of the hallmarks of the book is its feminist voice. As someone with Women's Studies undergraduate training, I found myself constantly questioning what feminism meant in terms of the voice in which I wrote. Zobeida Bonilla addresses the issue of "the all-embracing we" in her report in this journal. I, too, wrestled with the responsibility of the royal "we" as I wrote about what I termed "the royal v" ("v" for vulva and vagina, referring particularly to the anatomy section of the chapter).

I wondered: How has feminism changed across the history of the editions of *OBOS*? Would I succeed in attracting readers who label themselves as feminist? Would I succeed in attracting readers who eschew the term *feminist* but who respond to the voice or message of the book? With somewhat more perspective than I was able to have while writing the chapter, I constantly am in three places: looking back, being here, and looking ahead. I look back on the history of the book and the legacy that previous women in the Boston Women's Health Book Collective handed off to me. I sit here, eagerly awaiting the release of the new edition of the book, deeply concerned for women's health in this world, alternately frightened and hopeful at the state of the political health climate, both domestically and internationally. I look ahead to the future of *Our Bodies, Ourselves*, hoping that the place of the book is just as relevant for future generations of women from many walks of life as it has been for me.

References

Boston Women's Health Book Collective. 2005. *Our Bodies, Ourselves.* New York: Simon & Schuster.

———. 1998. *Our Bodies, Ourselves for the New Century.* New York: Simon & Schuster.

CHAPTER FIFTEEN

Medicine and Women's Studies: Possibilities for Enhancing Women's Health Care

ADRIANA CAVALCANTI DE AGUIAR

> At no time in the history of modern medicine have so many been there erod-
> ing the absolute authority of the male physician—economists, politicians,
> insurance companies, nurses, patients, humanists and women. He is losing
> control of his once sacrosanct world where he, and only he, dictated its mo-
> dus operandi.
>
> —Conley (1996, viii)

Despite cultural and economic distinctions, my home country, Brazil,
and the United States share common health needs. Problems that directly affect women's health are exacerbated by women's subordinate
position in society. Violence against women, sexually transmitted diseases, unwanted pregnancy, and the long-term management of chronic
diseases, among other public health problems, deserve attention in both
countries and challenge the health system and its professionals to engage
in dialogue with women.

This essay discusses contributions of feminist theory to the education
of health professionals in the United States and Brazil and grows from
my experience in Brazil as an educator, physician, and researcher. To
clarify my motivation for this study, I initially present some insights
grounded in Brazilian initiatives to educate health professionals and informed by feminist theory and pedagogy. Then I will analyze the benefits
for women's health care that might result from the integration of Wom-
en's Studies and medical education.

The relationship between patients and doctors has always been at the
center of my professional interest. After graduation from medical school
I started to work as a psychotherapist. I was soon convinced that the
most effective initiatives in the field of health are oriented toward prevention of additional problems and based on negotiation and exchange of
information. Meanwhile my attention was caught by a feminist initiative that aimed to promote health education for women. Developed at
the Oswaldo Cruz Foundation, the most important research institution
within the field of health in Brazil, courses offered for health professionals have employed innovative approaches to health education, moving
toward the integration of prevention and treatment of conditions through
a new understanding of the educational component of health care. These
courses contribute to a broader initiative, published by the Brazilian

Originally published in the spring 1998 issue (vol. 10, no. 1).

Ministry of Health as a federal program in 1983, known as Women's Comprehensive Health Care Program (PAISM) (Brazil Ministry of Health 1983). PAISM offers answers to women's health problems based on a holistic understanding of health, in contrast to the traditional emphasis on pregnancy and reproduction. PAISM aims to legitimize practices that encompass a new rationality within health care institutions in order to promote health and quality of life for women.

PAISM is based on a multidisciplinary approach to women's health and emphasizes educational activities with groups of clients, aiming to break the historical isolation of women and encouraging them to assume authorship over their lives and health. Accordingly, PAISM adopts "a new posture to be adopted by the health team, and consequently, a new approach to initiatives of professional training" (Brazil Ministry of Health 1983, 16). A challenge to the implementation of PAISM has been to encourage the development of training initiatives that question the rigid hierarchy within the health team and promote health professionals' creativity and leadership. The "absolute authority of the male physician" (Conley 1996, viii) is directly challenged. Because the proposal includes all kinds of professionals working in a team, and sees women as the active agents of their own health, the term *doctor-patient relationship* becomes obsolete. The proposal of integral health care, in its feminist conception, conceives the relationship between professional and client as an opportunity for transforming both subjects.

PAISM is inspired by the consciousness-raising groups of the feminist movement (Giffin 1994, 356) and Freirean pedagogy (Corrêa 1994). PAISM's small-group discussions and workshops are consistent with feminist pedagogies, see personal experiences as a key factor in knowledge production, and highlight the body as central in defining women's identity and political struggles. During the training, professionals are encouraged to learn how to listen to clients and exchange knowledge instead of prescribing recipes. Emotions play a crucial role in the process. The techniques include unconventional activities such as role-playing and body contact, recognizing the prior knowledge of the members of the groups. Some researchers consider this approach to be one of the major advances in public health care in Brazil (Gonçalves 1991; Aguiar 1992).

I have coordinated courses on women's health and education and trained health teams to implement PAISM in the Oswaldo Cruz Foundation as well as in the city of Niterói, in Rio de Janeiro State, from 1989 to 1995. In a previous study in a health district in Rio de Janeiro State (Aguiar 1992, 108) I documented changes in health professionals' professional relationships and personal lives after the training. I am convinced that the strategies used in PAISM trainings can and should be adapted to teach students in the formal professional education system. Nevertheless, the redefinition of authority and the sharing of decision making with clients do not seem attractive to those interested in maintaining privileges within the health system. In my previous study I observed that whenever physicians agree to participate in educational group activities, they often lecture, deviating from the premises of the program. Working with groups had, for some male doctors, the restricted connotation of "optimizing" the use of their time, enabling them to "teach" more women at the same time. The exchange of experiences and perspectives among the clients was not seen as either "educational" or necessary. Even today medical schools in Brazil hardly discuss PAISM's premises. However, rethinking medical education and medical curricula are crucial, since doctors are at the top of the hierarchy and are very influential in health care institutions.

Aware of the negative consequences of clinicians' traditional preparation and desiring to work toward improving professional training in the health field, I decided to pursue a doctoral degree in the United States, bridging feminism, health, and education. Feminist scholarship and debate around issues of health and education in the United States contrasts with the still peripheral status of the feminist debate in Brazilian academies. In addition, the literature and research produced in the United States have a major impact on health practices and beliefs in my country, helping to shape medical education and health care in that context.

Thus, this study is part of a larger attempt to rethink curricula in the field of health and medicine. Departing from the feminist critique of health care and medical education, I want to reflect on the entrance in medical schools of a new kind of student: women who majored in Women's Studies at the undergraduate level. I believe that the awareness they acquire during college may be an antidote to the alienation of medical training. These women will be able, hopefully, to keep their original intent of helping and communicating with people through a broader perspective on the social determination of diseases, which should enhance women's health care. I will discuss the need for collective reflection about the medical curriculum and pedagogy within and outside medical schools in order to train doctors who are sensitive and responsible to women's experiences and demands.

Women's Health Care

My experience as a medical doctor and health educator in Brazil simultaneously reinforces and denies the evidence of radical changes in women's health care. On the one hand, the women's movement has helped to introduce consciousness-raising groups in health centers, and the feminist analysis of the entanglement of gender, class, and race has raised crucial questions and proposed strategies to improve health care in general and women's health care in particular. On the other hand, a radical transformation demands time and organized efforts, since it encompasses changes in the training and education of health care professionals, an area that has proved impervious to feminist perspectives regarding health (Wear 1996).

One of the most compelling aspects of the feminist critique of health care involves the question of just what health care should be on a basic level. The feminist approach is "focused on wellness and health rather than disease and treatment" (Boston Women's Health Book Collective 1990, 653). Scholars have discussed how economic factors favor treatment as opposed to prevention, because health does not generate so much profit as illness (Camargo 1992, 201). Medical activities are not isolated from the larger medical-industrial complex of hospitals, clinics, the pharmaceutical industry, and the medical-equipment industry. This whole complex is at odds with the idea of health promotion and primary prevention advocated by feminists and public health professionals. In the famous feminist book *Our Bodies, Our Selves* (Boston Women's Health Collective 1990) the authors affirm:

> Policy-makers, usually male, have designed the system primarily for the convenience and financial gain of physicians, hospitals, administrators and the medical industries. *We believe that women, as the majority of consumers and workers, paid and unpaid, should have the major voice in health and medical care policy making in this country* [Emphasis theirs]. (653)

The Boston Women's Health Book Collective points out that women, who represent more than 50 percent of the population, are also a majority of the clientele and health providers,[1] but not of medical doctors. Thus, women are treated as objects of medical knowledge, which has ironically excluded them from research. Martin (1994b) describes the "disciplines of knowledge [that] ignore or misrepresent the experience and lives of women" (73). Considering males to be the norm (Jones 1996, 69), medical research has systematically excluded female subjects from research and extrapolated the results to women. "Almost everything that doctors and researchers claimed to know about women's health was based on research that had been conducted by men" (Howes and Allina 1994, 10). Known as "the new scholarship on women," a feminist critical scholarship has deconstructed the stereotypical images of females developed by men and proposed gender-sensitive research.

Women have also been the object of medicalization, which occurs when "medical people become the 'experts' on normal experiences or social problems" (Boston Women's Health Book Collective 1990, 656). Since women are supposed to look for physicians because of physiological life events (such as pregnancy and motherhood), they are more exposed to indoctrination. Medical care often extrapolates from science to value judgments, teaching women "how a good girl, a good wife, a good mother should behave" (Boston Women's Health Book Collective 1990, 657). The social control of women's bodies and sexuality has been a recurrent theme in the feminist literature (see, for example, Ehrenreich and English 1989).

Examples of incorrect or harmful medical advice and intervention regarding women abound. *Our Bodies, Out Selves* (1990, 652) offers a list of common problems faced by women who are not satisfied with the medical care they receive. Women have accused medical personnel of common attitudes such as not listening to them; withholding knowledge; lying to them; denying information about risks and negative effects of treatments; treating them poorly because of their race, sexual preference, age or disability; and administering unnecessarily mutilating treatments, among others. Some examples include, outrageous rates of unnecessary cesareans—up to 75 percent—(Marienskind 1981, 25) and unnecessary hysterectomies—up to 50 percent—(Ruzek 1978). What is known in the feminist literature as gender invisibility (see, for example, Rosaldo and Lamphere 1974) permeates daily health care. Howes and Allina (1994, 12) refer to an article published in the *New England Journal of Medicine* that demonstrates that women who see female physicians are "significantly more likely to be screened for breast and cervical cancer." Since these are two of the most prevalent types of cancer in females in the United States, it does not seem to be a simple coincidence, but an evidence of gender bias in health care.

Doctors' prejudices, power asymmetries between doctors and patients, and their lack of dialogue harm not only women's health but also that of poor people and people of color. Thus, we might expect that medical schools would be concerned with this evidence and eager to discuss it with students. However, attuned to a supposedly "scientific" or biological approach to the determination of diseases, medical curriculum deemphasizes social factors and their importance in determining illness and shaping the doctor-patient relationship. As a consequence,

> Partly through the sanctity of the private physician-patient relationship, medicine . . . also achieves social control by encouraging us to see personal problems as individual isolated experiences, rather than as problems we have in common with other women. (Boston Women's Health Book Collective 1990, 658)

Starting from the premise that women's health and illness are not only biologically but also socially determined, and that understanding the commonalties of their suffering may help women to struggle for welfare and adequate health care, I will in the next sections discuss some alternatives for a feminist approach to women's health care and medical training.

Gender and Medical Education

Many of the behaviors we complain about in physicians—their authoritarian manner, their insensitivity and condescension—can be traced back to their education and training as doctors.
                                    —Boston Women's Health Book Collective (1990, 663)

Wear (1996) confirms that "medical students entering medicine [are] full of energetic, altruistic idealism." However, "as the realities of power and authority become routinized in their education, their will to survive the moment often transcends their social conscience" (110).

Indeed, I myself experienced the dehumanizing training described in the literature. When I entered medical school in 1981 I had two main objectives: to help people who suffer and to enhance my self-knowledge and well-being. Medical school, I thought, would be the place where I would learn about human beings. However, within the first two years of the basic cycle I did not help anybody. Fragments of knowledge were taught in the disciplines without connection among them. The opportunity to help people was postponed to the third year. Then I started to work in a service that treats adolescents with severe conditions. Since I was just out of adolescence myself,[2] I felt the need for a collective discussion and reflection about our relationship as students to the clients. But I could not find much space for reflection inside medical school. Soon my closest friends and I started to be discriminated against by teachers because we refused to learn through practices that imposed pain and distress on patients who were already suffering.[3] During the oral exams in our clinical subjects, those teachers found the perfect situation for revenge. The grades we received on practical tests involving patients were often lower than on written tests, because some teachers did not stop asking questions, in an increasing degree of difficulty, until my friends and I could not answer them. I could generally resist being callous toward patients but not without developing an eating disorder. At that time I was not able to perceive discrimination from teachers because of my gender, but looking back I realize that I was much too opinionated for a "good" female student.

My experience as a student suggests similarities between the United States and Brazil in terms of medical training. Discussing the traditional medical curriculum, the Boston Women's Health Book Collective (1990) says,

> Medical schools ask students to absorb an enormous quantity of highly technical information in compressed form, largely through one-way lectures . . . Few could learn to think critically in this environment if they did not know how before medical school. (663)

Even those who were critical before would constantly be invited or forced to give up questioning things. Since the beginning of medical school, I was fortunate enough to participate in a "consciousness-raising" group of physicians who regularly met to reflect on their practice and training, which was a fundamental support in helping me resist the dehumanization of the doctor-patient relationship and the daily violence posed by medical training.

Medical training is still largely informed by what Freire (1985) called "banking education" (21). Ahistoric and acritical knowledge is "deposited" by teachers in students' minds, like money in banks. Focusing almost exclusively on illness, as opposed to health, much of the curriculum is about rare conditions and may be considered a waste of time and energy.[4] According to a woman physician quoted in *Our Bodies, Our Selves* (1990):

> The training program is disease-oriented, with life-threatening or rare conditions receiving the most attention . . . The day-to-day ills of the public are ignored as "minor problems." The promotion of health and the prevention of disease are neglected almost entirely. (663)

But why doesn't the medical curriculum emphasize knowledge necessary to help people to keep healthy or relieve the most common health problems? Economic reasons define the path toward specialization and the devaluation of primary health care and prevention. Besides, curricula are defined by specialists who want to maintain their status.[5]

In terms of financial and professional status, surgeons occupy the highest point in the hierarchy, with their practice of earning money through procedures that may involve the (sometimes unnecessary) mutilation of people's bodies. Primary health care, which demands complex reasoning and communication skills, is generally performed by women and is undervalued. Dickenstein (1996) affirms that

> women have been overly encouraged and mentored to enter primary care fields where they can enhance patient care by using their more acknowledged skills of better communication with patients. They have clearly and simultaneously been discouraged from applying to train in the more technical and higher remunerative fields of the subspecialties of surgery and medicine. (6)

Social as well as academic factors contribute to making female students and physicians unaware of these imbalances. Discussing the difference between educational equality and equal admission, Martin (1994d, 104) says that extending men's education to women, as in medical training, does not prevent "the training [from being] differently experienced by men and women," and she alerts us to the fact that fields where women predominate are "at risk of being downgraded in academic standing and resources" (104). This devaluation of women includes what Gilligan (1982) called their "ethics of care" (62–63), and what the Boston Women's Health Care Book Collective (1990) described as

> glaringly absent from medical training . . . —most of the values, concerns and skills often thought of as "feminine": nurturance, empathy, caring, sensitive listening . . . collaboration rather than competition . . . Women often complain bitterly of cold, abstract, impersonal or authoritarian doctors . . . These qualities may have less to do with the physician's original personality than with the one-sidedness of her or his training. (664)

Besides, "the very qualities medical reformers claim they are seeking in students [such as] sensitivity, empathy, honesty, humility—are instantly suspect if displayed by women, as signs of their possible clinical or intellectual incompetence" (Boston Women's Health Book Collective, 1990, 668).

The massive entrance of women into medical schools over the last decades has not reversed the exclusion of female perspectives and experiences from the medical curriculum (Jones 1996, 71). Moreover, according to Bickel (1996), despite the unquestionable advances made by the feminist movement, the dialogue among women about gender issues is still difficult within medical academies because even the tenured women who could exert leadership are afraid of being considered "troublemakers" (12). Wear and Bickel (1996) emphasize that "in a conservative environment a reputation as a feminist might impair a woman's effectiveness as a bridge-builder between the sexes and as an educator" (28). Duffin (1996) goes further to affirm that women doctors "tended to be silent and in some cases suspicious partners in the women's movement of the late twentieth century," and worse, that even those women physicians who were previously committed to feminism "began to turn away from pronounced feminism as they become successful practitioners: one commitment seems to have been increasingly incompatible with the other" (38).

This (un)equal medical education for women includes the absence of women's experiences as content of medical training. Conley (1996) affirms that both feminism and humanities are "foreign" and therefore avoided in the medical world. A humanist perspective is problematic since it "asks the unanswerable, forces physicians to think about that which is uncomfortable, because . . . unlike their traditional medical education, there is no 'right' answer" (vii). *Our Bodies, Our Selves* (1990) reaffirms that "the [medical] training usually does not challenge students to become more aware of the social and political realities affecting people's health or to work through their own sexism, homophobia, class bias, ageism and racism" (663).

Moreover, medicine defines a restrained range of pathologies into which doctors try to fit patients. "Cases" that do not present an identifiable, organic diagnosis, and therefore cannot be brought into a biomedical classification, are considered "functional" patients whose complaints are devalued. In the case of women, whose suffering often derives from their subordinate position within families, workplace, and society, they frequently cannot find adequate advice or feedback from doctors.

Women are associated with the undervalued sphere of social and biological reproduction. Martin (1994b) affirms that "marriage, childrearing, family life . . . involves difficult, complex, learned activities which can be done well or badly . . . The exclusion of education for reproductive processes . . . thus carries with it an unwarranted, negative value judgment about the tasks and activities, the traits and dispositions which are associated with them" (80). In the case of health care and health education, although women may no longer be restricted to the reproductive sphere, they are frequently responsible for it. The effects of gender stereotypes and the sexual division of labor on health, however, are not addressed in medical training.

The dichotomy between production (public) and reproduction (private) has consequences for women professionals and students, since "the patriarchic foundation of academic medicine prevents many of them from a meaningful integration of their professional and personal selves" (Wear 1996, ix). If they plan to be mothers and wives they will face huge problems. Klass (1996) affirms that "certain intensities of [medical] career are essentially incompatible with any kind of parenthood." The author is sarcastic: "[T]he influx of women into medicine, we can hope, will help us design medical careers for both men and women that will enable doctors to follow some of their own recommendations (reduce stress, . . . keep regular hours, spend time with your family)" (93). Using the metaphor of brainwashing, Our Bodies, Our Selves (1996, 664) attributes to doctors' medical training and future careers a great deal of responsibility for their well-known "high rates of mental breakdown, drug addiction, alcoholism, suicide and family disruption" (McCue 1982, 458).

Who has the power to introduce these themes in the conversation? Jones (1996) describes students' fear of contradicting their professors because they may "remember them when it comes time to give grades or do clinical work in a setting where ratings are more subjective" (7). In order to change women's peripheral position it seems necessary to find female role models, such as teachers and high-level administrators, who are engaged in the process of raising women's status. Low rates of women heads of departments, deans, even teachers, as documented by Klass[6] (1996), reinforce this concern. However, if men define the criteria for tenuring teachers, why would they choose more than a handful of women? Pressure from society in general and from the student body in particular is necessary.

The question thus remains: How is it possible to help women, as clients, students, and professionals, to pressure for dialogue and resist the devaluation and violence that medicine and its official knowledge offers them? How to make sure that women do not see each other through a male lens instead of as allies? In the next two sections I will try to make a contribution to this complicated discussion, taking off from my experience in Brazil and my fieldwork with women's studies concentrators in the United States.

Feminism, Women's Studies, and Medical Education

Becoming educated can be a journey of integration, not alienation . . . The general problem to be solved is that of uniting thought and action, reason and emotion, self and other.
—Martin (1994c, 211)

Discussing paradigms for curricula, Adrienne Rich (1979) defends initiatives already implemented in women's studies departments as "a breakdown of traditional departments and disciplines . . . [and of] the fragmentation of knowledge that weakens thought and permits the secure ignorance of the specialist to protect him from responsibility for the application of his theories" (143). Rich's ideas can be extrapolated to discuss the negative consequences of specialization within the medical field. Women's bodies are spread along clinical specialties, with, for example, their brains in neurology, their ovaries in gynecology, and their emotions in psychiatry; none of these is able to treat the complexity of women's suffering. Issues of sexuality, for example, are generally absent in medical schools, leaving doctors free to impose their own often conservative and normative biases.

Katz and Shotter (1996) propose that medical curricula teach students to deal with the patient's perspective on health and disease emphasizing their understanding of their world "and what it is like to them, trying in the face of their illness, to live in it" (921). We can read this advice as one that aims to reveal the healthy aspects of the patient's story, allowing doctor and patient to engage in a relationship that fosters the patient's healing capacities, situated in the web of culture and meaning in which the patient lives. These authors stress that it is "just within this unique [local] moral context that ill people organize, express, and experience their own unique forms of suffering" (925). They advocate that the medical consultation provide a dialogue that invites the patient to expand her knowledge and stimulate her sense of agency (923), and exemplify innovative training processes where "a routine medical examination embodying a medical sensibility became a relational rather than an alienating event, in which [the patient] came to feel involved and respected rather than objectified and pathologized" (924).

I believe the interdisciplinary approach of women's studies depart-ments may therefore enhance the awareness about the risks that affect women and other "minorities," as well as prepare professionals to de-velop a meaningful dialogue with the clients, starting from the clients' previous knowledge and beliefs. In this way effective strategies of health education and prevention could flourish, and the clients' informed com-pliance, based on understanding and agreement, could be achieved.

While reflecting upon the necessary relationship between feminism and health care, I was excited in my second year as a doctoral student of education at an Ivy League university to find out that some pre-medical students had been majoring in Women's Studies at the same university. In order to investigate the potential contribution of Women's Studies to medical education, in this section I want to discuss ideas that emerged in interviews with three undergraduate students, undertaken between Oc-tober and December 1996. All the interviewees are currently enrolled as Women's Studies concentrators, and are planning to go to medical school after college. The interviewees are in their early 20s, and come from a middle-class background. All three of them are Asian-American. The criteria for selection were based on the intention to apply for medical school and the availability to participate in the study.

The interviews lasted approximately one hour each and followed a semi-structured protocol, designed to investigate these students' perspectives about feminism and medicine, their reasons for choosing to concentrate in Women's Studies, and how they see the potential benefits and disadvan-tages this concentration poses to their prospective careers as doctors. The interviews were taped and entirely transcribed. After successive readings, I identified common themes and concepts, as well as peculiarities of each interview. I use the letters A, B, and C to identify the interviewees.

One of the questions addressed their interest in dealing with women's health care and how they define it, whether within the traditional spe-cialized and fragmented frame of gynecology or inserted in a larger social framework. Jones (1996) has quoted a second-year medical student who lamented the absence of a comprehensive approach to women's health: "We had a course in clinical medicine which included one-hour lectures on issues in medicine . . . Also included was 'women's health.' One hour. Women's health is not just a topic in medicine, it is medicine . . . As a woman I felt as if doctors were being taught that my health was unim-portant" (68). About this topic, one of the interviewees (A) declared:

> When I tell people I am very interested in women's health care [they say] "Oh! you want to be a gynecologist." No, not necessarily . . . Because when I say women's health care I don't just think reproductive health, I think interna-tional women's health care, I think public policy . . . I think women across class differences, across racial differences, you know, and I think maybe sort

of almost general practice but for women, and it always brings in political socioeconomic issues with them, I am not just interested in reproductive health, I am interested in women's health care.

But how would these young women operationalize this broader conception about women's health in concrete health care situations? Another interviewee (B) offers a suggestion that integrates medical appointments with educational activities and prevention:

> [O]ne of my ideals or my dreams is to have a women's clinic, which would be also a community clinic and would involve medical services, kind of like the strict biomedical services, but also there would be a library, there would be nutrition classes and exercise classes, and workshops, and it would be a way for people who are less advantaged to hook up with like social security and welfare, and counseling for abuse and drug addiction, and emotional trauma, and all those sorts of things, and also be involved with the community. That's kind of my ideal goal.

Part of the interview was devoted to discussing these young women's options for concentrating in Women's Studies, since I knew that pre-medical students tend to choose "scientific" concentrations such as biology and biochemistry. All of them were critical of the narrowness of medical training and willing to acquire a comprehensive perspective about health and illness. The reasons they presented included the following reflections:

> Women's Studies has helped me to question a lot of things and just not accept things at face level. I am always digging and trying to figure out why things are the way they are. And I know that especially with medical education in the United States it's so easy to go and be barraged with all this information and data and not critically examining why are they teaching me this and why I am learning this specific model rather than questioning: Is this the best thing that I could be learning, is this the best way we could be approaching things, what other questions are they leaving out, what other groups are they leaving out? Women's Studies has helped me to really start questioning things that I've been presented with. I guess going back to the medical education in this country, I guess a lot of what they teach in medical schools is based on studies done with men and done with men formulating the questions, and so I think I will gain more value having been a women's studies concentrator going in and seeing whether or not it's the best thing that could be there. (C)

The interviewees were also critical of the traditional choices pre-medical students make, concentrating in the sciences, which, from their perspective, accelerates the path toward the dehumanization of medical activity. One of them (A) declared:

> This brings up an interesting issue of the pre-medical education at least [here] and maybe the university system in America at large . . . It kind of fosters an environment that encourages students to only pursue science, which at least

in my mind medicine is not just science and it can never be, and never has been just science. It is very much an art and it is very much also that the issues of communication and doctor-patient relationship are absolutely essential and the fact that you can bring in the scientific knowledge, and a very concrete basis for diagnosis and prognosis and treatment is what makes the relationship so unique. So I think what happens with at least a lot of premedical students I know who are doing just science so they really sort of limit their worldview . . . As a doctor you are not just treating an organic disease, but you are treating a person's situation, a person who may be suffering as a result not only of this pathogen but also [because of] their economic condition, their condition because of their race, their condition as a result of their religion, their condition because of their gender.

Their choices in terms of concentration seem to reflect their wish to resist the alienation of medical doctors. Although aware of the possible prospective difficulties they may face, the interviewees seem satisfied with their decision. One explains her choice in the following terms:

I very definitely think that Women's Studies has made me more sensitive to a lot of issues I think I'll face as a doctor, certainly concerning women of different economic classes and certainly women from different cultures and certainly women who have different religious beliefs. To be able to address those issues with a great deal of humility as well as understanding and sensitivity, I think is absolutely essential, especially as we move into the future when medicine increasingly has to be more sensitive to people, all different kinds of people, that is not just medicine, scientific medicine is the Bible and is law, and it's imposed on a sort of passive patient but there is increasingly going to be a patient and a doctor who are interacting and the patient has a right to their input into the relationship as well. (A)

Katz and Shotter (1996) describe training processes that aim to teach medical students the ability to listen and open space for both doctor and patient to "become co-participants in the process of meaning creation. Privileging the voice of the patient in this way puts the conversation on a more equal footing—a talking *with* rather than a speaking for the patient" (929–30).

In some situations in both Brazil and the United States, the acknowledgment that inequalities of gender, race, and class lead to poor health (see Freudenberg et al. 1995) has engendered the idea of empowerment in initiatives of health education and prevention. Inspired by the work of Paulo Freire, "empowerment education is a strategy that involves people assuming control and mastery over their lives in the context of their social and political environment" (Freudenberg et al. 1995, 295). In this connection, one of the interviewees was very sensitive to the potentialities of the doctor-patient relationship regarding the patient's empowerment and autonomy:

One of the . . . key themes for me in my studies in Women's Studies has always been the idea of empowerment, the idea that the only way we will ever see real changing attitudes concerning women in our society is going to be . . . when women have the opportunity to determine for themselves what they will do with their bodies. And whether or not they make what we call the right or the wrong choice seems almost secondary to the fact that they choose that themselves, and that's very much how I hope . . . to practice medicine. It's not just me . . . prescribing stuff to the woman, it is very much like me discussing . . . I want to be in a relationship, almost like a friendship, a relationship of equals, that is not me with all this knowledge that she will never understand but it's me sharing my knowledge, what I can bring to her, and her bringing her knowledge of her own suffering to me, and having an exchange, and then, you know, the woman deciding what is best for her, and me giving my recommendations but not imposing. (A)

But hearing these young women's words we cannot forget to ask: Are there conflicts in their experience? Do they identify any potential hindrances attributable to their atypical path toward the medical degree? Surprisingly, all of them agree that the concentration in Women's Studies may be a positive factor when applying to medical school. As one of them believes:

In terms of medical school I don't think that they look negatively on women's studies concentrators, I think there is a recognition that it's broad . . . it is very interdisciplinary, and, if anything, I think it may help some women in admittance just because they are not just another bio major, they have something that sort of distinguishes them. (A)

Being associated with the stereotype of feminists ("bitchy," "unpleasant," "narrow-minded," "radical"), on the other hand, is a source of concern for them. They all affirm that the decision to go into medical school facilitated their option for concentrating in Women's Studies, because they could tranquilize their parents and friends into believing that, at the end, they would find an "objective" and "practical" profession.

But what may happen when these insightful young women enter medical school? It seems likely that they will join other medical students who have already suffered the disappointment of moving from an encouraging environment to a sexist one. As a second-year medical student expressed (cited in Jones 1996):

As classes started, I realized that my colleagues and classmates did laugh at tasteless and degrading jokes. People were openly homophobic and sexist, intolerant of all those different from them. I felt disappointed. Perhaps topics of gender, social orientation, and race could all be recognized as important topics of constant dialogue in our community. (67)

If gender-sensitive students do not find support to resist the objectification of women patients and their own invisibility within medical school, it becomes very difficult to hold the values they have once firmly believed. The compromises they will make in order to be fully credentialized may dry up their "desire to work for change" (Boston Women's Health Book Collective 1990, 666–67). The result is that many women end medical training "eager to prove that they can be as good as any male physician according to the male-centered criteria of the profession: clinical competence, emotional detachment and financial success" (Boston Women's Health Book Collective 1990, 668).

The exceptions to this process will be those who pay the price of isolation, acting as disturbing elements within traditionally male professions. However, Martin (1994d) reminds us: "It is hard, very hard, to be a living contradiction every minute and hour of every working day and night: the psychic costs are enormous, and the threat of ridicule is ever present" (111). The only effective way to oppose the lack of criticism of medical training for women, according to my experience, is to engage in support groups that discuss the historical, cultural, economic and educational bases of medicine, opening space for questioning the status quo and creating alternatives. In the next section I will discuss the importance of identifying and discussing the hidden curriculum of medicine, and how women can collectively find the strength to counteract it.

Consciousness Raising: A Feminist Alternative for Health Education and Professional Training

Conventional medical care . . . may be bad for our health because it emphasizes drugs, surgery, psychotherapy, and crisis action rather than prevention . . . [Rather], we believe in the healing powers within us—our ability to help one another by listening, talking, caring, touching—and in the power of small groups as sources of information sharing, support and healing.

—Boston Women's Health Book Collective (1990, 653)

The medical curriculum privileges biological aspects of disease causation, dismissing socio-cultural and economic ones. The medical discourse proclaims objectivity, but its practice suffers from the impact of subjective factors, which compose the physicians' "experience," and helps to define clinical conduct (Camargo 1992). Thus, the doctor's values and beliefs can hardly be separated from what she or he prescribes.

Because students are not stimulated to question things, they finish graduate school lacking scientific rigor (Camargo 1992) and biased toward certain types of clients. At the heart of some doctors' ideological perspectives are misogyny and sexism in professional training and health care. Because misogyny is transmitted in a non-explicit way, it may be considered part of a hidden curriculum in health education. As Martin (1994b) affirms, "the effects of an initiation into male cognitive perspectives constitute a hidden curriculum" (81), a curriculum that is not explicit but has its own learned content, including assumptions about women's identity, psychology, body, sexuality, and social roles. The challenge now is to build an alternative curriculum, "a curriculum which, through critical analysis, exposes the biased view of women embodied in the disciplines and which, by granting ample space to the study of women shows how unjust that view is" (81).

Martin (1994a) advocates that women engage in processes of consciousness raising in order to know the effects of hidden curricula on them, including lack of self-confidence and self-alienation. She explains that "once learning states are openly acknowledged so that the learners can readily become aware of them, even if they do not, the learning states can no longer be considered hidden" (161–62).

The Brazilian experience with professional training within health centers, according to PAISM's premises, demonstrates that health professionals may become aware of the collective pressure they suffer to reproduce sexual stereotypes. Employing training activities based on participation and integration between participants' minds and bodies, intellects and emotions, those educational groups inspired by the feminist movement have recast women's health care and team work:

> When we find a hidden curriculum, we can show it to those destined to be its recipients. Not that consciousness raising is any guarantee that a person will not succumb to a hidden curriculum. But still, one is in a better position to resist if one knows what is going on. Resistance to what one does not know is difficult, if not impossible. (Martin 1994a, 167)

Indeed, the consciousness-raising groups I am discussing are part of a larger reform concerned with improving access and the quality of health care, and can be considered counter-initiatives aiming at preparing professionals and clients to resist the sexism hidden in the curriculum of health educational activities. However,

> there is no guarantee that consciousness raising will insulate as successfully against learning states we do not want to and should not acquire. Certainly we must not view it as a substitute for institutional and societal reform. Yet, as the women's movement has shown, knowledge about what has happened or is happening to one can have powerful effects . . . when knowledge is shared and there is strong peer support, consciousness raising may be the best weapon individuals who are subject to hidden curricula have. (Martin 1994a, 168–69)

I join Martin (1994b) in her proposal for a new paradigm for education, a paradigm that is feminist in its critique of polarized oppositions: "one which would emphasize the development of persons and not simply rational minds; one which would join thought to action, and reason to feeling and emotion" (78). In this sense, the role of relationships is vital and health can be framed as a daily conquest, achieved through participation and debate.

Conclusion

> [S]eeing the value of group support and taking time for it are essential for change to occur in medical education. When women remain isolated from each other it is difficult for us to differentiate institutional from personal sources of impotence and alienation. It remains easier to blame ourselves for what is not rightly ours.
>
> —Brown (1996, 101)

Some important changes have already been set in motion by women's organizing to discuss health issues within the general society, within health services, and within the academy. The Brazilian experience demonstrates that significant gains in health care for women are possible, and that the hidden curriculum of dismissing women's values and experiences can be exposed. However, the scarcity of research on feminist perspectives on health, from a medical point of view, means that the issue is very much up in the air. As one of the interviewees points out, "insiders" in the medical world still have a crucial role to play. Since MDs do not tend to engage in feminist reflection, it is easy to condemn any critique as not scientific and not valid. Significantly reshaping women's health care requires interdisciplinary team work. In this respect, medical education can improve students' willingness to engage in collective reflection and team discussions. Israel and Velloso (1996) argue that

> regarding women's comprehensive health care . . . the construction of interdisciplinary work is a fundamental condition. It is necessary to break the fragmentation and isolation of knowledge, moving towards a non-compartmentalized perspective regarding the individual and her demands of health. (12)

I hope that this study adds some insights for those interested in improving women's health care through the reorientation of professional education. It will, hopefully, nourish the debate within and outside medical schools in both Brazil and the United States. As Duffin (1996) says, discussing her position as a feminist physician: "to remain silent about what I have observed would endorse forgetting" (45). We may be tempted to forget, but I believe that those who enter medical school aware of what will occur and attentive to other perspectives to deal with human suffering—as these women's studies concentrators may be—can make a difference in terms of our capacity to remember and redefine theory, politics, and women's health care.

Notes

I am grateful to Dr. Jane Roland Martin for her encouragement and helpful feedback on this paper and to Stephen Slaner for editorial assistance. This study received the support of the W.K. Kellogg Foundation.

1. According to the Boston Women's Health Book Collective (1990, 669), 83 percent of doctors were men but more than 80 percent of all health care workers were women.

2. In Brazil, medical school, which lasts six years, starts immediately after high school. In my third year of medical school I turned 20.

3. For example, repeatedly examining the same patient.

4. "Recall is poor after a short period, however, and many in academic medicine admit that much of this material, irrelevant to medical practice, has crowded out crucial skills and subject matter" (Boston Women's Health Book Collective 1990, 663).

5. "Specialists are not immune from putting their own needs and preferences above societal interests and tend to be slow to welcome individuals who are not like them, i.e., women and ethnic minorities" (Kanter 1977, cited in Bickel 1996, 15).

6. Klass (1996, 84) affirms that in 1987 two among 127 medical schools in the United States had women deans and there were only 78 female chairs of academic departments out of 2000.

References

Aguiar, A. (1992). *Integral health care for women in the Center-South Sanitary district: The professional's point of view.* Unpublished master's thesis, National School of Public Health, Oswaldo Cruz Foundation, Rio de Janeiro.

Bickel, J. (1996). Leveling the playing field: A national perspective on sexism and professional development in medicine. In D. Wear (Ed.), *Women in medical education: An anthology of experience* (11–20). Albany: State University of New York Press.

Boston Women's Health Book Collective (1990). *The new our bodies, our selves: A book by and for women.* New York: Touchstone Book.

Brazil Ministry of Health (1983). *Women's comprehensive health care program: Basis for programmatic action.* Brasilia, Brazil: Ministry of Health.

Brown, K. (1996). If the suit fits . . . In D. Wear (Ed.), *Women in medical education: An anthology of experience* (95–102). Albany: State University of New York Press.

Camargo Jr., K. (1992). (Ir) Racionalidade medica: Os paradoxos da clinica. *Physis: Revista de Saude Coletiva 11*(1): 203–27.

Conley, F. (1996). Foreword. In D. Wear (Ed.), *Women in medical education: An anthology of experience* (viii). Albany: State University of New York Press.

Corrêa, S. (1994). *Gênero reflexões conceituais, pedagógicas e estratégicas.* Recife: SOS Corporation.

Dickenstein, L. (1996). Overview of women physicians in the United States. In D. Wear (Ed.), *Women in medical education: An anthology of experience* (3–10). Albany: State University of New York Press.

Duffin, J. (1996). Lighting candles, making sparks, and remembering not to forget. In D. Wear (Ed.), *Women in medical education: An anthology of experience* (33–46). Albany: State University of New York Press.

Ehrenreich, B., and English, D. (1989). *For her own good: 150 years of the experts' advice to women.* New York: Anchor Books, Doubleday.

Freire, P. (1985). *The politics of education: Culture, power and liberation.* New York: Bergin and Garvey.

Freudenberg, N., Eng, E., Flay, B., Parcel, G., Rogers, T., and Wallestein, N. (1995). Strengthening individual and community capacity to prevent disease and promote health: In search of relevant theories and principles. *Health Education Quarterly, 22*(3):290–306.

Giffin, K. (1994). Women's health and the privatization of fertility control in Brazil. *Social Science and Medicine 39*(3): 355–60.

Gilligan, C. (1982). *In a different voice: Psychological theory and women's development.* Cambridge, MA: Harvard University Press.

Gonçalves, R. (1991). A saúde no Brasil: Algumas caracteristicas do processo histórico nos anos 80. *São Paulo em Perspectiva 5*(1): 99–106.

Howes, J., and Allina, A. (1994). Women's health movements. *Social Policy 6:* 6–14.

Israel, G., and Velloso, V. org. (1996). *Mulher e saúde: Práticas educativas em 11 municípios. Rio de Janeiro.* Núcleo de Estudos Mulher e Políticas Públicas: IBAM/MacArthur Foundation.

Jones, D. (1996). Father knows best . . . ? In D. Wear (Ed.), *Women in medical education: An anthology of experience* (59–74). Albany: State University of New York Press.

Kanter, R. (1977). *Men and women of the corporation.* New York: Basic Books.

Katz, A., and Shotter, J. (1996). Hearing the patient's voice: Toward a social poetics in diagnostic interviews. *Social Science and Medicine 43*(3): 919–31.

Klass, P. (1996). The feminization of medicine. In D. Wear (Ed.), *Women in medical education: An anthology of experience* (81–94). Albany: State University of New York Press.

McCue, J. (1982). The effects of stress on physicians and their medical practice. *New England Journal of Medicine 306*(8): 458–63.

Marienskind, H. (1981). An evaluation of cesarean sections in the United States (NIH Publication No. 82-2067). In *The new our bodies, our selves: A book by and for women*. New York: Touchstone Books, 1990.

Martin, J. (1994a). What should we do with a hidden curriculum when we find one? In *Changing the educational landscape: Philosophy, women, and curriculum* (154–69). New York: Routledge.

Martin, J. (1994b). The ideal of the educated person. In *Changing the educational landscape: Philosophy, women, and curriculum* (70–87). New York: Routledge.

Martin, J. (1994c). Becoming educated: A journey of integration or alienation? In *Changing the educational landscape: Philosophy, women, and curriculum* (200–211). New York: Routledge.

Martin, J. (1994d). The contradiction and challenge of an educated woman. In *Changing the educational landscape: Philosophy, women, and curriculum* (100–119). New York: Routledge.

Rich, A. (1979). Toward a woman-centered university. In *On lies, secrets and silence*. New York: Norton.

Rosaldo, M., and Lamphere, L. (Eds.). (1974). *Women, culture and society*. Stanford, CA: Stanford University Press.

Ruzek, S. (1978). *The women's health movement: Feminist alternatives to medical control*. New York: Praeger Publishers.

Wear, D. (Ed.). (1996). *Women in medical education: An anthology of experience*. Albany: State University of New York Press.

Wear, D., and Bickel, J. (1996). Women's programs at medical schools, and Feminism: What is the intersection? In D. Wear, (Ed.), *Women in medical education: An anthology of experience*. Albany: State University of New York Press.

CHAPTER SIXTEEN

Putting Our Heads Together: Academic and Feminist Approaches to Studying the Health of Women Workers

KAREN MESSING

The Canadian government recently[1] assembled a hundred or so professionals working on women's health, 99 percent of whom were women.[2] Symposium participants spent several days listening to presentations on, for example, the causes of women's heart attacks, the best way for a young woman to avoid sexually transmitted diseases, and the advantages and disadvantages of mammograms. Most presenters were health researchers from academia; others were from women's health clinics and action groups. At the end of the second day, people began to comment that they were not satisfied with the conference; something was lacking. Finally one woman identified the problem: Why were we all talking about women in the third person? What did it mean to us to say that "women" should or should not have mammographies or estrogen replacement therapy? How did a group of high-powered women feel about the results of the research on stress?

In my work on women's occupational health, I have often felt this sort of call to split my personality. Academics who do research on people must reckon with the context of scientific institutions whose traditions require the researcher to depersonalize and objectify research subjects. In addition, an academic who wants her research to result in social change must translate human problems into academic terms that are worthy of grant support; produce information that is publishable and at the same time useful to the people who have the problem; and propose solutions. This effort is made more complex when the project involves people of other social classes who are understandably mistrustful of academics, use a different language from that of university professors, and experience life situations whose constraints are not immediately obvious to academics.

These difficulties are most acute in the case of women academics who work on subjects that touch women's lives. Pressure to depersonalize women's needs and behaviors comes from scientific institutions with a long tradition of doing misdirected research on women.[3] Women researchers perceive institutionalized sexism; nevertheless, they are particularly sensitive to accusations of treating their scientific subjects in a subjective or emotional way. We, however, also feel pressure to treat

---

Originally published in the fall 1991 issue (vol. 3, no. 3).

women's problems sympathetically, since we frequently share the problems experienced by the women under study. Women academics experience biological constraints and social oppression, trouble with child-care, menstrual cramps, unequal contributions to household tasks, and sexual stereotyping. Like members of any oppressed group, we feel solidarity with our sisters. As good girls in academia, we know we are supposed to separate clearly our experiences as women and our roles as researchers in occupational health.[4] As feminists, we find it difficult. As scientists, we are increasingly wondering whether there is a creative way to use our subjectivity as a research tool. Some researchers recently have started to examine the possibility of taking advantage of their own knowledge that pertains to the situation of their subject, to create a context for their research results.[5]

I have been confronted with these questions while in a situation that was particularly favorable to playing out all available roles. Between 1978 and 1983 I held positions that required me to think about women's occupational health, as both an activist and a biologist. During these five years I was a member of the national women's committee of my union, the Confédération des syndicats nationaux (CSN), and I was responsible for suggesting union activity for the area of women's occupational health. I was part of a union group that developed positions on maternity leave, hazards during pregnancy, reproductive rights, protectionism, and physiological requirements of jobs in male and female employment "ghettos." We made suggestions on policy and on union practices, some of which were accepted by the entire union membership.[6] At the same time, in the context of a union-university agreement, I was and am still part of a research group, comprised mainly of women, which has done extensive research on women's occupational health.[7] We did research on genetic damage in women hospital workers exposed to ionizing radiation and on the health consequences of work in typical industrial "women's jobs." I eventually resigned from the women's committee, but the experience has been extremely valuable in orienting our group's research and in helping us to think about problems of subjectivity in academic research and about the proper use of academic resources by women militants.

The context in which we have been working is quite unusual in North America. The union context, the two-hundred-thousand-member CSN, represents a broad spectrum of public- and private-sector workers: hospital technicians, print and electronic journalists, assembly-line workers, lumberjacks, and secretaries. It offers a great many educational and support services to its members, including four full-time workers in occupational health and two in the women's service. Although it has never supported a political party, the union takes public progressive positions in all debates in the province; for example, it has voted officially to support socialism, Québec independence, free abortion on demand, and disarmament. It has had a very active women's committee for the past fourteen years, resulting in great progress in negotiating maternity leave, protection of pregnant women and fetuses, equal pay for work of equal value, and daycare. Since the CSN represents most of the public service workers, CSN contracts have been a source of advances for women over the past twelve years. Many advantages negotiated for women, in private-sector union contracts or passed as laws for all women, originated as proposals of the CSN women's committee or of its women's service.

It should be mentioned that the union-university agreement includes another union, to which university staff belong. The Fédération des travailleurs du Québec (FTQ) is a three-hundred-fifty-thousand-member union, the largest in Québec. It also represents all categories of workers, with more from the private sector than the CSN; is affiliated with the Canadian Labor Congress, which combines unions from other provinces; and is related to the American union, the AFL-CIO. Individual locals are financially independent. The FTQ has traditionally supported the Parti québécois, the social democratic pro-independence party. It has an active women's committee that groups representatives from the major categories of women workers and considers general questions relating to the membership as a whole, such as protection of pregnant workers, prevention of infertility, and equal access to employment.

The academic context is also somewhat unusual. The Université du Québec à Montréal (UQAM) was established in 1969 with a mandate to serve the community. It set up a committee for community service with representatives of women's and community groups; these representatives oversee the university's role in supporting teaching and research for the university community. Women's studies developed relatively early at UQAM. In 1977 a group of women professors formed the Groupe interdisciplinaire d'enseignement et de recherche sur la condition féminine (GIERF) (Group for Interdisciplinary Research and Teaching on Women) that developed a series of forty-five women's studies courses in various departments and now has a research center and an active seminar program.[8] This group has also acted as a lobby for the hiring of women professors and has worked closely with the women's committee of the professors' union to write language favorable to women into collective agreements. As a result the university had paid maternity leave, a number of daycare centers, affirmative action clauses, and nondiscriminatory health insurance before most other universities in North America.

Encouraged by faculty interest, the university developed its mandate for community service to include formal agreements with community groups. It hired employees specifically to formulate projects with women's groups, community groups, and unions. In 1977 an agreement was signed with the CSN and the FTQ that provided that the unions might request the services of professors to do education or research activities initiated and oriented by the unions.[9] In 1982 the university signed a similar agreement with Relais-femmes, an organization serving as a liaison with women's groups.[10] Subsequent collective agreements provided release time for educational and research activities and seed money for research projects. A professor of biology has done health education for the women's health center, a professor of economics has examined the role of women in family businesses, and a professor of literature has done a reading project in a community center. Unions have asked professors to do economic analyses, write histories of union activities, explain laws and suggest improvements to the laws, and do education and research in occupational health. A committee from the union or women's group orients the project and eventually evaluates it. In 1985–86, for example, faculty provided over five hundred contact-hours of educational sessions to more than five hundred participants in activities sponsored by the union-university agreement. The university supported forty research projects in progress with forty thousand dollars; outside funds provided another one hundred thousand dollars.[11]

The agreement with unions is nevertheless far from being an integral part of the day-to-day academic life of faculty. During the first ten years of its existence, twenty-three professors from eight departments, less than 5 percent of the faculty, were involved in educational projects and roughly the same number in research projects.[12] Although the university has shown its approval by financing educational activities in the form of fifty-four course equivalents and has put about thirty-five thousand dollars per year into research projects, many departments still consider research for granting agencies more respectable than research for unions. Some of the hesitation is due to traditional academic contempt for applied research, but much is due to prejudice against unions. In some cases, however, union-initiated projects, which have resulted in posing new questions, have led to grants from traditional granting agencies. The university community is impressed that about one hundred thousand dollars is received per year as grants for projects initiated through the agreement. This, of course, is a double-edged sword: such support pulls the professor from her original goal of fulfilling the request of the union, replacing that goal with a feeling of responsibility to the granting agency. In the absence of granting agencies with a specific mandate to fund community-initiated research, the centrifugal force is overwhelming.

Over thirty women's groups have benefited in some way from an intervention through the agreement with the university.[13] The number of faculty involved, however, is even less than the number involved with the union agreement; nine professors from seven departments participated in some way in 1986–88. All but one were from GIERF; thus, university resources are not fully available or are not fully used through this agreement, which is little-known at the university.

Our research group deals most often with a granting agency that functions differently from others in North America. In 1981 the Workers' Compensation Commission established a research arm, the Institut de recherche en santé et en sécurité du travail (IRSST) (Institute for Research on Occupational Health and Safety), with the mandate to support research that diminishes occupational health and safety risks. The board of directors of the IRSST is composed of 50 percent labor and 50 percent management. The regular functioning of the IRSST is assured by a "scientific council" composed of five scientists, who come from areas removed from occupational health and safety; four representatives from the CSN and FTQ unions; and four representatives from management. One of the union representatives, a founder of the CSN's women's committee, is now the vice president in charge of women's issues and public-sector negotiations.

For an academic accustomed to dealing with the usual granting institutions, it is unusual to deal with the IRSST. Decisions are made in a way that is similar to labor-management negotiations of union contracts, although scientists are consulted about the content of specific grant requests. The strong community representation means that the relevance of a proposal is critically important to its funding but also that the criteria for relevance change quite swiftly and unpredictably. In June 1986, for example, the institute decided, without warning, to cut support for all graduate students involved in health- rather than safety-related research. Many students who were in second or subsequent years of their programs were left stranded. They had not applied for other support, since there is a tradition of continuing support for students in good standing. The advantage of a research institution whose governing body is composed of representatives of the groups it wishes to support, however, is that the political character of research is recognized. In fact, the IRSST has supported research groups with union as well as management perspectives on occupational health. It has given our own research group the Centre pour l'étude des interactions biologiques entre la santé et l'environnement (CINBIOSE) (Center for the Study of Biological Interactions between Health and the Environment) ten years of generous support.

This group now does research on early detection of genotoxic and neurotoxic damage, as well as on the characteristics of "women's" work and the ergonomic and physiological constraints that restrict access to "men's" jobs.[14] This research is initiated in a formal and an informal context. The formal context originates with the university-union agreement: a union, such as the hospital workers or the poultry slaughterhouse workers, requests assistance in a specific area. University personnel help locate a scholar doing research in the relevant area and eventually assist the union in understanding the research results. Funds are initially provided by the university and, if necessary, through regular granting agencies. In practice roles are not so clearly defined. Since union-defined research questions are not necessarily recognized as interesting by academic standards, most professors do not spontaneously volunteer to participate in such research. Those who do are usually progressive, thus, these professors are interested in the union activity as well as the academic aspects of the research. The professor may encroach on the formal role of the unions in other ways. Unions do not develop needs that relate to the curricula vitae of university professors. The small number of scholars available receive requests on a wide variety of subjects in which few faculty are likely to have expertise. These researchers have the choice of learning an entirely new discipline every time a request is made or of reorienting union requests as a function of their specialty.

Also, granting agencies generally do not use the same priority scheme as unions when deciding on the level of interest of research proposals. Many researchers have trouble obtaining funds for union-initiated studies as these studies have been originally formulated and are faced with the conflict between the needs of the union and the requirements of peer review. They then may feel great pressure to redirect the original union request into something fundable. In the absence of substantial funding for community-based research, there is no way to respond directly to many union needs.[15] A great deal of our research comes about through informal contacts with unions with which we come in contact in educational sessions or unions I encountered through my work with the women's committee. In these cases, we become very involved with the union as well as the academic parameters of the research questions.

At the Université du Québec, therefore, a university context, a union context, a feminist context, and a granting institution create an unequaled opportunity for integrating academic research with feminist struggles inside and outside of the union movement. Our research group has grown in this very favorable environment. We are not only women studying women but also (except for the students) union members studying union members. As such we have sympathized actively with most of the groups we have studied. Of course we have been criticized for this attitude, but we have also profited so much from our double identity, both as feminists and as scientists, that we wonder if it is not an important way for gaining understanding of our subject matter. Listening sympathetically and empathetically has led us to new scientific and political understanding. And we have developed research methods and statistical tools as a result of this better understanding, to organize and to benefit from our subjective perceptions and other women's perceptions. Our scientific ideas have changed through our experiences as feminists. As a geneticist, I had a thorough training in embryology and teratology—the sciences that deal with pregnancy and fetal development. My preparation had shown me that the male and female reproductive systems are similar and that no working condition exists that is unsafe for pregnant women and safe for everyone else. I was, therefore, in favor of women working right up to the end of pregnancy and taking maternity leave once the child was born in order to rest after childbirth and spend time with the child. Working conditions, consequently, that make this situation uncomfortable or risky should be changed.[16]

In Québec in 1979, a law was passed providing for *retrait préventif*, or precautionary leave, for pregnant women holding jobs that posed a risk to them or the fetus. Job reassignment or, failing that, fully paid leave was available for such women for the duration of the pregnancy. The women's committee had many discussions on this subject, since a pregnant woman leaving a hazardous job would probably be replaced by another woman, or a man, who then would be exposed to the hazard. It would be more consistent with our knowledge of occupational risks and my understanding of male and female biology to insist that the employer remove the hazardous condition. And, of course, protectionist policies for women endanger women's jobs, since employers are reluctant to hire women who may take long leaves, when they can hire men who do not get pregnant. Thus, on principle, I was opposed to *retrait préventif* and should not have encouraged union members to take advantage of it.

As a member of the women's committee giving educational sessions on precautionary leave for pregnant women, however, I had a lot of contact with women for whom women's rights were an abstract issue, and uncomfortable working conditions and unreasonable employers were a daily reality. I had, after all, experienced my pregnancies when I was very young, in a relatively healthy environment far removed from the solvent fumes of the hockey stick factory or the violence of the psychiatric hospitals where some of our members worked. It was impossible for me to speak against precautionary leave for very long when so many unionized women regarded it as their only hope for getting through a pregnancy without paying for it in money or permanently impaired health.[17] In fact, I ended up supervising a large research project whose aim was to determine grounds for precautionary leave among hospital workers. This evolution was not one-sided. The information my colleagues and I could contribute influenced the positions of other feminists in the union, many of whom had very protectionist positions. Women who had thought that all pregnant women should have nine months of maternity leave came to realize that their impressions of pregnant women's fitness for work were based on women in very uncomfortable and risky jobs.

Our research has profited from the union-university contacts in other ways, especially from the constant challenges to our ideas. Listening to union members has enabled us to pursue lines of investigation we would never have considered. After listening to laundry workers describe the heavy loads they lift repeatedly, a task defined as "light" work, in very hot temperatures, Donna Mergler began an exploration of the physiological response to this kind of workload.[18] Nicole Vezina, another member of our research group, has become involved in the comparison of men's and women's jobs. The usual descriptions of heavy workloads have been developed for men's jobs and do not include the ergonomic constraints imposed by awkward postures or fast workspeed, which are typical of women's employment ghettos,[19] Vezina's research has resulted in legal decisions enabling supermarket cashiers to sit down, in easing the tremendous postural constraints on sewing machine operators, and in lowering the permissible temperature in kitchens. Work with the women's committees has resulted in developing ways to adapt traditional men's jobs in order to diminish risks for the average female body.[20] We also changed the focus of a research project after listening to hospital radiology technicians. Their descriptions induced us to put less emphasis on easily defined risk factors such as radiation exposure and more on lifting heavy patients and on a fast workspeed. In fact, talking to workers has enabled us to understand the great importance of workspeed in determining health symptoms.

Although we are stimulated by these scientific exchanges with workers, our excitement is not shared by all the scientists who review our work. When we write grant applications or articles about the use of worker input to generate hypotheses and yield new information, we are often reproached with the statement that we lack objectivity. We are thought to report uncritically the complaints of workers and even have been accused of using our academic titles simply to back up workers' grievances. In some sense this is true. Our research group has depended to some extent on questionnaires to tap the workers for information on their workplace and their health symptoms.[21] These questionnaires are usually developed after sympathetic listening to workers' descriptions of their workplace and their symptoms. In many cases this method is the only one available that permits us to learn about the symptoms that may plague most workers' lives, such as impotence, menstrual pain, or backache.[22] In addition, some variables, such as sharing of the domestic workload, may only be available through workers' reports.[23]

We think there should be a place in occupational health research for documentation and statistical description of workers' perceptions. Thus, we find ourselves making such obvious statements as, "Workers report that they work too quickly and that the more quickly they work the more they feel exhausted." This is because we think that when a large number of women are exhausted, scientists should listen to them. We also know that this obvious fact, women should not work so hard because they will get tired, has little influence on work schedules in factories or hospitals.

When scientists say the same thing, there may be a greater chance of changing working conditions. We spend a lot of time trying to back up the "subjective" with the "objective" measure of workplace-induced damage.[24] Some techniques include asking workers to report perceptions of other people ("Has anyone ever told you . . . , has a doctor ever prescribed . . ."). In some cases we have taken measurements of environmental variables and checked them against workers' perceptions. Other techniques involve correlating worker perceptions with laboratory tests of biological characteristics that are regarded, often erroneously, as less likely to be subjected to variation and interpretation than worker perception.[25] But we also have to ask ourselves about subjectivity and see whether or not using our intuitive identification with women workers is a valuable research tool. It would be a mistake, however, to treat the problem of subject/object as one that only touches women researching women; one of the challenges of science is to learn how to appropriately use this type of information. We, as scientists, have been developing this approach in the context of women's occupational health, but it is a problem for all whose research involves people.

In our work in the area of occupational health in close collaboration with women's and union groups, we have gained a knowledge of women's working conditions that could not have been obtained from any other source. This has enabled us to do research on questions of interest to women, questions not normally examined by other scientists. With women workers and their representatives, we have developed an approach geared toward making the knowledge we gain available to them. Sometimes we are afraid that our research results are not sufficiently used by the people who have asked for the studies. The wait between the appeal to our group and the response to what appears to the union as a simple question may take too long to meet the needs of the union. In the present economic context, when unions have all they can do to keep from folding entirely, taking time to work with us may be a luxury that overloaded union leaders cannot afford. But in general, we think, and have been told, that our contribution has helped the union to develop its analysis in many areas involving women's work.

It should be emphasized that we would never have had the energy to do all this without the time given to us in the university-union agreement, which allows course equivalents for educational activities and seed money for research. It seems to us that other universities could be convinced that they are supported by public funds and, therefore, by the money and labor of working women. These women have a right to access university resources, which more universities ought to provide in a form useful to the women and to the organizations these women have created to support themselves.

Notes

1. An earlier version of this essay appeared in *Women and Social Change: Feminist Organizing in Canada*, ed. Jeri Wine and Janice Ristock (Toronto: James Lorrimer Press).

2. Health and Welfare Canada, *Proceedings of the National Symposium on Changing Patterns of Health and Disease in Canadian Women, April 18– 20, 1988* (Ottawa: Minister of Supply and Services, 1989).

3. Sue V. Rosser, "Re-visioning Clinical Research: Gender and the Ethics of Experimental Design," *Hypatia* 4 (Summer 1989): 125–39.

4. Ruth Hubbard, *The Politics of Women's Biology* (New Brunswick, NJ: Rutgers University Press, 1990), 35–47.

5. Carol Gilligan, *In a Different Voice: Psychological Theory and Women's Development* (Cambridge, MA: Harvard University Press, 1982); Abby Lippman, "Prenatal Diagnosis: A Chance for Action-Research," *Resources for Feminist Research/Documentation sur la recherche féministe* 15 (November 1986): 65–66.

6. Confédération des syndicats nationaux (CSN), *Les femmes à la CSN n'ont pas les moyens de reculer* (Montréal: Service de la condition féminine, CSN, 1982); CSN, *Dix ans de luttes; les femmes à la CSN continuent d'avancer* (Montréal: Service de la condition féminine, CSN, 1984).

7. Donna Mergler, "Worker Participation in Occupational Health Research: Theory and Practice," *International Journal of Health Services* 17, no. 1 (1987): 151–67; Mergler, Carole Brabant, Nicole Vézina, and Messing, "The Weaker Sex? Men in Women's Jobs Report Similar Health Symptoms," *Journal of Occupational Medicine* 29 (May 1987): 417–21; Karen Messing, "Feminist Studies into Genetic Hazards in the Workplace," in *Despite the Odds: Essays on Canadian Women and Science*, ed. Marianne Ainley (Montréal: Vehicule Press, 1990), 349–58; "Do Men and Women have Different Jobs Because of their Biological Differences?" *International Journal of Health Services* 12, no. 1 (1982): 43–52; "Est-ce que les travailleuses enceintes sont protégées au Québec?" *Union médicale* 111 (March 1982); 1–6; "Are Women the Weaker Sex or Do They Just Have Hard Jobs? The Need for Research on Women's Occupational Health," *Chronic Diseases in Canada* 11 (March 1990): 27–29.

8. Groupe interdisciplinaire d'enseignement et de recherche féministes (GIERF), *Répertoire de tous les cours "Femmes, féminismes, rapport de sexes" offerts par 13 universités francophones du Canada* (Montréal: GIERF, 1989), 13–27.

9. Comité conjoint Université du Québec à Montréal (UQAM)-CSN-fédération des travailleurs du Québec (FTQ) *Le protocole d'entente UQAM-CSN-FTQ: Sur la formation syndicale* (Montréal: Services à la collectivité, UQAM, 1977).

10. UQAM, *Le protocole UQAM-relais-femmes* (Montréal: Services à la collectivité, UQAM, 1982).

11. Comité conjoint UQAM-CSN-FTQ, *Le protocole UQAM-CSN-FTQ: 1976–1986: Bilan et perspectives* (Montréal: Services à la collectivité, UQAM, 1988).

12. Comité conjoint UQAM-CSN-FTQ, *Le protocole UQAM-CSN-FTQ: 1976–1986.*

13. Marie-Hélène Côté, *Bilan des activités 1987–88 et perspectives pour la prochaine année* (Montréal: Services à la collectivité, UQAM, 1988).

14. Gillian Kranias, "Women and the Changing Faccs of Science," in *Despite the Odds,* 359–68.

15. Messing, "Feminist Studies."

16. Messing, "Le retrait préventif."

17. Pierre Bouchard and Geneviève Turcotte, "La maternité en milieu de travail, ou pourquoi les québécoises sont-elles si nombreuses à demander un retrait préventif?" *Sociologic et sociétés* 2 (1986): 113–28.

18. Brabant, Sylvie Bedard, and Mergler, "Cardiac Strain among Women Workers in an Industrial Laundry," *Ergonomics* 32, no. 6 (1989): 615–28.

19. Vézina, Daniel Tierney, and Messing, "When is Light Work Heavy? Components of the Physical Workload of Sewing Machine Operators Working at Piece Work Rates." *Applied Ergonomics* 23(4) (1992): 268–76.

20. Messing, Julie Courville, and Vézina, "Minimizing Risks for Women in Now Traditional Jobs," *New Solutions: A Journal of Environmental and Occupational Health Policy* (Spring 1991): 66–70; and Courville, Vézina, Messing, "Analysis of Work Activity of a Job in a Machine Shop Held by Ten Men and One Woman," *International Journal of Industrial Ergonomics* 1 (1991): 163–74.

21. Messing and Jean-Pierre Reveret, "Are Women in Female Jobs for their Health? Working Conditions and Health Symptoms in the Fish Processing Industry in Québec," *International Journal of Health Services* 13, no. 4 (1983): 635–47; Sylvie De Grosbois and Mergler, "L'exposition aux solvants

organiques en milieu de travail et la santé mentale," *Santé mentale au Québec* 10 (1987): 99–113; and Tierney, Patrizia Romito, and Messing, "She Ate not the Bread of Idleness: Exhaustion is Related to Domestic and Salaried Workload among Québec Hospital Workers," *Women and Health* 16 (January 1990): 21–42.

22. De Grosbois and Mergler, "Exposition aux solvants"; Mergler and Vézina, "Dysmenorrhea and Cold Exposure," *Journal of Reproductive Medicine* 30 (February 1985): 106–11.

23. Tierney, Romito, and Messing, "She Ate not the Bread."

24. Bedard, Brabant, and Mergler, "Thermal Discomfort and Seasonal Ambient Temperature in an Industrial Laundry" (presented at the Annual Meeting of the American Industrial Hygiene Association, Montréal, May 1988).

25. Messing, Ana Maria Seifert, Jocelyne Ferraris, Joel Swartz, and W. E. C. Bradley, "Mutant Frequency of Radiotherapy Technicians Appears to be Related to Recent Dose of Ionizing Radiation," *Health Physics* 57 (October 1989): 537–44.

Contributors

ADRIANA CAVALCANTI DE AGUIAR was affiliated with Oswaldo Cruz Foundation–EPSJV Rio de Janeiro State University at the time this article was written.

ZOBEIDA E. BONILLA, PHD, MPH, is assistant professor in the Department of Applied Health Science at Indiana University and senior program consultant for the Latina Health Initiative of the Boston Women's Health Book Collective. Her current work focuses on Latinas' health in the United States and the Caribbean, including maternal health, community-based participatory research, health disparities, qualitative program evaluation, anthropological methods in public health research, and *promotoras de salud* as a public health intervention.

SONDRA M. BRANDLER, DSW, was affiliated with the College of Staten Island of the City University of New York at the time this article was written.

ALICE J. DAN was a professor emerita of the University of Illinois at Chicago at the time this article was written.

HEATHER E. DILLAWAY is an associate professor of sociology at Wayne State University. She researches and teaches about women's health and structural inequalities (gender, race, class, age, and sexuality). Her current research focuses on how women's menopause experiences are shaped by their social locations and contemporary social contexts.

ANN M. FOX is an associate professor of English and the gender studies concentration coordinator at Davidson College. Fox's early scholarship traced the rise of feminist sensibilities in American commercial theater. More recently, her work centers on disability and theater. Fox and Lipkin have coauthored conference papers and an article in *Contemporary Theatre Review*. Her current study is on rereading twentieth-century American drama through the lens of disability studies.

M. BAHATI KUUMBA was associate director of the women's research and resource center and associate professor of women's studies at Spelman College at the time this article was written.

ELIZABETH SARAH LINDSEY received a master's in public affairs and urban and regional planning from Princeton University's Woodrow Wilson School. In 2005, she wrote the new chapter on sexuality and gender in the newest edition of the women's health classic, *Our Bodies, Ourselves*, and in 2006, she worked as a research consultant at the Triangle Project in Cape Town, South Africa, the oldest LGBT organization on the African continent. She works in the public sector, focusing on economic and small business development.

JOAN LIPKIN is the founding artistic director of That Uppity Theater Company in St. Louis, Missouri. As a playwright, lyricist, director, educator, and social activist, she has produced her work worldwide. She specializes in creating work about contemporary social issues for social service agencies and corporations and with marginalized populations, including people with disabilities, LGBT youth, adults and their families, women with cancer, and people with Alzheimer's. She has received numerous awards, including a Visionary, the James F. Hornback Ethical Humanist of the Year, a Frederick H. Laas Memorial, and Lifetime Achievement from Arts for Life, among others.

MARIANNE MCPHERSON, MS, MA, is a doctoral candidate in social policy at the Heller School for Social Policy and Management, Brandeis University. She holds degrees in public health, women's and gender studies, and psychology and has served as a program consultant to *Our Bodies, Ourselves*. Her interests concern gender and health policy, with a particular focus on adolescent reproductive health. She has conducted research on women's experiences with menstruation from menarche through early adulthood as well as on physician advocacy for reproductive health.

KAREN MESSING was affiliated with Université de Québec à Montréal at the time this article was written.

JENNIFER NELSON was an assistant professor in women's studies at the University of Redlands in Redlands, California, at the time this article was written.

CHRISTINE OVERALL is a professor of philosophy and University Research Chair at Queen's University, Kingston, Ontario. She was elected as a fellow of the Royal Society of Canada and is the author of five books, including *A Feminist I: Reflections from Academia; Thinking Like a Woman: Personal Life and Political Ideas* and *Aging, Death, and Human Longevity*. She is also the winner of the Royal Society's Gender Studies Award (2008).

LYNN ROBERTS is assistant professor and coordinator of community health education in the Urban Public Health Program at Hunter College. She has previously served as the director of community projects and training with the Hunter College Center on AIDS, Drugs, and Community Health and was the founding director of the Visiting Nurse Service of New York's First Steps Program, a comprehensive intervention program for substance-using mothers and their families in Harlem. She is a member of the *SisterSong* Women of Color Reproductive Health Collective's board of directors/management circle.

LORETTA ROSS is a co-founder and the national coordinator of the *SisterSong* Women of Color Reproductive Health Collective, a network founded in 1997 of eighty women of color and allied organizations that work on reproductive justice issues to fulfill a need for a national network that would organize women of color in the reproductive justice movement. *SisterSong* is headquartered in Atlanta, Georgia, and serves as a national organizing center for feminists of color. She is the co-author of *Undivided Rights: Women of Color Organize for Reproductive Justice,* written with Jael Silliman, Marlene Gerber Fried, and Elena Gutiérrez, and of "The Color of Choice" chapter in *Incite! Women of Color Against Violence.*

SUE V. ROSSER serves as dean of Ivan Allen College, the liberal arts college at Georgia Institute of Technology, where she is also professor of public policy and of history, technology, and society. She holds the endowed Ivan Allen Dean's Chair of Liberal Arts and Technology. She has edited collections and written approximately 120 journal articles on the theoretical and applied problems of women and science and women's health and is the author of eleven books.

ESTER R. SHAPIRO (Ester Rebeca Shapiro Rok) is associate professor in psychology and Latino studies at the University of Massachusetts, Boston, and research associate at the Mauricio Gaston Institute, where she directs the Health Promotion Research Group. She is a co-principal investigator for the Community Engagement Core of the NIH-funded HORIZON Center, a partnership between UMB & Harvard School of Public Health to reduce health disparities through community participation in gender-sensitive, culturally meaningful, and socially equitable public health research. Her scholarship and practice apply an integrative cultural and developmental systems model to understanding resources and barriers promoting or impeding positive development during family life cycle transitions, and participatory teaching and practice methods linking personal and social change for individuals, families, groups, and organizations.

ANDREA SMITH (UC Riverside, Media and Cultural Studies) is the author of *Native Americans and the Christian Right: The Gendered Politics of Unlikely Alliances.* She is also a co-founder of Incite! Women of Color Against Violence.

NANCY WORCESTER is a professor of gender and women's studies and continuing studies at the University of Wisconsin, Madison. She is a long-time women's health activist in England and the United States, coeditor with Mariamne H. Whatley of five editions of *Women's Health: Readings on Social. Economic, and Political Issues,* and one of the authors of the National Women's Health Network's book, *The Truth About Hormone Therapy: How to Break Free of the Medical Myths of Menopause.*

Index

ability identity, 207
ableism, 11, 207, 212, 213, 214
abortion: criminalization of, 42–45, 47;
  controversy over, 19; Hyde Amendment restrictions, 19, 50, 51, 58;
  rights vs. choice, 50; right to choose,
  51. *See also* March for Women's
  Lives
access to health care, 9, 100
Actual Lives (Austin, Texas), 222
Acuña, Eugenia, 78
African American women: birth control
  and abortion services, 33–34;
  breast-feeding, 35–36; empowerment
  and community development, 23–24;
  health problems, 39; history of health
  care in U.S., 25–27; medical abuses of,
  26; medical research on, 8; Tuskegee
  experiment, 26
age, chronological: for menopause
  diagnosis and treatment, 152–156; and
  reproductive aging, 137, 141–143, 159
age identity, 207
ageism, 11, 212, 213, 214, 216nn5, 9
aging women: aging as social construct,
  209–215; aging daughter's experience
  as caregiver for mother, 191; being
  treated as children, 199–200; as
  caregivers for aged relatives, 191–204;
  census data projections, 10, 192; filial
  expectations for caregiving, 193–195;
  filial role as caregivers performance,
  195–202; financial concerns for health
  care of, 200–201; foreign-born mothers' health care issues, 194; gerontological research and, 10; health care
  issues, 9–11; institutionalization of
  mothers, 195, 196, 197; old age redefined, 210; "passing for normal" or for
  younger, 213–214, 216n9; physical
  impairments, 213; social disablement,
  212–213. *See also* elderly women;
  menopause
Aguiar, Adriana Cavalcanti de, 12,
  248–267, 281

AIDS, 4, 114, 118–119; homophobia of
  health care workers, 124–125;
  research, 118–119, 127
ALAS. *See* Amigas Latinas en Acción
  Pro-Salud (ALAS)
ALAS/NCNV work group, 81, 83–84,
  88n12
alcoholism in homosexual population,
  120
American Indians. *See* Native American
  women
American Journal of Nursing, 23
Amigas Latinas en Acción Pro-Salud
  (ALAS), 73–74, 88n6
anatomy: chapter in *OBOS*, 241–247;
  self-exam or self-guide tour,
  243–244
anti-domestic violence / sexual assault
  movement, 46
anti–prison industrial complex movement, 44, 49
Anzaldúa, Gloria Evangelina, 17, 20n1
Asians and Pacific Islanders, 8
aspirin, and heart disease, 114
atherosclerosis prevention, 116
Avery, Byllye, 21n5

Baltimore Longitudinal Study on Aging,
  10
Bangladesh, 55
Banister, Katie Rodriguez, 226–227,
  233–236
Barnes, Helen, 32–34
Bart, Pauline, 169
Beauvoir, Simone de, 207
Bennett, Lisa, 225
Bickel, J., 255
black women: health care, historical
  literature on, 24; as midwives and
  health care workers, 25; prevalence of
  heart disease, 114; reproductive health
  problems, 38–39. *See also* African
  American women
Blenkner, Margaret, 194
body image, 97, 226